Veterinary Clinical Epidemiology

Third Edition

Ronald D. Smith

University of Illinois
College of Veterinary Medicine
Urbana, Illinois, U.S.A.

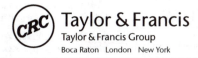

CRC Taylor & Francis
Taylor & Francis Group
Boca Raton   London   New York

A CRC title, part of the Taylor & Francis imprint, a member of the
Taylor & Francis Group, the academic division of T&F Informa plc.

Cover images (from left to right): A 17th-century illustration of a physician wearing protective clothing, including a mask, to protect against the plague. German engraving by Paulus Furst, Nuremberg, 1656. © Bettmann/CORBIS.

Death's Dispensary. George John Pinwell, 19th century. Philadelphia Museum of Art: The William H. Helfand Collection.

The Veterinarian. A Serious Case. Woodcut engraving by Ernst Bosch, 19th century. © Bettmann/CORBIS.

Dr. Ron Smith, a U.S. Peace Corps volunteer veterinarian in Ecuador, examines a calf afflicted with parasites. U.S. Peace Corps. 1969.

Cover design by Veronica Smith

Published in 2006 by
CRC Press
Taylor & Francis Group
6000 Broken Sound Parkway NW, Suite 300
Boca Raton, FL 33487-2742

© 2006 by Taylor & Francis Group, LLC
CRC Press is an imprint of Taylor & Francis Group

No claim to original U.S. Government works
Printed in the United States of America on acid-free paper
10 9 8 7 6 5 4 3 2 1

International Standard Book Number-10: 0-8493-1566-2 (Hardcover)
International Standard Book Number-13: 978-0-8493-1566-4 (Hardcover)
Library of Congress Card Number 2005005748

Library of Congress Cataloging-in-Publication Data

Smith, Ronald Dee, 1943-
   Veterinary clinical epidemiology / Ronald D. Smith.-- 3rd ed.
      p. ; cm.
   Includes bibliographical references and index.
   ISBN 0-8493-1566-2
   1. Veterinary clinical epidemiology. [DNLM: 1. Epidemiologic Methods--veterinary. SF 780.9 S657v 2005] I. Title.

SF780.9.S62 2005
636.089'44--dc22   2005005748

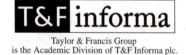

Taylor & Francis Group
is the Academic Division of T&F Informa plc.

Visit the Taylor & Francis Web site at
http://www.taylorandfrancis.com

and the CRC Press Web site at
http://www.crcpress.com

Preface to the First Edition

Medical knowledge is not static. Approaches to the diagnosis, treatment and prevention of disease change as new medical information is acquired. Much of this information is based on the observation of naturally or spontaneously occurring disease. The science of epidemiology evolved from the need to draw accurate conclusions from the study of health and disease in populations by controlling for bias, confounding and chance. Clinical epidemiology focuses on the application of epidemiologic methods and findings to medical decision-making. Results are usually directly applicable to patient care. Epidemiologic principles are also fundamental to critical interpretation of the medical literature.

This book is not intended to make epidemiologists out of veterinary students, but rather to show how experience with patients can be used to explore issues of importance in the practice of veterinary medicine. The decision to focus on clinical epidemiology in an introductory book for veterinary students was influenced by the following observations: (1) most veterinary graduates go into practice; (2) all practitioners are exposed to epidemiologic data from their patients, scientific meetings and the veterinary literature; and (3) the science of epidemiology plays a significant role in medical decision-making.

The first part of the book focuses on the application of epidemiology in medical decision-making at the individual and herd levels. The second part examines the epidemiology of disease in populations and outbreak investigation. Wherever possible, important concepts are illustrated with examples from the veterinary literature. Case studies appear throughout the book. A glossary of epidemiologic terms is also included.

It is the intent of the author that this book serve not only as a teaching resource, but also as a reference manual on the application of epidemiologic methods in veterinary clinical research. Readers' suggestions and contributions will be welcomed.

Ronald D. Smith, D.V.M., Ph.D.

Preface to the Second Edition

Since publication of the first edition of this book, the approaches and techniques of clinical epidemiology have become increasingly prominent in the veterinary literature. This second edition includes numerous updates throughout to reflect the increasing recognition of the role of clinical epidemiology as a basic science in clinical research. The chapters on the evaluation and use of diagnostic tests include expanded sections on likelihood ratios and ROC curves. The chapter on evaluating the cost of disease includes an expanded section on decision analysis. Many of the examples throughout the book have been updated with more recent examples from the veterinary literature.

During the revision process I have tried to maintain the basic focus of the book, e.g., the application of epidemiologic principles and techniques to problems regularly faced by veterinary practitioners. It is hoped that the book will help anyone working in the field of animal health to critically evaluate their own experiences and those of others, as reported in the medical literature and other forums.

Ronald D. Smith, D.V.M., Ph.D.

Preface to the Third Edition

The publication of the third edition of *Veterinary Clinical Epidemiology* coincides with an increased presence of epidemiologic concepts and methods in the practice literature, which continues to be the gold standard for the book's topical coverage. An underlying premise of the book is that patient-based research is epidemiologic research. Clinical epidemiology provides the scientific basis for the conduct and interpretation of patient-based research. It logically follows that the users of this information, veterinary students and practitioners, be skilled in its application to patient care. This approach to medical decision making is formalized in the practice of evidence-based medicine. Evidence-based medicine is increasingly important in an age where Internet-savvy consumers have ready access to an abundance of unfiltered animal health information and medical claims.

During the revision process I have tried to maintain the basic focus of the book, e.g., the application of epidemiologic concepts and methods to problems regularly faced by veterinary practitioners during the course of patient care. The patient may be an individual animal, a flock or herd, or any other defined animal population. Accordingly, the chapter sequence follows that of a case workup, initially at the individual patient level and later at the population level. However, the content has been packaged in such a way that educators can change the sequence of chapter coverage to suit their specific needs.

In preparing this edition, I have updated the numerous examples of epidemiology in veterinary practice appearing throughout the book. Examples come from around the world, and as a result, journal representation has been greatly expanded. There is increased coverage of hypothesis testing, survey design and sampling, and epidemiologic concepts related to the practice of evidence-based medicine. Some chapters, such as those dealing with the evaluation and use of diagnostic tests, risk assessment, causality, and statistics, have been extensively reorganized and rewritten to improve clarity. The identification of clinically relevant reports was facilitated by the Veterinary Information Network's (VIN) weekly "Clinical Updates from the Journals." Examples have been chosen that are exemplary of both epidemiologic methodology and issues of current importance in veterinary practice.

It is hoped that this book will help anyone working in the field of animal health to critically evaluate their own experiences and those of others, as reported in the medical literature and other forums. The numerous examples appearing in this and previous editions should be useful for instructors seeking examples of the application of epidemiology in veterinary practice.

A Note about the Cover: The sequence of historical images on the cover highlights progress in the application of epidemiologic concepts and methods to human and veterinary medicine. The first (*Plague Physician*: Paulus Furst, 1656) depicts a 17th-century plague physician whose protective clothing suggests an awareness of the transmissible nature of the disease at a time when much of medicine was guided by dogma rather than scientific reasoning. The second (*Death's Dispensary*: George John Pinwell, 19th century) marks the beginning of modern epidemiology, when the physician John Snow linked human cholera deaths in 19th-century London to sewage-contaminated water. At about the same time, early veterinarians, depicted in the third image (*The Veterinarian. A Serious Case*: Ernst Bosch, 19th century), drew on prior patient experience (epidemiologic data) to diagnose and treat animal diseases. The fourth image is a promotional photo taken during my U.S. Peace Corps service in Ecuador in the late 1960s, where I learned the relevance of epidemiology to patient care. The calf in the picture was suffering from a severe parasitic infection that could have been avoided by appropriate preventive strategies. As a result of this case, I conducted my first epidemiologic study: the chronology of various parasitic infections in young calves. The result was a preventive worming strategy that I implemented on many small farms like this one. The overall layout conveys the temporal sequence of these events against the intrinsic quantitative nature of the discipline of epidemiology. The cover was designed by Veronica Smith.

Ronald D. Smith, D.V.M., Ph.D.

Acknowledgments

I acknowledge the encouragement and support of Dr. George T. Woods, professor emeritus of epidemiology and preventive medicine, College of Veterinary Medicine, University of Illinois, who helped me recognize and pursue my true interests. It was he who sent me into the classroom, thereby planting the seed that led to this book.

I am indebted to the numerous veterinary students whose questions, critiques, and suggestions over the years have helped make the textual material more relevant and intelligible. My colleagues, Drs. Larry Firkins, Tony Goldberg, Uriel Kitron, Gay Miller, and Ron Weigel, have been very supportive by sharing their own experiences of the many ways in which epidemiology contributes to improving animal and human health.

I must recognize the contributions of the many fine veterinary researchers whose works are cited profusely throughout the text. I also want to acknowledge the excellent facilities, collection, and services provided by the Veterinary Medicine Library of the University of Illinois at Urbana-Champaign. This edition of the book relies much more on source articles from a variety of journals, and the ready access to the journals provided by the library was invaluable.

Finally, I thank Mr. John Sulzycki, Patricia Roberson, Randy Brehm, Jonathan Pennell, Richard Tressider, and the rest of the staff at Taylor & Francis, for their guidance and patience during the course of preparing this revision.

The task of preparing the third edition of this book was made easier by the continued understanding and support of my family: Lupe, Ronald, and Veronica.

The Author

Ronald D. Smith, D.V.M., Ph.D., is professor emeritus of epidemiology and preventive medicine in the College of Veterinary Medicine at the University of Illinois. He received his D.V.M. from Michigan State University in 1967 and his M.S. and Ph.D. degrees in veterinary medical science from the University of Illinois.

From 1967 to 1970, Dr. Smith served as a U.S. Peace Corps veterinarian in Ecuador, working primarily on preventive disease programs for cattle, swine, and horses. He joined the faculty of the University of Illinois College of Veterinary Medicine in 1974. Dr. Smith's research interests have focused on the epidemiology and control of vector-borne blood diseases of animals and veterinary medical informatics.

Dr. Smith has undertaken numerous consultancies throughout Central and South America on behalf of IICA, FAO, and IAEA. These consultancies have focused on the diagnosis, epidemiology, and control of vector-borne blood diseases of animals, and more recently veterinary medical informatics.

He has taught professional and graduate courses on veterinary epidemiology, food safety and public health, and medical informatics. Dr. Smith has presented numerous invited papers at international conferences and is the principal or coauthor of more than 90 scientific publications and scholarly works.

Contents

chapter 1

Introduction

1.1 Definitions

Over the years there have been many definitions of epidemiology. Some definitions follow:

1. "The study of the distribution and determinants of disease frequency in man" (MacMahon and Pugh, 1970).
2. "The study of the patterns of disease" (Halpin, 1975).
3. "The study of the health status of populations" (Schwabe et al., 1977).
4. "Epidemiology is nothing more than ecology with a medical and mathematical flavor" (Norman D. Levine, 1990, personal communication).
5. "The study of the distribution and determinants of health-related states or events in specified populations, and the application of this study to control of health problems" (*Stedman's Medical Dictionary*, 2000).

Common features of the above definitions are revealed if we consider their origin. The term *epidemiology* derives from three Greek words: *epi* ("about" or "upon"); *demos* ("populace" or "people of districts"); and *logos* ("word," thus science or theory). The term *epizootiology* is sometimes used in reference to comparable studies in animal populations. The distinction is useful when one wishes to describe the state of disease in human or animal populations specifically, particularly when discussing zoonotic disease. For most purposes, however, epidemiology is understood to refer to all animal populations, human and otherwise. Likewise, to avoid confusion, it is preferable to use the term *epidemic* in lieu of *epizootic*, and *endemic* in lieu of *enzootic* wherever possible (Dohoo et al., 1994). Thus, a simple **definition of epidemiology** that captures the spirit of earlier definitions and reflects the emphasis of this book is "the research discipline concerned with the distribution and determinants of disease in populations" (Fletcher et al., 1988).

This definition alone does not appear to provide sufficient grounds for creating a separate discipline. After all, laboratory researchers study disease in populations of animals, populations that may comprise hundreds or thousands of individuals. Furthermore, laboratory researchers address the same sorts of questions as do epidemiologists — questions such as the cause, clinical signs, diagnosis, treatment, outcome, and prevention of disease. An important distinction, however, is that epidemiologists study disease in its natural habitat, away from the controlled environment of the laboratory. Epidemiology deals with naturally or spontaneously occurring, rather than experimentally induced, conditions.

The foregoing definitions imply that epidemiology is concerned with the population rather than the individual. To a certain extent this is true. However, an understanding of health and disease in populations is fundamental to medical decision making in the individual.

1.2   Epidemiologic approaches

Epidemiology has its roots in disease surveillance and outbreak investigation. Many consider that epidemiology was born during the cholera investigations conducted by John Snow in London in the mid-1800s. However, examples of outbreak investigation can be documented as far back as the Greek and Roman eras (Morens, 2003). Over the years, a number of epidemiologic disciplines and associated methodologies have emerged. These categories are somewhat arbitrary, but illustrate some of the ways in which epidemiology contributes to veterinary and human medicine.

1.2.1   Quantitative epidemiology

Quantitative epidemiology strives to quantify the distribution of diseases and associated factors in terms of individuals, place, and time and explore potentially causal associations. Quantitative epidemiology is practiced at two levels: **descriptive** and **analytic**. Descriptive statistics may be expressed as numerator data (number of individuals), proportions, or rates, or in terms of central tendency and dispersion. Data-gathering methods include sampling and diagnostic techniques for detecting the presence of disease, surveillance techniques for monitoring disease activity, and record-keeping systems. The submission of patient encounter data from U.S. veterinary medical teaching hospitals to the Veterinary Medical Database (VMDB; http://www.vmdb.org/) is an example of a descriptive, data-gathering technique. Other examples are the monitoring and surveillance activities of the USDA's National Center for Animal Health (CEAH) Surveillance (http://www.aphis. usda.gov/vs/ceah/cnahs/) and microbiological surveillance by the Food Safety and Inspection Service's (FSIS) Pathogen Reduction/HACCP Implementation program (http: //www.fsis.usda.gov/oa/haccp/imphaccp.htm). Results are expressed as descriptive statistics. Historical surveillance data provide an especially useful point of reference for documenting changes in disease frequency from such diverse causes as new and emerging diseases or adverse reactions to new pharmaceuticals or vaccines.

Analytic epidemiology goes beyond the purely descriptive process to draw statistical inferences about disease occurrence and possible causal associations. Techniques employed include univariable and multivariable regression, clustered and spatial data analysis, survival analysis, decision analysis, risk analysis, mathematical modeling, and a variety of statistical tests of significance. These techniques may be used to help distinguish true causal relationships from those simply due to bias, confounding, or chance, a problem inherent to epidemiologic research.

1.2.2   Ecological epidemiology (medical ecology)

Ecological epidemiology focuses on understanding factors that affect transmission and maintenance of disease agents in the environment. These factors are sometimes referred to as the **agent–host–environment triad**. Ecological epidemiology provides the scientific foundation for past and present disease eradication programs. The successful eradication programs for Texas cattle fever (bovine babesiosis) and screwworm (*Cochliomyia hominivorax*) were conceived based on knowledge of the natural history of the respective diseases. Traditionally, ecological epidemiology has focused on the life cycle, or natural history, of disease. The integration of molecular biology into traditional epidemiologic research, e.g., **molecular epidemiology**, has provided new tools for studying disease occurrence at the molecular level.

1.2.3   Etiologic epidemiology

Etiologic epidemiology is primarily concerned with exploring causal relationships for diseases of undetermined origin. Other terms that have been used to describe this activity are medical detection, "shoe leather," and field epidemiology. One of the principal activities in this category is outbreak investigation. Investigation into the causes of food-borne disease outbreaks is a classic example of etiologic epidemiology. A variety of sophisticated analytic techniques have been developed to help assess the relative importance of multiple causes of disease.

1.2.4   Herd health/preventive medicine

Herd health/preventive medicine uses information from any or all of the sources mentioned previously to design optimal management, control, or preventive strategies. Sometimes this requires a formal risk analysis to determine the true impact of presumed risk factors. Economic considerations are often the basis for determining which strategy is most effective. The most effective strategy may not be the one that results in the lowest incidence of disease, but rather the one that results in the greatest profit. Veterinary practitioners must learn to think in these terms if they are to interact effectively with producers.

1.2.5   Clinical epidemiology

Clinical epidemiology may be defined as *the research discipline concerned with applying epidemiologic methods to questions directly relevant to the practice of medicine at the individual or herd/flock level.* The sorts of questions asked in the practice of medicine are listed in Table 1.1. The answers to these questions are of immediate relevance to disease diagnosis, risk appraisal, prognosis, and treatment. Study designs may be observational or experimental. Observational studies represent a formal approach to the inductive process by which practitioners turn their practical observations into experience. Experimental studies (clinical trials) evaluate the relative merits of various interventions such as therapeutic, surgical, or preventive approaches to a particular disease syndrome. Clinical epidemiology provides the tools to help practitioners apply their own experiences, the experiences of others, and the medical literature to medical decision making.

▼

Epidemiologists study disease in its natural habitat, away from the controlled environment of the laboratory. Clinical epidemiology focuses on the sorts of questions asked in the practice of medicine.

▲

1.3   Applications of epidemiology in veterinary practice

Epidemiology has been described as a basic science for clinical medicine (Sackett et al., 1991). Epidemiologic studies are often the only way of exploring clinical issues such as the accuracy of diagnostic tests, risk factor identification, cause of diseases of multiple or uncertain etiology, and disease prognosis with and without treatment. They also provide a means for studying rare conditions or complications of disease that would be difficult to induce experimentally. One's own patients represent an important source of epidemiologic data. The cumulative clinical experience captured in a patient database can be used to evaluate and improve patient care. Epidemiology also provides the tools for critical

Table 1.1 Clinical Issues and Questions in the Practice of Medicine

Issue	Question
Normality/abnormality	What are the limits of normality? What abnormalities are associated with having a disease?
Diagnosis	How accurate are the diagnostic tests or strategies used to find a disease?
Frequency/occurrence	What is the case definition for a disease; how common are each of the findings? What are the host and spatial and temporal distribution of the disease?
Risk/prevention	What factors are associated with the likelihood of contracting disease?
Prognosis	What are the consequences of having a disease? What factors are associated with an increased or decreased likelihood of recovering from disease?
Treatment/control	How effective is a therapeutic strategy and how does it change the future course of a disease? How can the risk and rate of spread of the disease be reduced? How useful are the available tools for diagnosis, treatment, control, and prevention?
Cause	What is the etiologic agent? What is its life cycle? What characteristics contribute to its pathogenicity and virulence? What factors determine the susceptibility or resistance of individuals to the disease? What conditions predispose populations to outbreaks?
Source/transmission	What is the source and reservoir mechanism of the causative agent? What are the periods of communicability? How is the agent spread from infected to susceptible individuals? What is the route of infection?
Cost	What is the impact of a disease in personal and economic terms?

Adapted from: Fletcher, R.H. et al., *Clinical Epidemiology: The Essentials*, 2nd ed., Williams & Wilkins, Baltimore, 1988. With permission.

evaluation of medical claims. Bias, methodological errors, invalid assumptions, and chance can lead to erroneous conclusions from clinical studies. As one author put it: "science is the currency of medicine and the standard by which therapeutic claims are judged" (Ramey, 2003a).

The relationship between epidemiology and clinical medicine has been formalized in the practice of **evidence-based medicine** (EBM), *the process of systematically finding, appraising, and using contemporaneous research findings as the basis for clinical decisions* (NLM, 2004). EBM consists of the following five steps (Sackett et al., 1997):

1. At each stage of the case workup, identify one or more clinically important information needs and convert them into answerable questions.
2. Track down, with maximum efficiency, the best evidence with which to answer the above questions.
3. Summarize and critically appraise the evidence found for scientific validity and applicability.

4. Apply the results of this appraisal to patient care.
5. Evaluate your performance at answering the questions.

Although it may not be necessary for a practitioner to follow these steps for every case, most would probably agree that medical claims should be supported by evidence derived from patient experience.

Example 1.1

The appropriate use of **complementary and alternative veterinary medicine** (CAVM) (AVMA, 2001) provides an opportunity to appreciate the implications of evidence-based medicine. Although CAVM options have been promoted for preventing or treating a broad range of animal ailments, there is a paucity of clinical studies (evidence sources) upon which to evaluate their efficacy and effectiveness (Ramey, 2003b). It is therefore difficult for CAVM-based medical claims to meet the criteria defined in steps 2 and 3 above. This does not mean that CAVM-based approaches do not work. It simply means that the choice of any therapeutic modality should be based on a critical evaluation of its scientific basis and evidence of a favorable outcome. If a client insists on adopting an alternative modality for which little or no clinical evidence exists, the practitioner should offer to assist in monitoring and evaluating the response in a critical but sympathetic way (Rollin, 2002).

An evidence-based review format has been adopted by the journal *Veterinary Dermatology* for systematic reviews of the medical/veterinary literature for the purpose of formulating the best approach to diagnosis and treatment of dermatologic diseases in animals. The Materials and Methods section of these reviews describes how the literature search was done, criteria for selection of references, data extraction, and quality assessment of the reports. Meta-analysis (quantitative systematic review) of pooled results may also be performed when several studies investigate the same intervention. The end result is a summary of the evidence for and against current treatment recommendations.

Example 1.2

The efficacy of 41 different pharmacological interventions used to treat canine atopic dermatitis (AD) was evaluated based on the systematic review of 40 prospective clinical trials enrolling 1607 dogs published between 1980 and 2002 (Olivry and Mueller, 2003). To be included, a clinical trial had to include at least five dogs with AD, defined as "a genetically predisposed inflammatory and pruritic allergic skin disease with characteristic clinical features and associated most commonly with IgE antibodies to environmental allergens." Studies that did not report at least one clinical outcome were also excluded. Studies were compared on the basis of design and methodological quality (randomization generation and concealment, masking, intention-to-treat analyses, and quality of enrollment of study subjects), benefit (improvement in skin lesions or pruritus scores) and harm (type, severity, and frequency of adverse drug events) of the various interventions. Meta-analysis of pooled results was not possible because of heterogeneity of the drugs evaluated. Consequently, a qualitative assessment of interventions, grouped on the basis of similar mechanisms of drug action, was performed. Study design, patient enrollment quality, nature of interventions, and main outcome measures were summarized in narrative or tabular form. An overall *grade of evidence quality,* based on study design and the number of subjects entered in active treatment groups, was also considered in the evaluation. The authors concluded that there was good evidence for recommending the use of oral glucocorticoids and cyclosporin for the treatment of canine atopic dermatitis, and fair evidence for using topical triamcinolone spray, topical tacrolimus lotion, oral pentoxifylline, or oral misoprostol. There was insufficient evidence available for or against recommending the prescription of oral first- and second-generation type 1 histamine receptor antagonists, tricyclic antidepressants, cyproheptadine, aspirin, Chinese herbal therapy, a homeopathic complex remedy, ascorbic acid, a benzoic acid derivative, papaverine, immune-modulating antibiotics or tranilast, and topical pramoxine or capsaicin. Finally, there was fair evidence against recommending the use of oral arofylline, leukotriene synthesis inhibitors, and cysteinyl leukotriene receptor antagonists. Interestingly, in 17 trials there was evidence that administration of a placebo resulted in a clinically relevant reduction in pruritis in some dogs with AD, presumably due to the seasonality of clinical signs in AD. Thus, clinical trials of any drug for treatment of AD must take into account the frequency and magnitude of a placebo effect.

1.4   Objectives

This text is intended to give you a working knowledge of veterinary epidemiology. Specifically, it (1) shows you how epidemiologic data are used in medical decision making, (2) familiarizes you with epidemiologic study designs that allow valid conclusions to be drawn while controlling for sampling bias and chance, and (3) helps you learn to review critically and extract useful information from the medical literature. This is not intended to be a methods book. Readers can consult the cited articles from which examples were taken to learn more about particular methods.

1.4.1   Development of medical decision-making skills

Medical curricula, both human and veterinary, tend to focus on the mechanisms of disease in the individual through the study of anatomy, physiology, microbiology, immunology, and other basic sciences. This fosters the belief that the correct diagnosis and treatment of disease depend entirely on learning the detailed processes of disease in the individual. In medical practice, we deal with uncertainties, expressed as probabilities or risk. Each member of a population affected by the same disease agent may display a unique combination of signs. The frequency distribution of signs exhibited by the affected population will influence the accuracy of your diagnoses, prognoses, and treatments. An understanding of this variability can help you choose and interpret diagnostic tests and make clinical decisions. A practical problem resulting from disease variability is that of case definition, the starting point for determining the effectiveness of new therapeutic regimens.

Example 1.3

Two properties of diagnostic tests that affect their performance are sensitivity and specificity. Sensitivity data frequently are not recognized as such when used to describe clinical findings in patients. Table 1.2 summarizes clinical pathologic findings among 15 dogs in which a diagnosis of leptospirosis was made based on serology, clinical signs, and history (Boutilier et al., 2003). Which finding provides better criteria for ruling out a diagnosis of leptospirosis: a

Table 1.2 Clinical Pathologic Findings of 15 Dogs Diagnosed with Leptospirosis

Case	Creatinine (mg/dl)	Urea Nitrogen (mg/dl)	Urine Specific Gravity	Alkaline Phosphatase (U/l)	Alanine Amino-Transferase (U/l)	γ-Glutamyl Transferase (U/l)	Total Bilirubin (mg/dl)	White Blood Cells (×10⁹/l)	Platelets (×10⁹/l)
1	**4.1**	29.6	**1.007**	67	21	5	0.1	13.2	339
2	**13.0**	**205.7**	**1.012**	97	33	15	0.6	**35.4**	315
3	**7.0**	**58.0**	**1.006**	30	19	8	0.4	9.0	555
4	**16.0**	**139.8**	**1.009**	53	15	16	0.3	**22.4**	223
5	**13.1**	**104.9**	**1.006**	67	22	4	0.5	**23.3**	192
6	**7.4**	**97.3**	**1.010**	52	22	7	0.3	15.1	320
7	**6.0**	**66.6**	**1.005**	64	29	7	0.3	9.0	230
8	**5.5**	**74.9**	ND	169	23	3	0.1	9.8	232
9	**11.5**	**330**	**1.010**	74	121	16	0.2	8.8	201
10	**7.6**	**114.8**	**1.010**	140	194	5	0.8	13.9	ND
11	0.9	11	1.019	**835**	**548**	**41**	**0.9**	4.7	193
12	0.4	9.2	ND	**1036**	**375**	**75**	**1.2**	10.7	351
13	0.2	8.7	1.021	**2176**	**2305**	**44**	**2.6**	25.5	399
14	**5.1**	**112.0**	**1.012**	**591**	**350**	**106**	**2.0**	15.8	196
15	**4.5**	**51.6**	**1.006**	**695**	**117**	**79**	**3.8**	**34.6**	324

Note: Abnormal values are noted in **bold**. ND = value not determined.
Source: Boutilier, P. et al., *Vet. Ther.*, 4, 178–187, 2003. With permission.

normal creatinine level or a normal white blood cell count? (*Hint*: See Chapter 4 for a clue.)

1.4.2   Learn epidemiologic methodology and how to analyze and present data

The science of epidemiology evolved from the need to study naturally occurring health and disease in populations. The study of health and disease away from the controlled environment of the laboratory increases the likelihood that bias, confounding, and chance will influence our findings. The tools of epidemiology include a variety of techniques for collecting, analyzing, and interpreting data. They enable one to draw accurate conclusions about populations by controlling for bias, confounding variables, and random error. Summary presentation of data as tables or graphs can help clarify relationships and trends.

A familiarity with descriptive and inferential statistics should be a prerequisite for veterinarians, who are continually faced with the risk of misdiagnosing a case. The design of animal disease surveillance programs is influenced by sampling and detection statistics. Private practitioners may be asked to participate in state and federal regulatory efforts and must understand their scientific basis. Accredited veterinarians are authorized to test animals for brucellosis, tuberculosis, and pseudorabies, and to sign health certificates for interstate movement.

Example 1.4

Chronic wasting disease (CWD) was diagnosed in 3% of 476 free-ranging white-tailed deer harvested during the 2001 hunting season in an area of Wisconsin where the disease is known to occur (Joly et al., 2003). Based on these findings, how many deer should be sampled from other parts of the state to be 95% sure of detecting CWD if the prevalence were the same? (*Hint*: See Chapter 9 for a clue.)

1.4.3   Learn to read the medical literature critically

Veterinary journals play an important role in keeping practitioners abreast of current medical knowledge. Examples are reports of new and emerging diseases, risk factors for disease and injury, and prognosis with or without medical intervention. The usefulness of this information ultimately depends on the adequacy of the study design and the analysis and interpretation of the data.

▼

A variety of study designs are used in clinical research. The poorest designs are so prone to problems of chance, bias, and confounding factors that the validity of their conclusions is marginal.

▲

A variety of study designs are used in clinical research (Smith, 1988) (Table 1.3). Each has inherent strengths and weaknesses (Table 1.4). The poorest designs are so prone to problems of chance, bias, and confounding factors that the validity of their conclusions is marginal (Dohoo and Waltner-Toews, 1985a–c). Given the effect that chance, bias, and confounding factors can have on the validity of conclusions derived from clinical research, students must learn to evaluate this important resource critically. The effectiveness of veterinary clinical research can be enhanced by choosing epidemiologic study designs appropriate for the clinical issue being examined, and through more rigid adherence to accepted norms for expressing the findings from such studies.

Table 1.3 Key for Classification of Study Designs

1. Subjects under study experienced experimentally induced disease, condition, or intervention	Experimental disease
Subjects under study experienced naturally occurring disease, condition, or intervention	Go to 2
2. Fewer than 10 animal units (individuals, herds, etc.) or outbreaks examined	Case report
Ten or more individuals or outbreaks examined	Go to 3
3. Cross-sectional: All observations on a given individual are made at essentially one point in time in the course of that individual's illness	Go to 4
Longitudinal: Subjects followed prospectively over a period of time; groups may be formed in the past (from records) or in the present	Go to 6
4. Comparison group absent	Case series
Comparison group present	Go to 5
5. Cases selected from an available pool of patients; noncases selected to resemble cases, but not necessarily members of the same population group	Case control study
Cases and noncases ascertained through random selection from a defined population	Prevalence survey
6. No intervention	Cohort study
Intervention	Go to 7
7. Comparison group absent	Uncontrolled clinical trial
Comparison group present	Go to 8
8. Nonrandom allocation of subjects into treatment and control groups	Nonrandomized controlled clinical trial
Random allocation of subjects into treatment and control groups	Randomized controlled clinical trial

Source: Smith, R.D., *J. Vet. Med. Educ.*, 15, 2–7, 1988. With permission.

Example 1.5

A study was conducted in a veterinary teaching hospital to identify risk factors for bite wounds inflicted on caregivers by dogs and cats (Drobatz and Smith, 2003). Eighty percent of case subjects (caregivers that had been bitten) were females. Can we conclude that women are at greater risk of being bitten than men? If not, what else do we need to know? (*Hint*: See Chapter 6 for a clue.)

Table 1.4 Relative Merits of Clinical Research Designs

Study Design	Limitations	Best Application
Case report	Temporal relationships; bias in case selection; statistical validity	Detailed description of uncommon diseases; surveillance
Case series	Temporal relationships; bias in case selection	Frequency of findings in a disease
Prevalence survey	Temporal relationships; measures prevalence, not incidence	Evaluation of diagnostic tests; incrimination of risk or causal factors; outbreak investigation
Case control	Temporal relationships; bias in selection of comparison group	Evaluation of diagnostic tests; incrimination of risk or causal factors; outbreak investigation; rare disease or diseases of long latency
Uncontrolled clinical trial	Time; ethical considerations; no comparison group	Prognosis with or without treatment
Nonrandomized controlled clinical trial	Time; ethical considerations; bias in selection of comparison group	Prognosis with or without treatment; evaluation of new treatments
Randomized controlled clinical trial	Time; ethical considerations	Prognosis with or without treatment; evaluation of new treatments
Experimental disease	Time; availability of animals or other animal models; cost	Proving relationship between risk or causal factors and disease; pathogenic mechanisms

1.5   Summary

Epidemiology is the research discipline concerned with the distribution and determinants of disease in populations. Epidemiology involves (1) the study of naturally occurring vs. experimentally induced disease, (2) the study of disease in the population vs. the individual, and (3) the detection of associations by inferential methods vs. the study of pathologic mechanisms.

Over the years a number of approaches and associated methodologies have emerged. Quantitative epidemiology attempts to describe and quantify the distribution of disease and associated risk factors in a population or defined geographic region. Ecological epidemiology focuses on understanding factors that affect transmission and maintenance of disease agents in the environment, e.g., its natural history. These factors comprise what is often referred to as the agent–host–environment triad. Etiologic epidemiology is primarily concerned with establishing causal relationships for diseases of undetermined origin. Herd health/preventive medicine endeavors to use information from any or all of the previously mentioned sources to design optimal management, control, or preventive strategies. Clinical epidemiology is the application of epidemiologic principles and methods to problems encountered in medical practice. It focuses on the substance of epidemiologic studies and their practical application in clinical settings.

The tools of epidemiology include a variety of techniques for collecting, analyzing, and interpreting data. They enable the investigator to draw accurate conclusions from population studies while controlling for bias, confounding, and random error. The relationship between epidemiology and clinical medicine has been formalized in the practice of evidence-based medicine (EBM), the process of systematically finding, appraising, and using contemporaneous research findings as the basis for clinical decisions. Because journals play such an important role in continuing medical education, students and practitioners must learn how to read modern medical journals critically. Because much of this information is gathered through epidemiologic study designs, a basic understanding of epidemiology is critical to their evaluation.

chapter 2

Defining the limits of normality

2.1 Introduction

> Personally, I have always felt that the best doctor in the world is the veterinarian. He can't ask his patients what is the matter … he's just got to know.

> **—Will Rogers**
> (Pediatricians would probably take issue with this.)

Although the way that we gather data may at times differ, the process of veterinary and human medical decision making is basically the same and consists of at least four steps. First, subjective data are collected, such as alertness, attitude, evidence of pain, etc. These data are based on our own observations and those of the owner. Objective data are also collected; indices include temperature, pulse, respiration, results of parasitologic examinations, complete blood counts, radiographs, etc. These data are then interpreted as either normal (within normal limits, unremarkable, noncontributory) or abnormal in light of our past experience and the medical literature, and we arrive at an assessment (or, in some cases, appreciation) of the problem. Depending on this assessment, we then devise a plan that may be a more complete workup, a rule-out of other possible diagnoses, a treatment, or client education (Sandlow et al., 1974).

▼

> Although the way that we gather data may at times differ, the process of veterinary and human medical decision making is basically the same and consists of at least four steps.

▲

At this point the astute reader will have realized that the acronym for this process (subjective data, objective data, assessment, and plan) is SOAP. SOAPs are part of the **problem-oriented medical records** system that provides a formal way of recording subjective and objective data about a patient. From these databases, patient problems are isolated and defined. All recognized problems, past and present, are assessed and listed as a problem list, and plans for the management of each problem are then recorded.

In this chapter we first review the properties of clinical measurements and their distributions within animal populations. Next we develop criteria by which abnormal values for clinical measurements are recognized, including normal reference ranges.

2.2   Properties of clinical measurements

Practitioners are continually collecting, categorizing, and quantifying biological data about their patients. In the hospital environment these data are categorized as patient history, clinical signs, and screening/definitive tests. The important point to remember is that clinical data alone mean nothing until interpreted in the context of expected values for the population. Clinical assessment is based on the degree to which patient data differ from population norms and match expectations for particular disease syndromes. The response to the treatment plan is assessed by the rate and degree to which clinical findings return to normal population values. In this section we examine the factors that influence the confidence we place in clinical measurements.

2.2.1   Signs and symptoms: objective vs. subjective data

The following are definitions from *Stedman's Medical Dictionary* (2000):

- A **sign** is "any abnormality indicative of disease, discoverable on examination of the patient; an objective indication of disease, in contrast to a symptom, which is a subjective indication of disease."
- A **symptom** is "any morbid phenomenon or departure from the normal in structure, function, or sensation, experienced by the patient and indicative of disease."

--------------------------▼--------------------------

Clinical data alone mean nothing until interpreted in the context of expected values for the population.

--------------------------▲--------------------------

It has been argued that because our patients cannot talk, veterinarians rely only on signs to assess the clinical condition and progress of patients. Animals are generally more stoic than humans and may not exhibit behavioral alterations until the condition has progressed quite far. Yet, our assessment of a patient's health may include subjective evidence that fits the definition of symptoms. Furthermore, we often use the terms *symptomatic* or *asymptomatic* to describe the presence or absence of evidence of disease.

It is important to recognize subjective data as subjective and ensure that measures have been taken to reduce the influence of personal bias in clinical measurements.

Example 2.1

Behavioral characteristics are an example of subjective data used to describe animals. Investigators (Hart and Miller, 1985) sought to develop breed behavioral profiles based on 13 traits (Table 2.1) as a guide for potential pet owners. In order to obtain profiles that were quantitative and free of personal biases, they surveyed 48 small-animal veterinarians and 48 obedience judges, randomly selected from directories so as to represent equally men and women, and eastern, central, and western regions of the U.S. The authors concluded that it is possible to obtain quantitative data that reflect objectively the consensus of authorities about differences in behavior among breeds of dogs. Some behavioral traits discriminated between breeds better than others. The authors attributed this ranking in part to early training and environment.

Table 2.1 Behavioral Characteristics Used as a Basis for Constructing Behavioral Profiles of 56 Dog Breeds (Ranked in Order of Decreasing Reliability Based on the Magnitude of the F Ratio)

	Behavioral Characteristic	F Ratio[a]
1.	Excitability	9.6
2.	General activity	9.5
3.	Tendency to snap at children	7.2
4.	Excessive barking	6.9
5.	Playfulness	6.7
6.	Obedience trainability	6.6
7.	Watchdog barking	5.1
8.	Aggression to dogs	5.0
9.	Dominance over owner	4.3
10.	Territorial defense	4.1
11.	Affection demand	3.6
12.	Destructiveness	2.6
13.	Housebreaking ease	1.8

[a] $p < 0.005$; see Chapter 9 for a more complete discussion of p values.

Source: Hart, B.L. and Miller, M.F., *J. Am. Vet. Med. Assoc.*, 186, 1175–1180, 1985. With permission.

2.2.2   Scales

Clinical data are of three types: nominal, ordinal, or interval. **Nominal data** can be placed into discrete categories that have no inherent order. Another name for nominal data is **categorical data**. Clinical phenomena that fall into this category are either inherent characteristics of an animal (e.g., name, species, breed, sex, and coat color) or discrete events (e.g., fracture, birth, death).

▼

Clinical data are of three types: nominal, ordinal, or interval.

▲

Ordinal data are categorical data with an obvious order that can be ranked, but the intervals are not uniform in size. Examples are degrees of depression, pain, or anxiety, degrees of dehydration or incoordination, and severity of respiratory sounds or cardiac murmurs. One student wrote in a canine patient's progress report: "On an alertness scale of 1 to 5, give him a 3."

Data that are ordered and for which the size of the intervals are equal are called **interval**. Another name of interval data is **continuous data**. Examples are weight, rectal temperature, packed cell volume, and leukocyte count. The size of the intervals depends on the precision of instruments used to make the measurements.

Most interval-level scales used in medicine have absolute (mathematically meaningful) zero points; e.g., a value of zero means absolute zero of the quantity being measured. Examples are body weight, heart and respiratory rates, blood chemistries and differentials, etc. A negative value is not possible. In some cases, such as the Fahrenheit or Celsius temperature scales, zero is simply an arbitrary point whose value happens to be called zero. On these scales zero does not represent an absolute absence of the factor being measured, and negative values are possible. Interval scales that have absolute zero points are sometimes referred to as **ratio** scales. Ratio scales permit the meaningful calculation of ratios. For example, if an animal's packed cell volume (PCV) increases from 10 to 20% in response to treatment, it is legitimate and meaningful to say that the PCV has doubled. If, on the other hand, the high temperatures on two successive days are 4 and 8°C, it makes no sense to conclude that the second day is twice as warm as the first because the zero point from which 4 and 8°C are starting out is only an arbitrary marker on a scale that potentially extends all the way down to about –273°C. In order to make such ratio judgments concerning temperatures, we would have to use a scale such as the Kelvin scale, whose zero point does mark an absolute zero level of temperature. Since ratio-level variables are treated the same as interval-level variables for all other statistical purposes, they will be considered as interval data throughout this text.

It is not uncommon for interval-level data to be reduced to the ordinal or categorical level in clinical records. For example, a hospital admission record may divide age and body weight into unequal interval classes (age: 0 to 2 weeks, 2 weeks to 2 months, 2 to 6 months, etc.; weight: 0 to 1 lb, 1 to 5 lb, 5 to 15 lb, etc.). These lower scales of measurement precision can be convenient for summarizing large amounts of information into clinically meaningful categories. However, useful information may be lost in the process. For example, a follow-up study of the prognostic values of animal age or weight for a specific condition may be impossible without precise interval-level data. Therefore, if time and other limitations permit, information should be recorded at the same level as it was measured.

Sometimes ordinal data are recorded on an interval-level scale and then analyzed statistically as if they were truly interval. This is an inappropriate conversion of data, as it may misrepresent the magnitude of differences among individual measurements. Furthermore, the raw data are often subjective in nature and do not meet the measurement and reproducibility criteria of interval-level data.

Example 2.2

Coprophagy, the ingestion of an animal's own feces or that of another of the same species, is considered to be a problem behavior in dogs that is both unattractive and unhygienic. The etiology of coprophagy in dogs is unknown, although several suggestions have been proposed, ranging from dietary or physiologic imbalance, unintentional reinforcement of the behavior by the owner, or a simple preference for the taste of certain kinds of feces. There is little empirical evidence on the benefits of any of the treatments that have been proposed. Wells (2003) conducted a clinical trial of two treatments for the prevention of coprophagy in 28 client-owned dogs with a history of coprophagy. Half were treated with a citronella spray collar that emits a cloud of spray together with an audible hiss under the dog's nose whenever the collar is triggered remotely by the owner. The remainder were exposed to sound therapy via a handheld alarm that emits a 115-dB screech whenever the trigger of the propellant spray is pressed, thereby interrupting the dog's behavior. To assess the relative efficacy of the treatments, owners rated the severity of their dog's feces eating for a week before the study began, during each of 3 weeks of treatment, and at the end of a fourth week, during which they had not been treated. Owners watched from an inconspicuous site in the yard and counted the number of stools the dog ingested in relation to the number available for ingestion. Severity of coprophagy was scored on a scale ranging from 1 to 4, where 1 indicated 0 to 25% of available feces were eaten, 2 indicated 26 to 50%

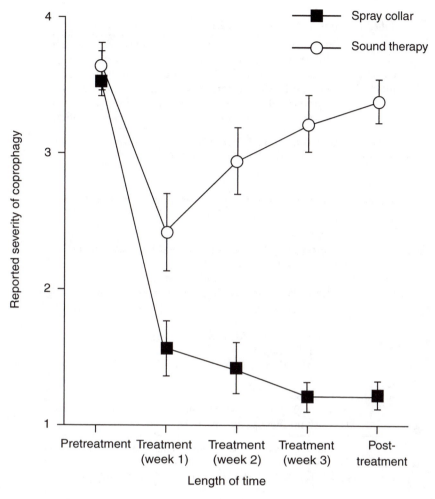

Figure 2.1 Mean (se) reported severity of coprophagy (1 = lowest level, 4 = highest level) exhibited by dogs that were treated with a spray collar or sound therapy, before, during, and after treatment. (From Wells, D.L., *Vet. Rec.*, 153, 51–53, 2003. With permission.)

of available feces were eaten, 3 indicated 51 to 75% of available feces were eaten, and 4 indicated 76 to 100% of available feces were eaten. This scoring system is a clear example of converting broad ordinal data (0 to 25%, 26 to 50%, etc.) to a fixed interval scale (1, 2, etc.) with a concomitant loss of precision. The potential discrepancy between the original (percentage) data and the converted score can be appreciated by considering that owner scores of 26 and 50% (a 24% difference) would both be recorded as 2, whereas an owner assessment of 25% coprophagy (only 1% less than 26%) would be recorded as 1. An evaluation of the converted scores reveals a significantly lower incidence of coprophagy during the first week of both treatments, but in the dogs treated by sound therapy its incidence subsequently increased (Figure 2.1). The behavioral problem appears to have been reduced most effectively in the dogs treated with the spray collar, and continued to decrease during the period of treatment. However, the true magnitude of the difference between treatments is difficult to assess without comparing the original percentage-based data. The error bars depicted in Figure 2.1 may not accurately reflect the true difference between treatment groups.

Table 2.2 Clinical Assessment of Anemia in the Dog and Cat

Nominal	Breed, sex, diet, history of drug administration or recent infection, existence of a heart murmur or hemorrhages
Ordinal	Color of mucous membranes, grade of heart murmur
Interval	Age, cardiac and respiratory rates, packed cell volume, complete blood count, frequency distribution of erythrocyte morphologic types, total plasma protein

Source of data: Straus, J.H., in Fenner, W.R., Ed., *Quick Reference to Veterinary Medicine*, J.B. Lippincott Co., Philadelphia, 1982, pp. 383–398.

Table 2.3 Clinical Stages of Tumors of the Canine Prostate Gland

T	Primary tumor
	T0 = no evidence of tumor
	T1 = intracapsular tumor, surrounded by normal gland
	T2 = diffuse intracapsular tumor
	T3 = tumor extending beyond the capsule
	T4 = tumor fixed or invading neighboring structures
N	RLN[a]
	N0 = no evidence of RLN involvement
	N1 = RLN involved
	N2 = RLN and juxta-RLN involved
M	Distant metastasis
	M0 = no evidence of distant metastasis
	M1 = distant metastasis detected

[a] RLN = regional lymph nodes. RLN include external and internal iliac nodes; juxta-RLN include lumbar nodes. b = bony involvement.

Source: Turrel, J.M., *J. Am. Vet. Med. Assoc.*, 190, 48–52, 1987. With permission.

The differences among nominal, ordinal, and interval-level variables can be appreciated in Table 2.2, which summarizes the clinical assessment of canine and feline anemia.

2.2.3   Clinical staging

Clinical staging is another expression of the degree of abnormality. Separation of patients based on the severity of their condition is necessary before comparing such things as diagnostic tests, prognosis, and response to treatment.

One internationally recognized form of clinical staging is the TNM Classification of Tumours in Domestic Animals (Owen, 1980), which was established by an international consultation sponsored by the World Health Organization (WHO) Programme on Comparative Oncology. The staging criteria were modeled after a classification system established in 1968 for tumors in humans. The principal purpose of international agreement on clinical staging of animal tumors is to provide a method of conveying clinical observations without ambiguity. The system arose from the fact that survival rates were higher for localized, compared with disseminated, tumors. Before establishment of the TNM staging system, these groups were often referred to as early cases and late cases, implying some regular progression with time.

The uniformity of clinical staging among practitioners varies, depending in large part on the subjectivity of the criteria used. For example, contrast the relatively rigid TNM criteria for classification of canine prostate tumors (Turrel, 1987) (Table 2.3) with criteria

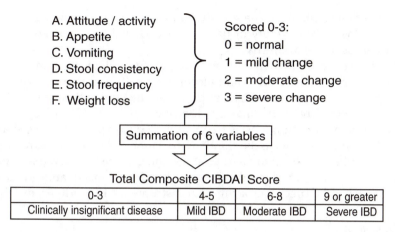

A. Attitude / activity
B. Appetite
C. Vomiting
D. Stool consistency
E. Stool frequency
F. Weight loss

Scored 0-3:
0 = normal
1 = mild change
2 = moderate change
3 = severe change

Summation of 6 variables

Total Composite CIBDAI Score

0-3	4-5	6-8	9 or greater
Clinically insignificant disease	Mild IBD	Moderate IBD	Severe IBD

Figure 2.2 Criteria for assessment of canine inflammatory bowel disease activity index (CIBDAI). (From Jergens, A.E. et al., *Vet. Intern. Med.*, 17, 291–297, 2003. With permission.)

proposed for assessing the severity of canine inflammatory bowel disease (Jergens et al., 2003) (Figure 2.2; example below). Clinical staging is necessary, but definitions are only as good as the criteria used to construct them. Furthermore, clinical staging is based on the present state of knowledge, and most systems will require modification in the future.

Example 2.3

Inflammatory bowel disease (IBD) in dogs is a chronic gastrointestinal tract disorder of unknown cause and ill-defined pathogenesis. Human correlates include Crohn disease and ulcerative colitis. The severity of IBD is highly individualistic and may differ considerably among canine patients. Accurate staging of the degree of illness (activity) is hampered by the variability of clinical signs. Jergens et al. (2003) developed a canine IBD activity index (CIBDAI) scoring system for assessing canine IBD activity and validated its clinical application by correlating it to objective laboratory and histologic indices of intestinal inflammation. The severity of six salient gastrointestinal signs were scored 0 to 3 by a gastroenterologist based on the magnitude of their alteration from normal in a given IBD patient. These scores were then summed, yielding a total cumulative CIBDAI score that reflected clinically insignificant disease or the presence of mild, moderate, or severe IBD (Figure 2.2).

2.2.4   Validity and reliability

Validity and reliability are terms that have been used to describe the quality of clinical measurements. **Validity** (or accuracy) describes the degree to which a measurement reflects the true status of what is being measured. **Reliability** is a measure of the repeatability or reproducibility of a clinical measurement. Reliability is sometimes referred to as **precision**.

Validity and reliability are relatively easy to establish when measurements can be compared with some accepted standard. Examples are blood chemistry measurements in which instruments are calibrated with known standards. Another example may be serodiagnostic tests in which subsequent culture or necropsy may confirm the presence of disease. Validity and reliability are more difficult to establish for other clinical measurements that rely on our senses and for which no physical standards exist. Examples might be the validity of our estimate of the severity of pneumonia based on auscultory findings vs. necropsy, or the reproducibility of pain scores assigned to patients by different clinicians, e.g., **interobserver variability**.

Validity may be independent of reliability. Repeated serologic tests on a serum sample, for example, may give consistently valid (accurate) results, but titers may vary considerably about the true value. In contrast, an improperly functioning thermometer can be very reliable, but systematically off the mark (inaccurate).

The **coefficient of variation** (CV) is frequently used to express the precision of clinical measurements. The CV is equal to the standard deviation of a set of measurements divided by their mean, and is usually expressed as a percentage. The CV therefore represents the percentage variation of a set of measurements around their mean, and provides a useful index for comparing the precision of different instruments, individuals, or laboratories.

2.2.5 Variation

There are two major sources of variation in clinical measurements. One is associated with the act of measurement itself, while the other is associated with biological variation within and among individuals. Clinicians should be aware of potential sources of variation to avoid erroneous conclusions about data in a given situation.

2.2.5.1 Measurement variation

Measurement variation may be due to variation in the way samples are handled and processed, the performance of the instruments being used, or the observers themselves. It can be thought of as the variation recorded during repeated measurements of the same parameter in an individual, irrespective of other members of the population.

Example 2.4

The Schirmer tear test is used routinely in evaluating the adequacy of tear production in animals that have signs of keratoconjunctivitis. Hawkins and Murphy (1986) evaluated the clinical importance of observed discrepancies in the absorptive capacity of tear test strips. Major inconsistencies in the ability of test strips to absorb water were found within one lot of tear strips from a single manufacturer. The variability in the tear strips examined could influence the clinical diagnosis of keratoconjunctivitis sicca and the subsequent interpretation of response to treatment, as well as the interpretation and repeatability of research data.

2.2.5.2 Biological variation

Biological variation can manifest at all levels of an animal population. The histopathologic description of a biopsy, for example, may vary depending on the region of the affected lesion or the organ from which it is taken. Clinical measurements vary over time within an individual. In some cases this variation may be cyclic, such as hormone levels, heartworm microfilarial counts, or body temperature. In others it varies with each patient.

Veterinary medicine is unique in that practitioners deal with disease at both the individual and herd levels. Although the effects of biologic variation on herd data can be moderated by taking larger sample sizes, there is little the practitioner can do to reduce the effects of biological variation when interpreting tests on individual patients. As a rule, rigid adherence to test protocols is the single most important way to reduce overall test variation.

Example 2.5

Nutrient foramina are common findings in skeletal radiography. Location and radiographic appearance of these foramina are usually uniform and bilaterally symmetrical. Foramina that appear in unusual locations may be misdiagnosed as fractures. Losonsky and Kneller (1988) examined bilateral metacarpopha-langeal radiographs in 100 Standardbred horses. Left and right proximal pha-langeal foramina were symmetrical in 45 horses, but were asymmetrical in the remaining 55 horses. Of 200 proximal phalangeal foramina (in 100 horses), 78 were in the dorsal cortex, 61 were in the palmar cortex, and 61 were not visible radiographically. A significant ($p = 0.05$) effect of age or sex could not be determined. Dorsal nutrient foramina are those most commonly mistaken for fractures, presumably because of the length and vertical direction of the de-creased density line. In 36 (63%) of 57 Standardbreds with dorsal nutrient foramina, these foramina were unilateral in the proximal forelimb phalanx. The authors concluded that radiographic comparison of the opposite limb would not have been a valid guideline for determining normality in more than half of these horses.

2.2.5.3 *Reducing the effects of variation*

In an effort to reduce variation, it may be useful to distinguish **random variation** from **systematic variation**, or **bias**. Random variation results from the chance distribution of measurements, such as erythrocyte counts in different microscope fields, around an aver-age value and will not significantly alter our interpretation of the true status of what is being measured. Inaccuracy due to random variation can be reduced by taking a larger sample size. On the other hand, systematic variation, such as erythrocyte counts reported by different technicians, may consistently be biased. In these cases, use of a correction factor may be indicated. This is what we are actually doing when we blank an instrument, such as a spectrophotometer, or when we adjust the scale of a chart recorder. As long as these corrections are made carefully and systematically, the validity of the data is not compromised.

Reference ranges for clinical measurements should be determined and expressed by age intervals for each species. For example, plasma protein values are very low in dogs at birth, elevate to the levels seen in the dam after the puppies have nursed, gradually drop during the second 6 months of life, then begin to elevate again after the first year. Maximum levels for this parameter in dogs are reached at about 7 to 10 years, after which the animal will have gradually decreasing values. Leukocyte differential counts in cattle are similar to those in dogs and cats from birth to weaning. After that, they change drastically in the bovine and lymphocytes become the predominant peripheral leukocyte.

2.3 Distributions

The adage that a picture is worth a thousand words (or numbers) is nowhere more true than in the expression of population data. Data that can be measured on an interval scale, whether continuous or discrete, can be expressed as a **frequency distribution**. The fre-quency distribution may be presented as a table or as a graph, referred to as a **histogram** or frequency polygon. Frequency distributions may take many forms, but all include at least one scale representing the range of possible values in a distribution, usually divided into intervals, and a second scale depicting the number or proportion of the population that falls within each interval.

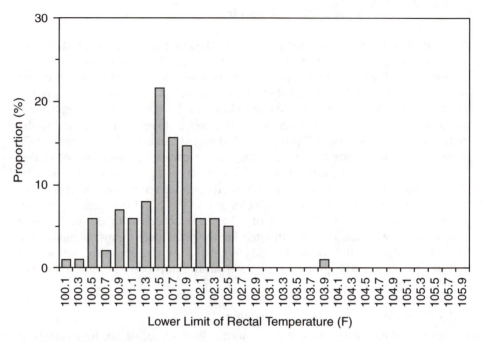

Figure 2.3 Frequency distribution of rectal temperatures in normal dogs.

Example 2.6

A typical histogram is depicted in Figure 2.3, which presents the distribution of 102 normal canine body temperatures. The size of each interval on the abscissa (x-axis) is 0.2°F. We could have chosen any other interval, as long as it was not smaller than that used to actually record the measurements. The scale on the ordinate (y-axis) depicts the proportion of dogs in each interval. Note that x-axis intervals are retained in the histogram even for temperature values in which the count is zero. Histograms should not be confused with **bar charts**, which differ from histograms in that intervals for values in which the count is zero are omitted. Bar charts are useful for displaying the counts for values of both ordered and nonordered variables.

2.3.1 Basic properties of distributions

Although Figure 2.3 represents a summary of 102 temperature readings, it is convenient to further summarize this data, particularly if we wish to compare it with other temperature distributions. Two basic properties of distributions can be used to summarize this data: **central tendency**, or the middle of the distribution, and **dispersion**, an index of the spread of the data. There are various ways of expressing central tendency and dispersion. These are summarized in Table 2.4 along with their advantages and disadvantages.

▼

Two basic properties of distributions can be used to summarize data: central tendency and dispersion.

▲

Table 2.4 Expressions of Central Tendency and Dispersion for Frequency Distributions

Expression	Definition	Advantages	Disadvantages
Measures of Central Tendency			
Mean	Sum of values for observations ÷ number of observations	Well suited for mathematical manipulation	Easily influenced by extreme values
Median	The point where the number of observations above equals the number below	Not easily influenced by extreme values	Not well suited for mathematical manipulation
Mode	Most frequently occurring value	Simplicity of meaning; the only way to describe the center of ordinal data.	Sometimes there are no or many "most frequent" values
Measures of Dispersion			
Range	From lowest to highest value in a distribution	Includes all values	Greatly affected by extreme values
Standard deviation	The absolute value of the average difference of individual values from the mean[a]	Well suited for mathematical manipulation	For non-Gaussian distributions, does not describe a known proportion of the observations
Percentile, decile, quartile, etc.	The proportion of all observations falling between specified values	Describes the known proportion of observations without assumptions about the shape of the distribution	Not well suited for statistical manipulation

$$[a] \quad \sqrt{\frac{\Sigma(X - \bar{X})^2}{N-1}}$$

Source: Fletcher, R.H. et al., *Clinical Epidemiology: The Essentials*, 3rd ed., Lippincott Williams & Wilkins, Baltimore, 1996. With permission.

2.3.2   Shapes of naturally occurring distributions

2.3.2.1   Unimodal, bimodal, and multimodal

The frequency distribution for a variable can have one or more measurement values with the maximum frequency, or **mode**. The shape of a distribution can be characterized in part by the number of modes it has. A distribution with only one modal value is unimodal; with two modal values, bimodal; etc. In general, a distribution with more than one mode is called multimodal.

2.3.2.2   Symmetry, skewness, and kurtosis

Another characteristic of the shape of a distribution is **symmetry** (or its converse, skewness). These properties are reflected in the relationship between the mean, median, and

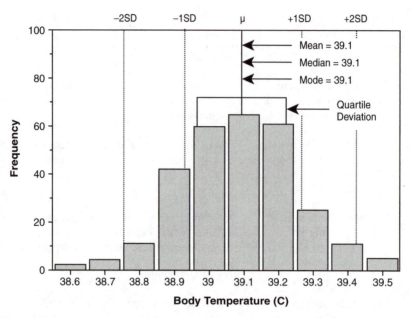

Figure 2.4 Frequency distribution of rectal temperature values for a cat over a 24-hour period. (Data courtesy of Dr. R.M. Weigel, College of Veterinary Medicine, University of Illinois. With permission.)

mode of a distribution. In symmetrical distributions, the mean, median, and mode are equal. In positively skewed distributions, the mean is greater than the median, due to extreme values at the upper values of the distribution (often referred to as skewed to the right). In negatively skewed distributions, the mean is less than the median, due to extreme values at the lower values of the distribution (skewed to the left). **Kurtosis** describes the peakedness of a data distribution, e.g., whether the shape of the distribution is relatively short and flat, or tall and slender, or somewhere in between.

Figure 2.4 shows the frequency distribution of body temperatures taken over a 24-hour period for a single cat. This distribution is unimodal and symmetric, with the mean, median, and mode all coinciding (at 39.1°C). Figure 2.5 shows the frequency distribution of heart rate values for the same cat over the same 24-hour period. This distribution is positively skewed, with the mean greater than the median.

2.3.2.3 Factors influencing the shape of frequency distributions

Actual frequency distributions for many clinical measurements of animal populations change with characteristics such as age, sex, plane of nutrition, and, in food-producing animals, stage of production.

Example 2.7

Figure 2.6 depicts the frequency distribution of blood urea nitrogen (BUN) levels among 47 dairy herds (Payne et al., 1970). The data are only a portion of a battery of blood chemistry test results that were systematically collected from representative members of dairy herds to produce metabolic profiles (Stevens et al., 1980). The histograms actually represent the distribution of herd means. This is appropriate because the producer and veterinarian are often interested in herd performance rather than the health of individual animals. The metabolic profiles are used as a diagnostic aid to help identify metabolic

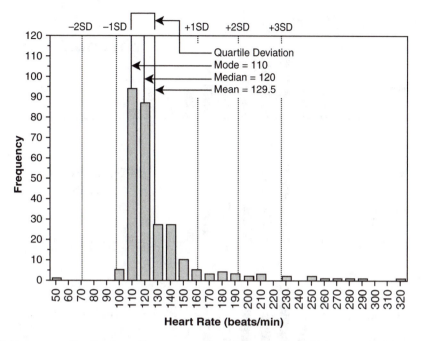

Figure 2.5 Frequency distribution of heart rate values for a cat over a 24-hour period. (Data courtesy of Dr. R.M. Weigel, College of Veterinary Medicine, University of Illinois. With permission.)

problems in dairy herds that can then be corrected through improved feeding practices.

In this example the shape of the distribution curves vary with performance. For example, the distribution of BUN values of dry cows is broad and relatively flat, whereas that of middle-yield cows is skewed to the right. Thus, the timing and choice of population samples must be taken into consideration to avoid bias in test results.

2.3.3 The normal distribution

At this point it is important to draw a distinction between the naturally occurring distributions discussed above and the **normal or Gaussian distribution**, the symmetrical bell-shaped curve that is frequently used as the standard that biological data are assumed to fit. The normal distribution (Figure 2.7) is a mathematical or theoretical model that describes the distribution of repeated measurements of the same physical properties by the same instrument. The dispersion of these measurements thus represents random variation alone. Because the frequency distribution for many continuous random variables in biology *approximate* a normal distribution, the latter is frequently used as a mathematical or theoretical model for calculating central tendency and dispersion. In clinical epidemiology it is frequently used to calculate the limits of normality.

The mathematical representation of the normal distribution is not discussed here, but some consequences of the mathematical formulation for the shape and other distribution properties of the normal distribution should be mentioned. The normal distribution is unimodal, with the mean equal to the median equal to the mode. It is symmetrical, meaning that within a given number of **standard deviation** (SD) units from the mean, there will be the same proportion of values in the positive direction as in the negative direction. Approximately two thirds of all values will be within ±1 SD of the mean,

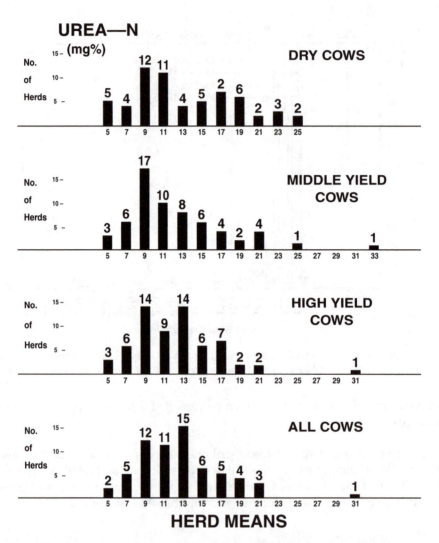

Figure 2.6 Distribution of results for urea in metabolic profile tests on 47 dairy herds. (From Payne, J.M. et al., *Vet. Rec.*, 87, 150–157, 1970. With permission.)

approximately 95% of values will be within approximately ±2 SDs of the mean, and approximately 99% of values will be within approximately ±3 SDs of the mean in a normal distribution.

2.4   Reference ranges and the criteria for abnormality

We now come to a crucial point: Given the variety of clinical measurements and dispersion inherent in animal data, how do we determine what is normal and what is abnormal? The distribution of clinical values among normal and diseased individuals frequently overlaps.

Example 2.8

In Figure 2.8 the frequency distribution of body temperatures for a group of clinically normal dogs (from Figure 2.3) is superimposed on that for dogs

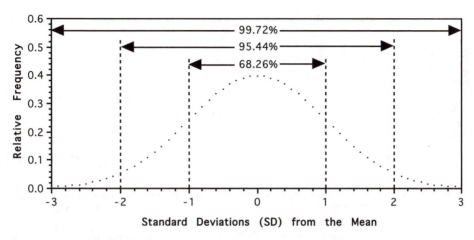

Figure 2.7 Percentages under the normal (Gaussian) curve at various standard deviations.

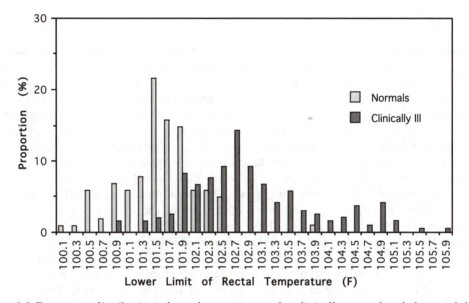

Figure 2.8 Frequency distribution of rectal temperatures for clinically normal and abnormal dogs.

exhibiting various signs of respiratory or gastrointestinal infection, such as runny eyes and nose, harsh lung sounds, coughing, diarrhea, and lethargy. Not only is the shape of each histogram different, but there is a significant degree of overlapping of normal with abnormal.

▼

When there is no clear division between normal and abnormal, three criteria have proven useful: being unusual, being sick, and being treatable.

▲

When there is no clear division between normal and abnormal, three criteria have proven useful: being unusual, being sick, and being treatable (Fletcher et al., 1996).

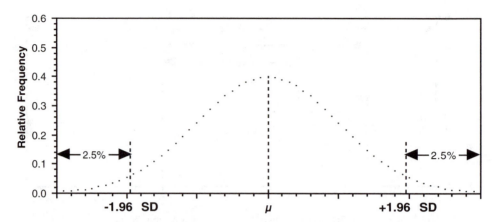

Figure 2.9 Mean (µ) and critical values (±1.96 SD) for the 95% confidence interval, under a two-tailed test of significance, where abnormality is associated with either high or low values, as blood leukocyte counts.

2.4.1 Abnormal as unusual

The criteria for abnormality may be approached statistically. One approach assumes that normal clinical values exhibit a Gaussian distribution. Thus, if we arbitrarily define the cutoffs (e.g., **critical values**) between normal and abnormal to be the mean ± 1.96 SDs, then 95% of the reference values would be within the normal range and 5% outside (2.5% on each end of the distribution). In the example of normal canine body temperatures (Figure 2.3), the mean or average temperature (µ) was 101.6°F with an SD of ±0.6°F. Application of these criteria would yield a maximum normal temperature of 102.8°F.

These criteria are the basis for **two-tailed tests of significance**. This approach is fine if we do not want to specify abnormality as being above or below our normal range, e.g., a *nondirectional hypothesis of normality* (Figure 2.9). Sometimes a **one-tailed test of significance** is more appropriate, as when we wish to define where fever begins. In this case we are not interested in the bottom of the normal range, but rather the top, e.g., above normal body temperature. The one-tailed approach still defines normal as 95% of reference values, but the 5% abnormals all come from the right-hand side of the bell-shaped curve (Figure 2.10). As a result, the normal/abnormal cutoff would be shifted to the left (critical value = +1.645 SD), resulting in a more conservative estimate of normal. The one-tailed approach would yield a maximum normal temperature of approximately 102.6°F.

There are two limitations to the statistical approach to defining normality. First, if we define the normal range as comprising 95% of the reference population, then 5%, or 1 in 20, would fall outside of the normal range. Since the entire reference population was normal to begin with, these would be **false positive results** for the condition that we are measuring. The likelihood of false positives increases when multiple test panels are interpreted. As more tests are added to a panel, it becomes more likely that a normal individual will have at least one false abnormal result. If we were to extend the normal range to include 99% of the reference population, then the likelihood of classifying true disease individuals as normal, e.g., **false negative results**, increases.

The second important limitation to the statistical approach to normality is that mean and SD determinations assume that the data being analyzed follow a Gaussian (i.e., bell-shaped or normal) distribution. The normal distribution represents only random variation, whereas clinical measurements are subject to many other sources of variation. As a result, if distributions of clinical measurements from many individuals resemble normal curves, it is largely by accident. The canine temperature data in Figure 2.3 approximate the normal

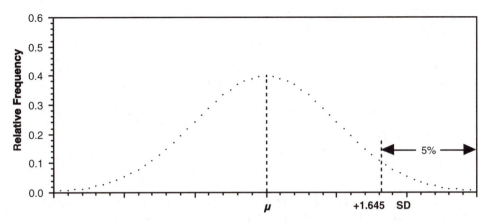

Figure 2.10 Mean (μ) and critical values (+1.645 SD) for the 95% confidence interval, under a one-tailed test of significance, where abnormality is associated with high values, as body temperatures.

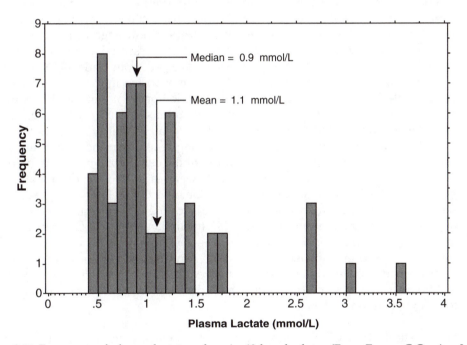

Figure 2.11 Frequency of plasma lactate values in 60 beagle dogs. (From Evans, G.O., *Am. J. Vet. Res.*, 48, 131–132, 1987. With permission.)

distribution. Other data, such as canine plasma lactate values (Figure 2.11), do not. It is often assumed, as a matter of convenience, that clinical measurements are normally distributed.

Before making an assumption of normality, one should determine whether the distribution can in fact be approximated by a normal curve. This may be done simply by constructing a histogram of the data and looking for obvious departures from a normal distribution, such as skewing. A more formal approach would be to perform a **chi-square goodness-of-fit test**. If the data are not normally distributed, then one could define normal as the 2.5 to 97.5% percentile range of the cumulative distribution. This approach is independent of the shape of the distribution curve and provides an attractive alternative

Table 2.5 Reference Values (Expressed as %) for Selected Cell Types
in Normal Canine Bone Marrow Aspirates

Cell Type	Mean	SD	95% CI[a]	Median	$X_{0.25}$–$X_{0.975}$
Erythroid cells	45.0	9.81	25.77–64.23	45.7	22.0–63.9
Myeloid cells	43.7	8.68	26.69–60.71	43.6	28.6–65.0
Lymphocytes	6.39	3.75	–0.96 to 13.74	5.25	1.73–19.6
Basophilic normoplasts	5.06	2.66	–0.15 to 10.27	4.55	1.30–12.7

[a] 95% confidence intervals were calculated as the mean ± 1.96 SD.

Source of data: Mischke, R. and Busse, L., *J. Vet. Med. A Physiol. Pathol. Clin. Med.*, 49, 499–502, 2002.

for determining critical values. By this method the cutoff for the upper 2.5% of the normal distribution for canine temperatures (see Figure 2.3) would be 102.6°F.

Example 2.9

Assessment of bone marrow aspirates is an important tool in the diagnosis of a number of canine ailments, including canine pancytopenia, myeloproliferative disorders, and detection of micrometastases. Knowledge of the normal physiological range of different bone marrow cells is essential for the interpretation of abnormal bone marrow aspirates received from patients. Normal reference ranges for canine marrow differentials reported in the literature are usually based on the mean and standard deviation or the median and overall range of observed values. Typically, a small number of animals are used. Mischke and Busse (2002) studied the cellular composition of bone marrow aspirates from 92 clinically healthy dogs receiving general anesthesia for routine surgery. Results were reported as percentiles of the cumulative distribution. In addition, means ± standard deviation (SD) were estimated for comparative purposes. Table 2.5 lists the mean, SD, median, and 95% reference ranges for selected marrow cells. Reference ranges were calculated as both the 2.5 to 97.5% percentile range and the mean ± 1.96 SD (Gaussian method). Of particular interest is the discrepancy in reference ranges obtained by the two methods. In some cases, the Gaussian method yields a negative number for the lower limit, probably because the original data are skewed (compare the respective means and medians). In these cases, the percentile distribution method must be used to define the normal reference range.

The statistical approach to normality is useful in many situations; but in others, different criteria are needed.

2.4.2   Abnormal as associated with disease

This approach relies on calling abnormal those findings that are regularly associated with disease, disability, unproductivity, or death. An example might be the different classes of heart murmurs associated with valvular defects, or the pinging sound one hears on auscultation of the abdomen of cows suffering from displaced abomasum. This approach is fundamental to the evaluation of diagnostic tests, where the frequencies of findings in cases and noncases of a disease are compared. This concept will be discussed extensively in the next two chapters.

Table 2.6 Distribution of Deaths and Culls among Calves according to Percentage of Serum Gamma Globulin

Group	No. of Calves	Gamma Globulin (%)	Deaths	Culls	Total Loss	Loss (%)
	1	1.1–6.2	8	4	12	16.40
	2	6.3–12.0	2	1	3	4.10
	3	12.1–19.3	1	1	2	2.73
	4	19.4–46.7	0	1	1	1.35
	Total		11	7	18	6.14

Source: House, J.A. and Baker, J.A., *J. Am. Vet. Med. Assoc.*, 152, 893–894, 1968. With permission.

Example 2.10

Table 2.6 presents the results of a study (House and Baker, 1968) designed to establish the normal/abnormal cutoff for serum gamma globulin levels based on risk of disease. Calves receive almost all of their maternal antibody by nursing rather than by transplacental transfer. Because serum gamma globulin levels are considered to indicate colostral absorption, serum gamma globulin levels were measured in 293 calves 3 to 6 days of age at calf-rearing units. The median percentage of gamma globulin for all calves was 12.1, with a range of 1.1 to 46.7%. The percentage of gamma globulin in experimentally deprived calves is reported to range from 1.5 to 3.0%. As normal values had not been established, the calves were allotted to four equal-sized groups (quartiles) based on the percentage of gamma globulin, and their performance was monitored. The results show that the percentage of loss (deaths and culls) increases as the percentage of gamma globulin decreases, and that gamma globulin levels below approximately 7% should be considered abnormal. Application of these criteria would result in 25% of calves being considered abnormal vs. only 5% using the statistical approach described previously.

2.4.3   Abnormal as detectable or treatable

For some conditions, the level of disease at which intervention is practical may determine whether a particular clinical measurement is considered abnormal. The decision to treat is usually based on evidence from clinical trials. The definition of treatability frequently changes with the accumulation of new knowledge. Consider, for example, parasitism in horses. As the efficacy of anthelmintics for equine strongyles has increased, the egg per gram (EPG) counts tolerated by owners and practitioners have steadily declined. A comparable phenomenon has occurred over the years with drug and chemical residues. As the sensitivity (e.g., absolute sensitivity or detection limits) of assays and instruments has improved, the tolerable level of many substances in animal tissues, fluids, and products has decreased.

In food animal medicine abnormality may be defined as the point at which treatment is economically justified. This point, termed the **economic threshold**, is dependent on the cost of treatment and the economic gain that can be expected. To be effective in these situations, a veterinarian must be knowledgeable in economic analysis as well as in medicine.

2.5   Summary

The process of medical decision making consists of four components: collection of (1) subjective and (2) objective data, (3) assessment of the situation, and finally (4) a plan of action. There are three principal scales used for measuring clinical phenomena: nominal, ordinal, and interval. Nominal data can be placed into discrete categories that have no inherent order. Another name for nominal data is categorical data. Ordinal data are categorical data with an obvious order that can be ranked, but the intervals are not uniform in size. Data that are ordered and for which the sizes of the intervals are known are called interval or continuous data.

Validity and reliability are terms that have been used to describe the quality of clinical measurements. Validity (or accuracy) describes the degree to which a measurement reflects the true status of what is being measured. Reliability is a measure of the repeatability or reproducibility of a clinical measurement. Reliability is sometimes referred to as precision. Validity and reliability are relatively easy to establish when measurements can be compared with some accepted standard. Validity and reliability are more difficult to establish for clinical measurements that rely on our senses and for which no physical standards exist.

There are two major sources of variation in clinical measurements. Measurement variation is associated with the act of measurement itself and may be due to the performance of the instruments being used, the observers themselves, or both. Biological variation can manifest at all levels of an animal population. As a rule, rigid adherence to test protocols is the single most important way to reduce overall test variation.

Two basic properties of distributions can be used to summarize interval data: central tendency, or the middle of the distribution, and dispersion, an index of the spread of the data. The most common measures of central tendency and dispersion are the mean and SD, respectively. The frequency distribution for a variable can have one or more measurement values with the maximum frequency, or mode. A distribution with only one modal value is unimodal; two modal values, bimodal; etc. In general, a distribution with more than one mode is called multimodal. Another characteristic of the shape of a distribution is symmetry (or its converse, skewness). These properties are reflected in the relationship between the mean, median, and mode of a distribution. In symmetrical distributions the mean, median, and mode are equal. In positively skewed distributions, the mean is greater than the median (skewed to the right), while in negatively skewed distributions, the mean is less than the median due to extreme values at the lower range of the distribution (skewed to the left). The median, rather than the mean, is often used to represent the middle of a skewed distribution.

Actual frequency distributions for many clinical measurements of animal populations change with characteristics such as age, sex, plane of nutrition, and, in food-producing animals, stage of production. The normal distribution is a mathematical or theoretical model that represents random variation alone. It is frequently used to estimate the limits of normality.

Three criteria have been used to distinguish normal from abnormal: (1) being unusual, (2) being sick, and (3) being treatable. Being unusual assumes that abnormal values occur outside of an arbitrary normal range, usually defined as 95% of recorded values. A disadvantage of this approach is that approximately 5% of normal individuals would be classified as abnormal on any single test. Being sick relies on calling abnormal those findings that are regularly associated with disease, disability, unproductivity, or death. Being treatable defines abnormal as the level that is detectable and worth treating.

chapter 3

Evaluation of diagnostic tests

3.1 *Introduction*

Diagnostic tests play a major role in medical decision making. In the clinical setting, the results of a diagnostic test may be used to decide whether to initiate or withhold treatment and, if treatment is chosen, to determine the level of treatment. Diagnostic tests are also applied at the herd level to determine the frequency of disease within the herd, to identify the cause of a disease process, and, sometimes, to select those animals that should be culled.

A diagnostic test does not have to be laboratory based, but it should provide information on which decisions can be made. Test results may be reported using any of the three scales described earlier: nominal, ordinal, or interval. A serologic test, for example, may be interpreted as either positive or negative (nominal), strong or weak positive (ordinal), or reacting up to a given dilution of serum or titer (interval).

A distinction must be made between diagnostic and screening test scenarios. **Diagnostic testing** is used to distinguish between animals that have the disease in question and those that have other diseases on the differential list (White, 1986). Diagnostic testing begins with diseased individuals. **Screening** is used for the presumptive identification of unrecognized disease or defect in apparently healthy populations. Screening begins with presumably healthy individuals. The same test, examination, or procedure may be used for either purpose. The distinction is necessary because of the nature of the population used to standardize the test and the effect of disease prevalence on the interpretation of test results.

This chapter discusses how the properties of diagnostic tests are evaluated and expressed. Chapter 4 presents guidelines, or rules, for their application in medical decision making. Techniques employed for the evaluation of diagnostic tests are summarized in Table 3.1.

▼

A distinction must be made between diagnostic and screening test scenarios. Diagnostic testing begins with diseased individuals, whereas screening begins with presumably healthy individuals.

▲

3.2 *Test accuracy*

Test accuracy is the proportion of all test results, both positive and negative, that are correct. Another term for accuracy is **validity**. Accuracy is often used to express the overall

Table 3.1 Techniques for the Evaluation of Diagnostic Tests

Test Parameter Being Evaluated	How Measured	How Expressed
Validity	Two-by-two table	Sensitivity, specificity, positive and negative predictive values, accuracy
Optimum cutoff	Response operating characteristic (ROC) curve	Positive/negative cutoff value
Comparison of tests	Fixed cutoff: pretest/posttest curve	Posterior probability ÷ prior probability
	Continuous variable: response operating characteristic (ROC) curve	Likelihood ratio at different levels of the test; area under the curve
Clinical utility	True positive rate ÷ false positive rate; false negative rate ÷ true negative rate	Likelihood ratio for a positive or negative test
	Decision analysis[a]	Testing and treatment thresholds

[a] See Chapter 14.

performance of a diagnostic test. Because accuracy answers the question "What is the likelihood that the test result is correct?" this test property is of great interest.

The accuracy of diagnostic tests falls on a continuum. As a general rule, as tests become more accurate, they also become more tedious, invasive, and costly. The choice of simpler tests over more elaborate and accurate diagnostic strategies must be made with the realization that some risk of misclassification exists, which is justified by the feasibility and cost of the simpler tests. The choice of a particular test requires a balance between the risk of making an incorrect diagnosis and the relative cost of false positive and false negative results (Dubensky and White, 1983). As a result, diagnostic testing is frequently approached in stages, substituting simpler tests for more rigorous ones, at least initially.

Example 3.1

The diagnostic strategy for tumors of the mammalian lymphoid and hemopoietic tissues includes several tests varying in cost and accuracy. These tumors include canine malignant lymphoma, feline lymphosarcoma and leukemia, and bovine leukosis. For example, bovine leukosis may initially be suspected based on relatively nonspecific evidence such as unthriftiness, visual swelling of lymph nodes, morphologic appearance of circulating leukocytes, and changes in blood biochemical parameters. A serologic test for bovine leukosis virus (BLV) infection may next be performed to ensure that the animal in question has been exposed to the virus, thus increasing the likelihood that the animal is truly suffering from BLV. Finally, a lymph node biopsy may be performed to determine the true cause of lymph node enlargement. The proof of the diagnosis, or gold standard, will come after you have convinced the owner of your diagnosis and a necropsy is performed.

For economic reasons, the diagnostic strategy for the avian leukosis complex, or Marek's disease, a similar neoplastic disease of poultry, would be quite different. Because the economic value of individual birds is insignificant, a sample of afflicted birds from the flock would be necropsied immediately to determine the disease status of the flock.

3.2.1   The standard of validity (gold standard)

Ideally, all diagnostic tests should be backed by sound data comparing their accuracy with an appropriate standard. The **gold standard**, sometimes called the definitive test, refers to the means by which one can determine whether a disease is truly present. Its function is that of a quality control device. The gold standard provides the basis for determining the value of diagnostic tests, treatment strategies, and prognoses. In some cases, a simple microbiologic culture or blood smear is sufficient to confirm the presence or absence of disease. In others, more elaborate, risky, and expensive tests must be used, each with its own inherent accuracy.

▼

> The gold standard is a quality control device that provides the basis for determining the value of diagnostic tests, treatment strategies, and prognoses.

▲

Postmortem examination, or necropsy, is often regarded as the ultimate confirmational test. A well-performed necropsy is an instrument of quality control and a supplier of data on disease processes and the accuracy of diagnosis and treatment (Holden, 1985). However, many disorders cannot be confirmed even at necropsy, because they stem from subtle biochemical or neurologic alterations measurable only in the living animal.

3.2.2   Postmortem examination as a diagnostic test

Postmortem examination is used more frequently as a diagnostic tool in veterinary medicine than in human medicine (Kent et al., 2004). Besides its value as a quality control device for monitoring the accuracy and interpretation of other diagnostic tests, postmortem examination offers a number of other benefits. When combined with patient history, it can provide information on the efficacy and toxicity of therapeutic agents, permit the detection of conditions that may have been important but were either clinically inapparent or obscured by the most prominent disease, and help to monitor the influence of environmental factors on physiologic processes. In addition, postmortem examination is a highly effective method for exploring the variable manifestations of animal diseases.

Slaughter checks are part of the diagnostic and surveillance programs performed by food animal practitioners for their clients (Cooper and Helman, 1999). **Organoleptic** (sight, smell, and touch) inspection of animal carcasses continues to be a part of new slaughter inspection models in the U.S. that include (1) risk-based allocation of inspection resources, (2) statistically based sampling strategies, and (3) a livestock and poultry disease reporting system (Cates et al., 2001).

Example 3.2

Studies in human medicine have reported discrepancies of 6 to 65% when clinical and postmortem diagnoses were compared. Despite these discrepancies, autopsy rates in human hospitals have declined over the years. Kent et al. (2004) reviewed the medical records of 623 hospitalized dogs that died or were euthanatized and necropsied at a veterinary teaching hospital in 1989 and 1999 to determine whether there has been a comparable decline in the necropsy rate and the level of agreement between clinical and pathologic diagnoses. The authors found that there was a significant ($p < 0.001$) decline in the necropsy

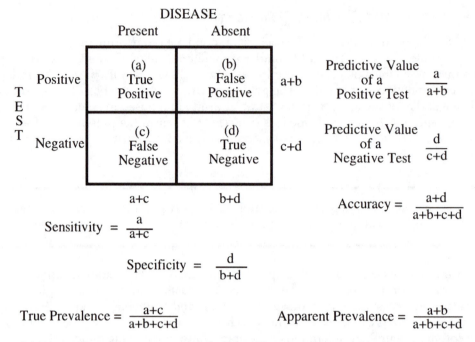

Figure 3.1 Diagnostic test outcomes and definitions. There are four possible test outcomes: two are correct and two are incorrect. Values for all four outcomes are used to estimate test sensitivity, specificity, predictive values and accuracy, and the true and apparent prevalence of disease in the population.

rate, from 58.9% of in-hospital deaths in 1989 to 48.3% in 1999, and that disagreement between clinical and pathologic diagnoses occurred in approximately a third of the cases in both 1989 and 1999. The highest proportion of discrepancies between clinical and pathologic diagnoses were in dermatology, emergency and critical care, and internal medicine; the lowest were in oncology and ophthalmology. The authors conclude that despite the continual improvement of diagnostic methods, the accuracy of diagnoses had not improved significantly over this period, and that necropsy is the best method to assess overall diagnostic accuracy.

3.3 Properties of diagnostic tests

The performance characteristics of diagnostic tests can be evaluated by using the two-by-two table depicted in Figure 3.1. Data must be obtained for all four cells.

3.3.1 Sensitivity and specificity (true positive and negative rates)

Two special terms are traditionally used to describe the characteristics of a test. **Test sensitivity** is defined as the likelihood of a positive test result in patients known to have the disease (pT+/D+). It is sometimes referred to as the **true positive rate**. Test sensitivity has also been referred to as **operational sensitivity** to distinguish it from **analytic sensitivity**, a term used to express the detection limits of an assay. **Test specificity** is the likelihood of a negative test result in patients known to be free of the disease (pT−/D−). It may also be referred to as the **true negative rate**.

Table 3.2 Hematologic and Serum Biochemical Findings in Cats with Chronic Renal Disease

Clinicopathologic Finding	% of Cats	Clinicopathologic Finding	% of Cats
Hematologic findings		**Biochemical findings (continued)**	
Hyperproteinemia (>8.0 g/dl)	61.6	Hypokalemia (<3.6 mEq/l)	29.7
Lymphopenia (<1200/µl)	56.9	Hyponatremia (<149 mEq/l)	29.7
Nonregenerative anemia (PCV<27%)	41.1	Hyperglycemia (>125 mg/dl)	23.5
Leukocytosis (>20,000/µl)	27.4	Increased anion gap (>35 mEq/l)	18.6
Leukopenia (<6000/µl)	4.1	Hypocalcemia (<8.3 mg/dl)	14.8
Hypoproteinemia (<6.0 g/dl)	2.7	Hypercalcemia (>10.5 mg/dl)	11.5
		Hypoalbuminemia (<2.3 g/dl)	11.1
Biochemical findings		Hyperalbuminemia (>3.6 g/dl)	9.3
Azotemia (creatinine >1.8 mg/dl)	96.9	Hypernatremia (>162 mEq/l)	7.8
(BUN >35 mg/dl)	95.8	Hyperkalemia (>5.4 mEq/l)	6.2
Hypercholesterolemia (>155 mg/dl)	72.5	Hypochloremia (<105 mEq/l)	4.8
Decreased CO_2 combining power (<15 mEq/l)	62.7	Hyperchloremia (>135 mEq/l)	3.2
Hyperphosphatemia (>7.1 mg/dl)	58.3		

Source: DiBartola, S.P. et al., *J. Am. Vet. Med. Assoc.*, 190, 1196–1202, 1987. With permission.

Example 3.3

Case series are excellent sources of data on the sensitivity of a particular test or finding. The frequency of clinicopathologic findings associated with chronic renal disease in cats in Table 3.2 (DiBartola et al., 1987) demonstrates the effect of biological variation on test sensitivity. Sensitivity data such as these provide useful criteria for ruling out diseases on a differential list. For example, among serum biochemical findings, azotemia was present in 97% of affected cats, whereas hyperchloremia was present in only 3.2%. Thus, if a patient presented with clinical signs suggestive of chronic renal disease (lethargy, anorexia, weight loss), normal blood creatinine levels would provide a better basis for ruling out the diagnosis than would normal chloride levels. One caveat in this study is that it is not clear how chronic renal disease was confirmed in the cats (gold standard).

3.3.2   False positive and negative rates

Two additional rates may be derived from the preceding test characteristics. The **false positive rate** is the likelihood of a positive test result in patients known to be free of the disease (pT+/D−) and equals (1 − specificity). The **false negative rate** is the likelihood of

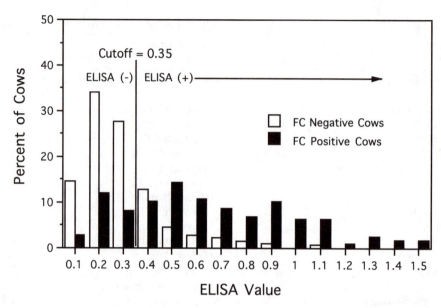

Figure 3.2 Frequency distribution of 404 ELISA values for 264 *M. paratuberculosis* fecal culture (FC)-negative and 140 fecal culture-positive cattle. Any ELISA value of 0.35 (35% of the optical density of the positive reference serum) is considered positive, and any value of <0.35 is considered negative. (From Spangler, C. et al., *Prev. Vet. Med.*, 13, 197–204, 1992. With permission.)

a negative result in patients known to have the disease (pT–/D+) and equals (1 – sensitivity).

In summary, sensitivity and the false negative rate describe how the test performs in patients with a disease, whereas specificity and the false positive rate describe how the test performs in patients without the disease.

Example 3.4

The significance of the comparisons in Figure 3.1 can be appreciated by inserting data collected during the evaluation of an enzyme-linked immunosorbent assay (ELISA) for antibody to *Mycobacterium paratuberculosis*, causative agent of paratuberculosis, or Johne's disease of cattle. The true infection status of the cattle (gold standard) was determined by fecal culture (Spangler et al., 1992). Figure 3.2 depicts the frequency distribution of 404 ELISA values recorded for 264 culture-negative and 140 culture-positive cattle. The optimum cutoff value was set at 0.35, corresponding to the point where the sum of diagnostic errors (total false positive plus false negative diagnoses) was minimized. Test performance at this cutoff is evaluated in Figure 3.2. Serologic test sensitivity was 72.9%. The infected cattle that were not detected (27.1%) are referred to as false negatives. Serologic test specificity was 84.8%, with 15.2% false positive results. Any shift in the ELISA cutoff criterion to the left (increasing test sensitivity) or right (increasing test specificity) in Figure 3.2 would require a recalculation of test parameters summarized in Figure 3.3.

3.3.3   Predictive values

Although a test's sensitivity and specificity are important properties, clinicians should be more concerned with a test's **predictive value**, i.e., the probability that a test result reflects

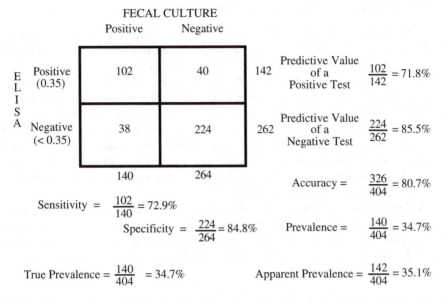

FECAL CULTURE

	Positive	Negative			
E L I S A Positive (0.35)	102	40	142	Predictive Value of a Positive Test	$\frac{102}{142} = 71.8\%$
Negative (< 0.35)	38	224	262	Predictive Value of a Negative Test	$\frac{224}{262} = 85.5\%$
	140	264			

Sensitivity = $\frac{102}{140} = 72.9\%$

Specificity = $\frac{224}{264} = 84.8\%$

Accuracy = $\frac{326}{404} = 80.7\%$

Prevalence = $\frac{140}{404} = 34.7\%$

True Prevalence = $\frac{140}{404} = 34.7\%$

Apparent Prevalence = $\frac{142}{404} = 35.1\%$

Figure 3.3 Evaluation of an ELISA for the detection of antibody to *M. paratuberculosis*. In this example, any ELISA value of 0.35 (35% of the optical density of the positive reference serum) is considered positive, and any value of <0.35 is considered negative. (Source of data: Spangler, C. et al., *Prev. Vet. Med.*, 13, 197–204, 1992. With permission.)

the true disease status (see Figure 3.1). **Positive predictive value** is the probability of disease in an animal with a positive (abnormal) test result (pD+/T+). **Negative predictive value** is the probability that an animal does not have the disease when the test result is negative (pD−/T−). Whereas sensitivity and specificity can be regarded as absolute properties of a test (with the possible exception described in the example below), predictive values are relative, varying with the likelihood, or **pretest probability**, of disease in the individual being tested. The pretest probability of disease may be based on patient history, the clinician's experience with similar patients, or the prevalence of the condition in the population from which the individual was drawn. For a full discussion of prevalence, see Chapter 5.

Example 3.5

Strictly speaking, prevalence of disease cannot influence test sensitivity and specificity in the way that it affects predictive values. However, there are situations in which test sensitivity and specificity may differ between populations of high and low prevalence. For example, the sensitivity of antigen tests for canine heartworm has been shown to increase with increasing worm burdens (Courtney et al., 1988). Courtney and Cornell (1990) have discussed how the distribution of different types and intensity of heartworm infection (patent, immune-mediated occult, unisex occult, immature occult, high and low worm burdens) may differ among canine populations in regions of high and low endemicity or among different classes of dogs, thereby affecting the overall sensitivity of the test. Consequently, test sensitivity based on a study of Florida dogs, where worm burdens are high, may be much higher than one could expect in regions of low endemicity. In a similar fashion, antibody titers to a disease agent may be higher among animals residing in areas with a high prevalence of that disease, thereby affecting the sensitivity and specificity of antibody tests.

3.3.4   *The effect of prevalence on predictive values*

Diagnostic tests are used in populations with widely differing disease frequencies. As indicated previously, prevalence per se has no effect on test sensitivity or specificity, but predictive values may vary considerably. As the prevalence of infection decreases, the positive predictive value also decreases, but the negative predictive value increases.

The predictive value of diagnostic results can be improved by selecting more sensitive or specific tests. A more sensitive test improves the negative predictive value of the test (fewer false negative results). A more specific test improves the positive predictive value (fewer false positive results). However, because prevalence commonly varies over a wider range than sensitivity or specificity, it is still the major factor in determining predictive value. Therefore, improved sensitivity and specificity cannot be expected to result in a dramatic improvement in predictive value.

The decline of the predictive value of a positive test with decreasing prevalence is of special concern in test and removal programs for disease eradication among food-producing animals. Use of a serologic test of low specificity (and therefore low positive predictive value) could result in excessive culling of disease-free individuals from a herd.

Example 3.6

The ability to test milk samples from individual cows for antimicrobial residues is essential for the determination of labeled withholding periods. Because there are no rapid assays intended for testing milk from individual cows, it has become commonplace to use assays approved for commingled milk testing for this purpose. Gibbons-Burgener et al. (2001) determined the likelihood of false positive results when testing posttreatment milk samples from each of 92 cows with mild clinical mastitis by use of three commercially available assays labeled for use with commingled milk. Posttreatment samples were collected the first time cows were milked, following the completion of the labeled withholding period. The results of high-performance liquid chromatography performed on each sample, interpreted in light of FDA-established tolerance levels for each antimicrobial in individual milk samples, served as the gold standard. Sensitivity, specificity, and positive and negative predictive values (PPV and NPV, respectively) were determined for each assay. Sensitivities of the three tests ranged from 62.5 to 91.67%, and specificities from 84.7 to 97.6%. Although the NPVs of the three tests were all above 98%, PPVs were low, ranging from 20.8 to 55.6%. The low PPVs were due to the low prevalence of violative resides in the sample population (3.7 to 6.9%, depending on the antibiotic), leading the authors to conclude that none of the assays would be useful for detecting violative antimicrobial residues in individual milk samples from cows treated for mild clinical mastitis.

3.3.5   *Likelihood ratios*

The **likelihood ratio** is an index of diagnostic utility that expresses the likelihood that a given finding on the history, physical, or laboratory examination would occur in an animal with, as opposed to an animal without, the condition of interest (Sackett, 1992). By "finding" we mean the presence (or absence) of any sign or any of the levels of a laboratory test result, such as an ELISA value.

The likelihood ratio is calculated from the same two-by-two table used to calculate other aspects of test performance (Figure 3.4). The **likelihood ratio for a positive test** is

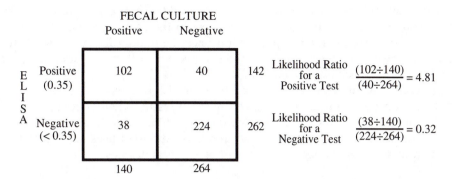

Figure 3.4 Calculation of positive and negative likelihood ratios from data presented in Figure 3.2 on an ELISA test for *M. paratuberculosis* antibody in cattle. The likelihood ratio for a positive test (cutoff) = sensitivity ÷ (1 – specificity), or true positive rate ÷ false positive rate. The likelihood ratio for a negative test (< cutoff) = (1 – sensitivity) ÷ specificity, or false negative rate ÷ true negative rate. (Source of data: Spangler, C. et al., *Prev. Vet. Med.*, 13, 197–204, 1992. With permission.)

the ratio of the true positive rate (pT+/D+) divided by the false positive rate (pT+/D–), or equivalently, sensitivity/(1 – specificity). The **likelihood ratio for a negative test** is the ratio of the false negative rate (pT–/D+) divided by the true negative rate (pT–/D–), or equivalently, (1 – sensitivity)/specificity. The ideal diagnostic test would yield a likelihood ratio of infinity for a positive test (e.g., 100%/0%) and a likelihood ratio of 0 for a negative test (e.g., 0%/100%). A likelihood ratio of 1 for either a positive or negative test means the test result conveys no information. In the paratuberculosis test example shown in Figure 3.4, the likelihood ratio for a positive test is 4.81 (72.86%/15.15%), meaning that an ELISA value of 0.35 is almost five times as likely to occur in an *M. paratuberculosis*-infected animal than an uninfected animal. The likelihood ratio for a negative test is 0.32 (27.14%/84.85%), meaning that an ELISA value of <0.35 is about one third as likely to occur in an infected vs. uninfected animal. The likelihood ratio does not convey the actual likelihood of disease in an individual, only the likelihood that the test result would occur in an individual with, vs. an animal without, the disease.

The likelihood ratio offers several advantages over other methods of reporting test performance. Because the likelihood ratio is derived from test sensitivity and specificity only, it is unaffected by disease prevalence, making it an especially stable expression of test performance. The likelihood ratio is also useful for interpreting test results that fall on a continuum, such as serologic titers or serum biochemical values, where the likelihood of disease increases the more measurements deviate from normal. For example, by expanding the levels of *M. paratuberculosis* test results from 2 (as in the two-by-two table above) to 10 (as in Table 3.4), the range of likelihood ratios is widened from 15-fold (0.32 to 4.81) to 327-fold (0.15 to 49.03). In this way test results become more useful for ruling diseases in and out because we are utilizing information that would otherwise be lost if results were expressed in terms of a single positive/negative cutoff. Finally, the likelihood ratio can be used in conjunction with the pretest probability of disease to estimate the likelihood of disease given a positive or negative test result. This application of the likelihood ratio will be discussed in the next chapter.

3.3.6   Accuracy, reproducibility, and concordance

Accuracy, reproducibility, and concordance are other terms used to describe diagnostic test performance. As stated above, **accuracy** (or validity) is the proportion of all tests, both positive and negative, that are correct (see Figure 3.1). The numerical limits of test accuracy are its sensitivity and specificity. Accuracy is often used to express the overall performance of a diagnostic test. However, its value is subject to the same constraints as predictive value and is correct only for the population used to standardize the test. As disease prevalence changes, so does accuracy of the test (except for the special condition where test sensitivity and specificity are equal).

Reproducibility (also known as reliability or precision) refers to the degree to which repeated tests on the same sample(s) give the same result, whereas **concordance** is the proportion of all test results on which two or more different tests agree. An important attribute of test concordance is that as the number of different tests applied to the same sample increases, the likelihood of agreement on all tests decreases.

Example 3.7

Schwartz et al. (1989) evaluated the interlaboratory and intralaboratory agreement of Lyme disease test results among four independent laboratories for serum specimens from 132 outdoor workers in New Jersey. The measurement of agreement employed, the kappa statistic, ranged from 0.45 to 0.53 among the four laboratories, representing low levels of agreement. Of 20 sera reported as positive by at least one laboratory, 85, 50, and 30% were reported positive by two, three, and four laboratories, respectively. The kappa statistic is discussed in Chapter 9.

3.4   Interpretation of tests whose results fall on a continuum

3.4.1   Trade-offs between sensitivity and specificity

The frequency distribution of test results in normal and diseased animal populations, particularly when measured on an interval scale, forces us to make a trade-off between sensitivity and specificity. Figure 3.5 depicts the distribution of rectal temperatures for the two populations of dogs discussed earlier (see Figure 2.8), with a normal/abnormal (negative/positive) cutoff line superimposed. Because the two distribution curves overlap, moving the cutoff point to the left increases the sensitivity of the test, i.e., the probability of detecting a diseased individual, but decreases the specificity. Moving the cutoff to the right has the opposite effect. There is no way to adjust the cutoff so that sensitivity and specificity are improved at the same time.

▼

The frequency distribution of test results in normal and diseased animal populations, particularly when measured on an interval scale, forces us to make a trade-off between sensitivity and specificity.

▲

Example 3.8

Earlier in this chapter data collected by Spangler et al. (1992) during the evaluation of an ELISA for *M. paratuberculosis* infection in cattle were used to illustrate how test performance at a fixed cutoff would be estimated (Figure 3.3). This cutoff was chosen by the investigators because it was the point at which the sum of diagnostic errors (false positives plus false negatives) was minimized. Since the ELISA results were originally recorded on a continuous

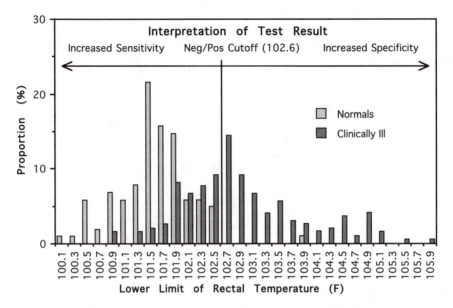

Figure 3.5 Frequency distribution of rectal temperatures from normal and abnormal dogs to demonstrate the effect of moving the negative/positive cutoff on the sensitivity and specificity of a diagnostic test.

scale, it is possible to evaluate test performance over the entire range of recorded readings. The results of this analysis are summarized in Table 3.3. The sensitivity of the ELISA in diagnosis of *M. paratuberculosis* infection decreased from 100 to 19% as the cutoff value for a positive test (as a percent of the OD [optical density] of the positive reference serum) was increased from <10 to 90%, while specificity increased from 0 to 99.6% over the same range of cutoff values. Regardless of the cutoff point, a risk of misdiagnosis will always exist. In this example, increasing the cutoff criterion for a positive test decreased test sensitivity but increased specificity. Decreasing the cutoff would have the opposite effect.

The effect of test sensitivity and specificity on predictive values can be appreciated by studying the number of false negative and false positive diagnoses in Table 3.3, which illustrates an important point: tests of low sensitivity increase the likelihood of false negative results, whereas tests of low specificity increase the likelihood of false positive test results.

3.4.2 *Receiver operating characteristic (ROC) curve*

For test results that fall along a continuum, e.g., ELISA cutoffs for *M. paratuberculosis* infection (Table 3.3), test performance can be depicted graphically by plotting a **receiver operating characteristic (ROC) curve** (also called response operating characteristic curve), which compares the true positive rate, or sensitivity, on the vertical axis with the false positive rate (1 – specificity) on the horizontal axis. ROC analysis is the standard method to demonstrate the covariation of test sensitivity and specificity, and provides a simple method for evaluating a test's ability to discriminate between health and disease over the complete spectrum of operating conditions (cutoffs). ROC analysis can be used to select cutoffs or to compare diagnostic tests.

Table 3.3 Effect of Cutoff on the Performance of an ELISA Test
for *M. paratuberculosis* Infection in Cattle

ELISA Cutoff[a]	Fecal Culture		Sensitivity (%)[b]	Specificity (%)[c]	False Negative[d]	False Positive[e]	Sum
	Number Positive	Number Negative					
<10	3	39	100	0	0	264	264
10	16	91	98	15	3	225	228
20	11	73	86	49	19	134	153
30	14	33	79	77	30	61	91
40	20	11	69	89	44	28	72
50	15	7	54	94	64	17	81
60	12	5	44	96	79	10	89
70	9	3	35	98	91	5	96
80	14	1	29	99	100	2	102
90	26	1	19	99.6	114	1	115
Totals	140	264					

[a] ELISA values expressed as a percent of the optical density of the positive reference serum.

[b] Sensitivity = $\dfrac{\text{No. ELISA(+)/fecal culture(+)} \geq \text{cutoff}}{\text{total fecal culture(+)}}$

[c] Specificity = $\dfrac{\text{No. ELISA(+)/fecal culture(–)} < \text{cutoff}}{\text{total fecal culture(–)}}$

[d] Number of false negative diagnoses at each cutoff = $(140) \times (1 - \text{sensitivity})$.

[e] Number of false positive diagnoses at each cutoff = $(264) \times (1 - \text{specificity})$.

Source of data: Spangler, C. et al., *Prev. Vet. Med.*, 13, 197–204, 1992. With permission.

A ROC curve for the data in Table 3.3 is depicted in Figure 3.6. Each point on the ROC curve defines a set of operating characteristics for the test based on sensitivity and specificity. Tests that discriminate well approach the upper left corner of the ROC curve. The ROC curve for less discriminatory tests falls closer to the diagonal (dashed line) running from lower left to upper right. The diagonal line reflects test values that are uninformative, e.g., where the true positive rate equals the false positive rate. Reliance on test results is no better than tossing a coin. The area under the ROC curve (AUC) provides a measure of overall test performance. According to guidelines proposed by Swets (1988), the AUC can be used to distinguish among noninformative (AUC = 0.50), less accurate $(0.50 < \text{AUC} \leq 0.70)$, moderately accurate $(0.70 < \text{AUC} \leq 0.90)$, highly accurate $(0.90 < \text{AUC} < 1.00)$, and perfect (AUC = 1.00) tests.

The astute reader will note that the ROC curve is really only a series of likelihood ratios (true positive rate vs. false positive rate), using a range of cutoff values as the criteria for test interpretation. Because likelihood ratios are independent of disease prevalence, the ROC curve is a basic tool for assessing and using diagnostic tests (Zweig and Campbell, 1993).

3.4.3   Two-graph ROC analysis

A disadvantage of ROC analysis is that it is not possible to read the cutoff value for a selected combination of sensitivity and specificity directly from the ROC plot. **Two-graph receiver operating characteristic (TG-ROC) analysis** solves this problem. In TG-ROC, test sensitivity and specificity are plotted as separate dependent variables against cutoff values as the independent variable (Greiner et al., 1995).

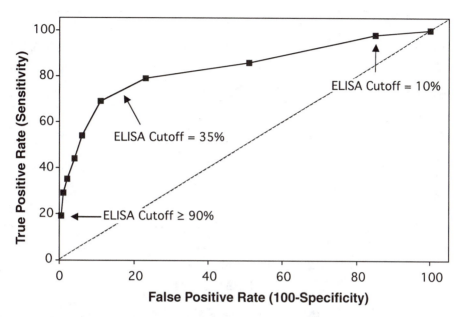

Figure 3.6 ROC curve for an ELISA for the diagnosis of *M. paratuberculosis* infection in cattle. The diagonal line reflects test values that are uninformative, e.g., where the true positive rate equals the false positive rate. See Table 3.3 for corresponding sensitivity and specificity values. (Source of data: Spangler, C. et al., *Prev. Vet. Med.*, 13, 197–204, 1992. With permission.)

A TG-ROC plot of data in Table 3.3 is depicted in Figure 3.7. The covariance of test sensitivity and specificity in response to positive/negative cutoff is readily apparent in this plot. Test sensitivity and specificity are maximized by selecting the ELISA positive/negative cutoff that corresponds to the point where the two lines intersect. The vertical (dashed) line represents the positive/negative cutoff chosen by the authors, corresponding to 35% of the positive control ELISA value. This cutoff favors test specificity at the expense of test sensitivity, but results in the lowest number of diagnostic errors, as there were more disease-free than infected animals in the study population.

3.4.4 Selecting a cutoff

Positive/negative cutoffs are used to simplify the diagnostic process by defining the level of a test result that is required to establish or reject a diagnosis. In defining the optimal cutoff one strives to reduce the consequence of false negative or false positive test results. Ideally, the choice of a positivity criterion should include a consideration of (1) the distribution of results in two different populations — normal patients and patients with disease, (2) the prevalence or likelihood of disease in the population from which individuals being tested come, and (3) the cost of false positive and false negative test results.

▼

Tests of low sensitivity increase the likelihood of false negative results, whereas tests of low specificity increase the likelihood of false positive test results.

▲

The most direct approach is to select the cutoff resulting in the lowest total number of diagnostic errors (false positive diagnoses plus false negative diagnoses). The actual prevalence of disease must be known or estimated. At a disease prevalence of about 50%,

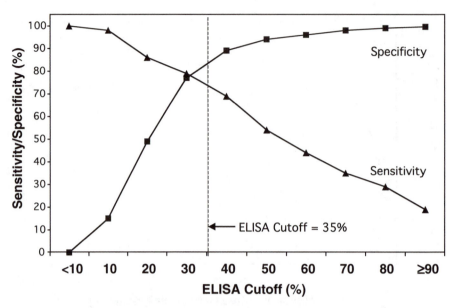

Figure 3.7 TG-ROC plot for ELISA for the diagnosis of *M. paratuberculosis* infection in cattle. Original data appear in Table 3.3. The covariance of test sensitivity and specificity in response to positive/negative cutoff is readily apparent in this plot. Test sensitivity and specificity are maximized by chosing the ELISA positive/negative cutoff at the point corresponding to the intersection of the two lines. The vertical (dashed) line represents the positive/negative cutoff chosen by the authors, corresponding to 35% of the positive control ELISA value. This cutoff favors test specificity at the expense of test sensitivity, but results in the lowest number of diagnostic errors, as there were more disease-free than infected animals in the study population. (Source of data: Spangler, C. et al., *Prev. Vet. Med.*, 13, 197–204, 1992. With permission.)

the optimum cutoff is the point on a ROC curve closest to the upper-left-hand corner, where test sensitivity and specificity are maximized; e.g., (sensitivity + specificity)/2 attains its highest value (Sackett et al., 1991). In TG-ROC this corresponds to the point where the sensitivity/specificity lines intersect.

In the *M. paratuberculosis* example (prevalence = 34.7%), the lowest total number of diagnostic errors occurs at an ELISA cutoff of approximately 35% of the positive reference value, represented by the vertical (dashed) line on the TG-ROC plot (Figure 3.7). This cutoff favors test specificity at the expense of test sensitivity, but results in the lowest number of diagnostic errors, as there were more disease-free than infected animals in the study population.

This approach does not take into account the relative cost of false positive vs. false negative diagnoses, which can be factored in by simply multiplying the relative or absolute cost by the respective number of false negative and false positive diagnoses and summing the result for each cutoff. For example, if false negatives are more costly than false positives, then test sensitivity should be increased to compensate for this difference. We are willing to accept an increase in the number of false positive results because of the relatively greater penalty for a false negative result.

3.5   Comparison of diagnostic tests

3.5.1   For tests with fixed cutoffs

The accuracy of a test with a fixed positive/negative cutoff is dependent upon the test's sensitivity, specificity, and the likelihood (pretest probability) of disease in the patient or

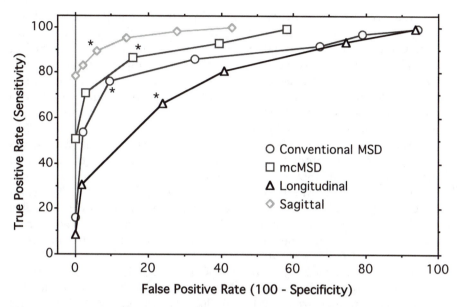

Figure 3.8 ROC curve for conventional MSD and mcMSD and sagittal and longitudinal ratio values at C6. Areas under the curve are sagittal, 0.9783; mcMSD, 0.9305; conventional MSD, 0.8305; longitudinal, 0.7970. The cutoff or operating points (MSD or ratio value) that maximize both sensitivity and specificity are identified with an asterisk. (Source of data: Moore, B.R. et al., *Am. J. Vet. Res.*, 55, 5–13, 1994. With permission.)

population. Although test accuracy varies with pretest probability, the range of variability is much less than that of a test's positive or negative predictive values. Whereas test accuracy cannot be less than its sensitivity or specificity, predictive values can range from 0 to 100%. Despite its variability, accuracy is a convenient way to compare the overall performance of a diagnostic test, particularly if a common value for pretest probability is used in the comparison.

3.5.2 For test results that fall on a continuum

The evaluation of tests whose results fall on a continuum differs from that for tests with a fixed cutoff because there is no predetermined normal vs. abnormal cutoff for the test result. Using **ROC analysis** (Greiner et al., 2000), in which AUCs are calculated over the range of each test's operating conditions, the magnitude and statistical significance of differences among tests can be compared and superior tests identified. Another advantage of ROC analysis is that it permits comparison of tests that use different measurement scales. For example, in Figure 3.8 (see example below) test results are measured in millimeters (conventional minimum sagittal diameter (MSD) and magnification-corrected MSD (mcMSD)) and as a ratio (sagittal and longitudinal ratio).

Example 3.9

Cervical stenotic myelopathy (CSM), also known as wobbler syndrome or equine sensory ataxia, is the leading cause of spinal ataxia of horses in most parts of the U.S. Spinal ataxia results from spinal cord compression caused by malformation of the cervical vertebrae and narrowing of the vertebral canal, most frequently involving C5 to C7. The disease usually occurs within the first 1 to 2 years of life. Although definitive antemortem diagnosis requires myelographic examination, cervical radiographs, which permit calculation of the vertebral canal's MSD (in millimeters), may be useful for screening patients. The value of survey radiography in CSM is still controversial, due in part to the effect of magnification in radiographs of standing horses. Moore et al. (1994) compared three methods of vertebral canal diameter assessment that minimize (mcMSD) or eliminate (sagittal and longitudinal ratio) the effects of radiographic magnification with the conventional MSD method in CSM-affected and unaffected horses. Disease status (gold standard) was established by a combination of myelography, histologic examination of the spinal cord, and neurologic examination. ROC curves for vertebral sites C4 through C7 were generated to compare the ability of conventional MSD, mcMSD, sagittal ratio, and longitudinal ratio methods to discriminate between CSM-affected and unaffected horses. To facilitate comparative and statistical analysis, each ROC curve was quantitatively assessed by calculating the area under the curve. The sagittal ratio method was the most accurate for distinguishing between CSM-affected and unaffected horses at vertebral sites C5, C6, C7, and overall. Figure 3.8 compares the results obtained at C6. It is clear that the sagittal ratio ROC curve has the highest sensitivity/specificity combination over its entire operating range. Areas under the curve are sagittal ratio, 0.9783; mcMSD, 0.9305; conventional MSD, 0.8305; and longitudinal, 0.7970. The cutoffs or operating points (MSD or ratio value) that maximize both sensitivity and specificity for each method are identified with an asterisk. The authors caution that the actual cutoff for establishing a diagnosis of CSM will depend, in part, on the consequences of misdiagnosis (for example, euthanasia vs. follow-up myelography).

3.6   Sources of bias in the evaluation of diagnostic tests

3.6.1   Relative vs. true sensitivity and specificity

Many times it is not possible to determine the true disease status of animals used for test standardization. However, the relative sensitivity and specificity of a diagnostic test can be estimated by comparing test results with those obtained using an accepted standard test that has been in use for many years. This approach might be used by a private practitioner to compare a heartworm serodiagnostic test with the traditional Knott's test in client-owned dogs. When there is no gold standard, the comparison of overall performance of one test relative to another is a measure of **concordance** rather than accuracy. Comparisons of the relative accuracy of one test over another are valid only when the true health status of test animals can be determined.

The argument could be made that the evaluation of an ELISA test for *M. paratuberculosis* infection in cattle described earlier in this chapter really measured relative vs. absolute test performance, because the gold standard, fecal culture, is itself prone to error. However, the rigid criteria used by the authors to define absence of infection (negative herd history for 15 years and negative herd fecal culture, or absence of signs and negative results on at least three cultures) make it unlikely that misclassification significantly affected the results of the study.

3.6.2   The spectrum of patients

Test sensitivity and specificity must be determined in the appropriate population. To establish a test's efficacy for ruling out a diagnosis, sensitivity should be examined in a broad range of patients with the disease. Similarly, to rule in a disease, a test's specificity should be established in a broad range of patients without the disease (Ransohoff and Feinstein, 1978).

The challenge in the diseased group is to discover whether (and when) the test yields false negative results. The diseased group should include individuals covering the spectrum of clinical and pathologic findings and those with complications that might yield false negative results. The distribution of infection stages in the population used to evaluate the test can also affect measurements of test performance. For example, the sensitivity of an ELISA test for *M. paratuberculosis* infection of cattle is known to increase from approximately 25% to almost 90% as the disease progresses through the three successive stages of infection. Thus, estimates of test sensitivity may vary greatly depending on the age distribution and infection history of herds used to evaluate the test (Collins and Sockett, 1993).

The challenge in the comparison group is to determine whether (and under what circumstances) the test yields false positive results. When evaluating a screening test, apparently healthy animals should be used as the nondiseased group. If the same test were to be evaluated in a diagnostic testing scenario, the nondiseased group should consist of animals that do not have the disease for which the test is being evaluated, but have other diseases that compete with the disease of interest in the differential diagnosis (White, 1986).

Example 3.10

Dubensky and White (1983) evaluated the use of total plasma protein (TPP) in the diagnosis of traumatic reticuloperitonitis (TRP) in 169 dairy cattle. Sixty-three cows with surgically confirmed TRP served as cases, while 106 cows surgically explored for other abdominal diseases that might be confused with TRP during differential diagnosis were controls. The presenting clinical signs in the two groups were similar and included anorexia, abdominal pain, bloat, colic, dehydration, depression, diarrhea, decreased milk production, fever, increased or decreased heart rate, and weight loss. The surgical diagnoses (gold standard) for the control group included at least 12 distinct disease syndromes that should be on the differential list with TRP (Table 3.4).

3.6.3 Bias in associating test results with disease

Several forms of bias may occur when the status of a test as positive or negative and the status of disease as present or absent are not made independently (Ransohoff and Feinstein, 1978).

Workup bias occurs when the results of a test affect the subsequent clinical workup needed to establish the diagnosis of a disease. If a diagnostic test yields a positive result, we are more likely to pursue the diagnosis, increasing the probability of detecting the disease if it is really present. On the other hand, a negative test result may cause us to limit follow-up testing, increasing the probability of missing the disease, if present.

Review bias occurs when the results of a test affect the subjective review of the data that establish the diagnosis. For example, a positive serologic test result may affect the subjective interpretation of thoracic radiographs used to support a diagnosis of occult heartworm disease.

Incorporation bias occurs when the diagnostic test being evaluated, or a related test, is also used to support the diagnosis of the disease. As a result, the case for their use in ruling out disease would be weakened.

Table 3.4 Surgical Diagnosis of 106 Cattle in the Control Group with Clinical Findings Consistent with Traumatic Reticuloperitonitis

	Diagnosis	No. of Animals
1	Intussusception/intestinal obstruction	16
2	Peritonitis	14
3	Vagus indigestion/bloat	13
4	Abscess	
	Abdomen	2
	Abomasum	1
	Liver	6
	Omasum	1
	Ruminoreticulum	2
5	Abomasal ulcers	11
6	Johne's disease	10
7	Lymphosarcoma	3
8	Fatty Liver	3
9	Indigestion	2
10	Distended small intestine	2
11	Diarrhea	1
12	Unknown	19
	Total	106

Source: Dubensky, R.A. and White, M.E., *Can. J. Comp. Med.*, 47, 241–244, 1983.

3.7 Statistical significance

Often journal articles report that a diagnostic test was able to detect a statistically significant difference between control and infected groups. The magnitude of this difference may not be great enough to be clinically useful in the individual, however. In some cases, statistical significance is achieved only by using relatively large numbers of animals. If smaller numbers are used, a statistically significant difference may not occur.

3.8 Summary

Diagnostic tests play a critical role in the medical decision-making process. A distinction must be made between diagnostic and screening test scenarios. Diagnostic testing is used to distinguish between animals that have the disease in question and those that have other diseases on the differential list. Diagnostic testing begins with diseased individuals. Screening is used for the presumptive identification of unrecognized disease or defect in apparently healthy populations. Screening begins with presumably healthy individuals. The same test, examination, or procedure may be used for either purpose.

Test accuracy is the proportion of all tests, both positive and negative, that are correct. It is often used to express the overall performance of a diagnostic test. The gold standard refers to the means by which one can determine whether a disease is truly present. It provides a standard with which the performance characteristics of diagnostic tests can be evaluated. Test sensitivity is defined as the likelihood of a positive test result in patients known to have the disease. Test specificity is the likelihood of a negative test result in patients known to be free of the disease. Test sensitivity is sometimes referred to as operational sensitivity to distinguish it from absolute sensitivity, a term used to express the detection limits of an assay. Two additional rates may be derived from the preceding test characteristics. The false positive rate is the likelihood of a positive test result in patients known to be free of the disease. Tests of low specificity increase the likelihood of false positive test results. The false negative rate is the likelihood of a negative result in patients known to have the disease. Tests of low sensitivity increase the likelihood of false negative results. Taken together, sensitivity and the false negative rate describe how the test performs in patients with a disease, whereas specificity and the false positive rate describe how the test performs in patients without the disease.

The probability that a test result reflects the true disease status of an individual is called the predictive value of the test. Positive predictive value is the probability of disease in an animal with a positive (abnormal) test result. Negative predictive value is the probability that an animal does not have the disease when the test result is negative (normal). Whereas sensitivity and specificity can be regarded as absolute properties of a test, predictive values are relative, varying with the likelihood, or pretest probability, of disease in the individual being tested. The pretest probability of disease may be based on patient history, the clinician's experience with similar patients, or the prevalence of the condition in the population from which the individual was drawn.

Other terms may be used to describe test performance. The likelihood ratio is an index of diagnostic utility that expresses the likelihood that a given finding on the history, physical, or laboratory examination would occur in an individual with, as opposed to without, the condition of interest. Reproducibility refers to the degree to which repeated tests on the same sample(s) give the same result, whereas concordance is the proportion of all test results on which two or more different tests agree.

Clinical values in normal and diseased animal populations usually overlap, particularly when measured on a continuum. Consequently, there is no way to adjust the positive/negative cutoff so that sensitivity and specificity are improved simultaneously. The optimal cutoff can be determined by selecting the cutoff yielding the lowest total number of incorrect diagnoses at a given pretest probability (or prevalence) of disease. ROC curve analysis and two-graph ROC analysis can be used to identify the optimum cutoff. These analyses can be made more clinically relevant by incorporating the relative cost of false positive and false negative test results in the analysis.

The comparison of tests with fixed cutoffs can be accomplished by examining their respective accuracies. For tests whose results fall on a continuum, their ROC curves can be compared.

Three sources of bias in the interpretation of diagnostic tests are (1) improper standards of validity, (2) the spectrum of patients, and (3) prior knowledge of the health or disease status of individuals. Estimates of diagnostic test accuracy are only valid when the true health status of test animals can be determined. If an existing test is used in place of a gold standard, then relative, rather than true, sensitivity and specificity are measured, and the level of agreement between the tests is called concordance rather than accuracy. Bias in the spectrum of patients occurs when the characteristics of the population to be tested differ from those used to standardize the test. Prior knowledge of the disease status of an individual may influence the effort expended to establish a diagnosis, whereas knowing a test result may influence the subjective review of data used to establish a diagnosis. When the diagnostic test being evaluated is also used to support the diagnosis of the disease, the test's performance may appear better than it really is.

chapter 4

Use of diagnostic tests

4.1 Introduction

The value of diagnostic tests depends in part on the way in which they are used. Probably the worst approach to medical diagnostics is to perform every conceivable test on a patient, in the hope that something will show up. This would be a waste of hospital and patient resources and would needlessly expand rather than reduce the differential list. Indiscriminate testing at the herd level tends to reduce the predictive value of tests and can lead to unnecessary culling in disease eradication programs. Chapter 3 dealt with the nuts and bolts of diagnostic tests. This chapter focuses on strategies that can be used to increase the efficiency of the diagnostic process.

▼

Probably the worst approach to medical diagnostics is to perform every conceivable test on a patient, in the hope that something will show up.

▲

4.2 Calculation of the probability of disease

In the previous chapter a number of indices of test performance were discussed. These include test sensitivity, specificity, predictive values, likelihood ratio, etc. Although these indices are useful for expressing how well a test performs individually and in comparison with other tests, they do not directly answer the most fundamental question arising from their use: *What is the likelihood of disease in this individual given a positive or negative test result?* The following section describes a number of ways for answering this question.

4.2.1 From a two-by-two table

The likelihood of disease for a given test result (known as the **posttest probability** of disease) can be estimated directly from the two-by-two table used to evaluate the test's performance. The **likelihood of disease given a positive test result** is, by definition, the test's positive predictive value. **The likelihood of disease given a negative test result** is equal to 100 − negative predictive value (when expressed as a percentage). There is an important caveat to using a two-by-two table in this way. As predictive values are very sensitive to the prevalence (or pretest probability; see below) of disease, it is important that the true prevalence of disease embodied in the two-by-two table (see Figure 3.1) be representative of the population from which the individual being tested was drawn.

4.2.2   Use of Bayes' theorem

The mathematical relationship among pretest and posttest probabilities and test results was described hundreds of years ago in **Bayes' theorem** (see Kramer, 1988). Bayes' theorem provides a theoretical framework for the calculation of posttest probabilities from information that we already know (*a priori*) about the implications of a diagnostic test. Using Bayesian analysis, the posttest probability of disease given a *positive* test equals

$$\frac{\text{true positives}}{\text{all positives}} = \frac{\text{pD} \times \text{sensitivity}}{\text{pD} \times \text{sensitivity} + [(1 - \text{pD}) \times (1 - \text{specificity})]}$$

and the posttest probability of disease given a *negative* test equals

$$\frac{\text{false negatives}}{\text{all negatives}} = \frac{\text{pD} \times (1 - \text{sensitivity})}{\text{pD} \times (1 - \text{sensitivity}) + [(1 - \text{pD}) \times (\text{specificity})]}$$

In these equations, the pretest probability of disease (pD), test sensitivity, and test specificity must be expressed as a proportion (rather than a percentage).

4.2.3   Use of the likelihood ratio to calculate posttest probabilities

4.2.3.1   Conversion between the probability of disease and the odds of disease

Regardless of the scale used to report test results (positive/negative or level of a test result), the way in which the likelihood ratio is used to estimate the likelihood of disease is the same. The basic mathematical relationship is represented by

$$\text{pretest odds} \times \text{likelihood ratio (LR)} = \text{posttest odds}$$

Because this equation is based on the odds of disease, we need to convert disease probability to odds and back again. The conversion between probability of disease and odds of disease is basically a question of converting a rate (probability) to a ratio (odds), and vice versa. In a rate, the numerator is also included in the denominator. Thus, if the prevalence (or probability) of canine heartworm infection is 20%, then 1 in 5 dogs (or 0.20 in 1) is infected. In a ratio, the numerator is not included in the denominator. In the above example, the ratio of infected to uninfected dogs would be 1 to 4 (or 0.25 to 1). The relationship between probability and odds of disease is expressed mathematically as:

$$\text{odds of disease} = \frac{\text{probability of disease present}}{1 - \text{probability of disease present}}$$

$$\text{probability of disease} = \frac{\text{odds of disease}}{\text{odds of disease} + 1}$$

Thus, if the probability of heartworm infection is 20%, then the odds of heartworm infection would be $0.2 \div 0.8 = 0.25$ (to 1). If the odds of heartworm infection is 0.25 (to 1), then the probability of heartworm infection is $0.25 \div 1.25 = 0.20$.

Table 4.1 Use of the Likelihood Ratio to Estimate the Posttest Probability of Infection of Cattle with *M. paratuberculosis* for a Positive or Negative Test Result

Test Result	Pretest Probability of Disease	Pretest Odds of Disease	Likelihood Ratio	Posttest Odds of Disease	Posttest Probability of Disease
Positive test result (ELISA 0.35)	0.35 =	0.54 ×	4.81 =	2.60 =	0.72
Negative test result (ELISA < 0.35)	0.35 =	0.54 ×	0.32 =	0.17 =	0.15

Note: The pretest probability of infection is 35%, the prevalence of fecal culture-positive cattle in the test population.

Adapted from data in Figure 3.4.

4.2.3.2   Calculation of the posttest probability of disease

To illustrate how the likelihood ratio can be used to estimate posttest probabilities, let us return to the use of an enzyme-linked immunosorbent assay (ELISA) test for diagnosis of *Mycobacterium paratuberculosis* infection in cattle (Chapter 3). At the optimal cutoff the likelihood ratio for a positive test (ELISA 0.35) was 4.81 and for a negative test (ELISA < 0.35) was 0.32. Table 4.1 depicts the results for a positive and negative test result, assuming a pretest probability of infection of 35% (prevalence of fecal culture-positive cattle in Figure 3.3).

A positive test result would increase the likelihood of *M. paratuberculosis* infection from 35 to 72%, but a negative test result would decrease the likelihood of infection to only 15%. Whenever possible, it is best to express the likelihood ratio for each level of a test result, rather than above or below an arbitrary cutoff. For example, if the actual ELISA value were 0.85 (likelihood ratio = 26.40), then the posttest odds of infection would be 26.40 × 0.54 = 14.26, increasing the posttest probability to 93%. This information is lost if test results are simply reported as positive or negative based on an arbitrary cutoff.

4.2.3.3   A nomogram for applying likelihood ratios and Bayes' theorem

Fagan (1975) offered a solution to Bayes' theorem in the form of a nomogram, a variation of which is depicted in Figure 4.1. The nomogram effectively depicts the relationship among the pretest and posttest probabilities of disease and the likelihood ratio. The pretest and posttest odds have also been included in the nomogram to help clarify the relationship between probability and odds of disease. Although not as precise as the formulas discussed earlier, the nomogram provides a simple method for estimating the posttest probability of disease from the pretest probability for any level of a test result.

Consider, for example, the data in Table 4.1. To estimate the posttest probability of *M. paratuberculosis* infection for a positive test result, simply anchor a straightedge along the left y-axis at a point approximating the 35% pretest probability of disease. Next, pivot the straightedge until it also lines up with a likelihood ratio of approximately 4.81. The straightedge should cross the right y-axis at about 72%, which is the posttest probability of disease. The same technique can be used to estimate the posttest probability of disease for a negative test result (likelihood ratio = 0.32), or for an ELISA value of 0.85 (likelihood ratio = 26.40).

4.2.3.4   Estimating posttest probability of disease from the magnitude of a test result

For test results that fall on a continuum, there is a correlation between the magnitude of the test result and the likelihood (probability) of disease. The relationship between measured test values and the corresponding likelihood ratios can be represented mathematically through a fitted regression line. In Table 4.2 likelihood ratios have been calculated

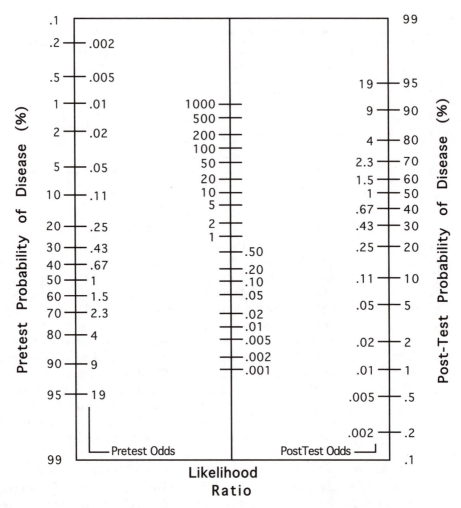

Figure 4.1 A nomogram for applying likelihood ratios and Bayes' theorem to the estimation of the posttest probability of disease. (From Fagan, T.J., *N. Engl. J. Med.*, 293, 257, 1975. With permission.)

over the range of ELISA values registered by animals who were shedding or not shedding *M. paratuberculosis* in their feces (Spangler et al., 1992). In Figure 4.2 an exponential equation has been fitted to the data. This equation can be used to estimate the likelihood ratio directly from any measured ELISA value, thereby directly estimating the probability of disease. The high r^2 value (0.989) demonstrates the strong positive correlation between the amount of serum antibody to *M. paratuberculosis* and the likelihood of fecal shedding ($r^2 = 0.989$), which is probably a reflection of the way in which ELISA values were expressed, e.g., as a proportion of the positive control. Knowing the magnitude of the ELISA OD value would be useful not only for interpreting a test result as positive or negative, but also for prioritizing cows for culling from the herd.

4.2.4 Use of posttest probabilities in medical decision making

Besides its inherent value as an expression of the likelihood of disease, the posttest probability can be used to rank the likelihood of diagnoses on a differential list or to reconcile a series of test results, where the posttest probability after one test becomes the

Table 4.2 Relationship between ELISA Optical Density (OD) and Likelihood of Fecal Shedding of *M. paratuberculosis* in Cattle

| | Fecal Culture | | |
ELISA Cutoff	Number Positive	Number Negative	Likelihood Ratio[a]
<10	3	39	1.00
10	16	91	1.15
20	11	73	1.70
30	14	33	3.40
40	20	11	6.47
50	15	7	8.43
60	12	5	11.50
70	9	3	18.48
80	14	1	37.71
90	26	1	49.03
Totals	140	264	

Note: ELISA values are expressed as a percent of the optical density of the positive reference serum.

[a] Likelihood cutoff =

$$\frac{\text{No. ELISA(+) / fecal culture(+)} \geq \text{cutoff} \div \text{total fecal culture(+)}}{\text{No. ELISA(+) / fecal culture(-)} \geq \text{cutoff} \div \text{total fecal culture(-)}}$$

Source of data: Spangler, C. et al., *Prev. Vet. Med.*, 13, 197–204, 1992. With permission.

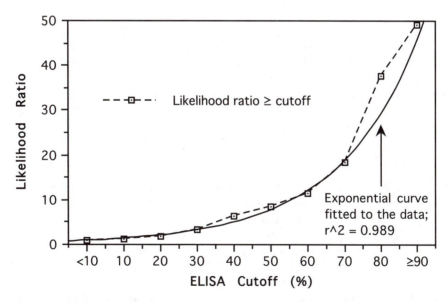

Figure 4.2 Exponential curve fitted to data from Table 4.2. Likelihood ratios were based on the proportion of *M. paratuberculosis* fecal culture-positive and -negative cows whose ELISA values were greater than or equal to a given cutoff. The solid line is an exponential curve fitted to the data. (Source of data: Spangler, C. et al., *Prev. Vet. Med.*, 13, 197–204, 1992. With permission.)

Table 4.3 Aspects of Multiple Test Strategies

Considerations	Multiple Test Strategy		
	Parallel Testing	Serial Testing	Herd Retest
Interpretation of test strategy	Positive diagnosis requires only one positive test result	Positive diagnosis requires that all test results be positive	Positive diagnosis requires only one positive test result
Effect of test strategy	Increase sensitivity	Increase specificity	Increase sensitivity at the herd level
Greatest predictive value	Negative test sequence	Positive test sequence	Negative test sequence
Application	Rule out a disease	Rule in a disease	Rule out a disease
Purpose; clinical setting	Rapid assessment of individual patients; vaccination clinics, emergencies	Time not crucial; avoid excessive testing of groups of animals; test and removal programs	Time not crucial; test and removal programs
Comments	Useful when there is an important penalty for missing a disease, i.e., false negative results	Useful when there is an important penalty for false positive results	Useful when there is an important penalty for missing a disease, i.e., false negative results

new pretest probability for the next test. This sequential approach works as long as certain conditions are met. Most importantly, either the test(s) must be conditionally independent (i.e., the sensitivity and specificity of the second test must not depend on the results of the first) or all conditional dependencies must be explicitly described (i.e., the probability of the second test being positive, given both disease and a positive result for the first test).

4.3   Multiple tests

Diagnoses are seldom made on the basis of a single test. **Multiple testing** is common in the veterinary hospital and in the field. The interpretation of multiple test results depends on the sequence in which they are conducted and the way in which their results are integrated. This section discusses the principles by which multiple tests are interpreted. Table 4.3 summarizes the factors to be considered in ordering and interpreting multiple tests.

4.3.1   Parallel testing

In **parallel testing**, two or more different tests are run on a patient or herd, usually at the same time. A positive diagnosis requires that only one of the test results be positive. A common example of parallel testing is the initial screening of outpatients during vaccination clinics. Typically, a careful physical examination is conducted and the temperature, pulse, and respiratory rate are recorded. The degree of overlap in the distribution for these parameters among normal and sick animals is considerable.

Diagnostic tests are usually done in parallel when rapid assessment of the patient's condition is necessary, as in emergency or hospitalized patients, or emergency care patients where the health status of the patient will determine whether a subsequent procedure can be performed. *The net effect of parallel testing is to ask the patient to prove that it is healthy.*

Parallel testing is particularly useful when the clinician is faced with the need for a very sensitive test but has available only two or more relatively insensitive ones. By using

Table 4.4 Sensitivity, Specificity, and Positive (pD+/T+) and Negative (pD–/T–) Predictive Values of Serum Alkaline Phosphatase and Gamma Glutamyl Transferase Activities When Interpreted Individually and in Parallel in Cats with Liver Disease

Test	Sensitivity (%)	Specificity (%)	Positive Predictive Value (%)	Negative Predictive Value (%)
ALP	50	93	96	36
GGT	86	67	90	59
ALP and GGT	94	67	91	77

Source: Center, S.A. et al., *J. Am. Vet. Med. Assoc.*, 188, 507–510, 1986. With permission.

the tests in parallel, the net effect is a more sensitive diagnostic strategy with a higher negative predictive value. On the other hand, specificity and positive predictive value are lowered. Only animals that have negative results on all tests are considered to be truly free of disease. The price is evaluation or treatment of some patients without disease.

Example 4.1

Cats with hepatobiliary disorders often have vague clinical signs until the disease process is advanced (Center et al., 1986). High serum activities of certain liver enzymes often provide the first laboratory evidence of liver disease and may suggest the type of pathologic process developing in the liver. The diagnostic value of serum gamma glutamyl transferase (GGT) was compared with serum alkaline phosphatase (ALP) activity for the detection of liver disease in the cats. Sixty-nine cats (male = 36, female = 33) were examined because of suspected hepatic disease or because hepatic disease was considered after initial clinical observations. The diseased group consisted of 54 cats with histologically confirmed liver disease, while the control group consisted of 15 cats initially suspected of hepatic disease but subsequently found to be free of substantial histologic abnormalities of the liver. The study showed that GGT activity had superior sensitivity, but lower specificity, than ALP activity (Table 4.4). The best sensitivity and negative predictive value (pD–/T–) was achieved by determining GGT and ALP activities simultaneously (in parallel). Therefore, the authors recommended that both tests be used in parallel to rule out the possibility of hepatobiliary disease in the cat.

A disadvantage of parallel testing is that as the number of tests included in the testing strategy increases, the risk of false positive diagnoses also increases. If the clinician orders enough tests, a new abnormality will be discovered in virtually all healthy patients. The reason is obvious if we recall that the normal range of values is usually defined to include 95% of the normal population. Thus, as the number of unrelated tests performed in parallel increases, the chance that the patient will be normal on all tests decreases. On the other hand, normal results on parallel tests increase the likelihood that the patient is truly normal. Parallel testing is usually used on an individual patient basis rather than on groups of animals, such as litters, kennels, or herds.

4.3.2 Serial testing

In **serial testing**, two or more different tests are run on a patient or herd, but all test results must be positive for a positive diagnosis to be made. *The net effect is to ask the patient to* *prove that it is truly affected by the condition being sought.* Serial testing maximizes specificity and positive predictive value, but lowers sensitivity and negative predictive value. We can be more confident in positive test results, but run an increased risk that disease will be missed.

Serial testing may be used during the course of a diagnostic workup, where rapid assessment of patients is not required, or when some of the tests are expensive or risky (these tests being employed only after simpler and safer tests suggest the presence of disease). CONSULTANT, <http://www.vet.cornell.edu/consultant/consult.asp>, a computer-based veterinary diagnostic support system, employs a serial test strategy to generate a differential list from findings entered by the user. As the number of findings increases, the number of diseases that share all of the findings decreases, resulting in a progressively shorter differential list.

Serial testing is also an integral part of disease control programs. Typically, screening tests are followed by confirmatory tests of positive herds or animals to reduce the likelihood that healthy animals are needlessly culled from the herd. The Cooperative State–Federal Bovine Tuberculosis Eradication Program is an excellent example of serial testing. Begun in 1917, the program has nearly eradicated bovine tuberculosis from the U.S. livestock population. Accredited veterinarians play a key role in the program by applying the primary diagnostic test, the caudal fold test (CFT), on a routine basis to herds. This is the official tuberculin test for routine screening of individual cattle, dairy goats, and herds of such animals in which the tuberculosis status of the animals is unknown. The test measures the cellular reaction of cattle to the intradermal injection of purified protein derivative (PPD), which is extracted from *Mycobacterium bovis* organisms. Results are recorded as **negative** or **suspect**. Suspect animals are then retested by a state or federal regulatory veterinarian using the comparative cervical test (CCT) to differentiate responses caused by mammalian tubercle bacilli and those induced by other mycobacteria. The CCT in cattle is performed by injecting *Mycobacterium avium* and *M. bovis* PPD tuberculins into separate sites in the skin of the neck. The difference in size of the two resultant responses usually indicates whether tuberculin sensitivity is caused by infection with bovine type bacilli rather than an avian type, by *M. paratuberculosis*, or by a transient sensitization to other saprophytic mycobacteria in the environment. These organisms are responsible for some of the false positive tuberculin reactions that are a major problem in areas where tuberculosis has been nearly eliminated. Results may be negative, suspect, or **reactor** (positive).

The proportion of reactors with no gross lesions detected on postmortem examination can be greatly reduced by the use of the CCT. However, it is much more tedious, difficult to interpret, and expensive than the caudal fold test. Consequently, it is not used as a primary screening test. To confirm a diagnosis of tuberculosis, it is necessary to isolate and identify the etiologic agent. Cultural results usually require 6 to 8 weeks.

Example 4.2

The state of Michigan lost its bovine tuberculosis (bTb) disease-free status when a bTb-positive bovine was identified in 1995. In response, a tuberculosis control program was initiated that included testing of all cattle in the state that were older than 12 months. A **serial skin testing protocol** was used that employed the CFT as a **screening test**, followed by retesting of suspects (CFT responders from herds of unknown bTb status) with the comparative cervical test (CCT). Cattle that responded to the CFT and were from herds of positive bTb status were classified as **reactors** and removed from the herd without further testing.

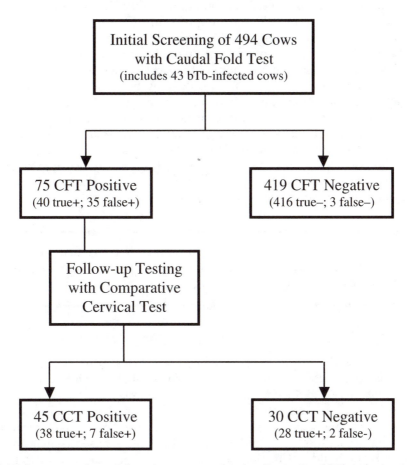

Figure 4.3 Performance of a serial testing strategy for the diagnosis of bTb infection in naturally exposed cattle. Initial screening employed the highly sensitive (93.02%) CFT. Test-positive cattle were subsequently tested with the more specific CCT. (Source of data: Norby, B. et al., *J. Vet. Diagn. Invest.*, 16, 126–131, 2004. With permission.)

Norby et al. (2004) evaluated the performance of the CFT and CCT alone and in series (CFTCCT$_{SER}$) in 494 naturally exposed cattle in seven bTb-infected herds. Mycobacterial isolation and polymerase chain reaction (PCR) used **in parallel** (Isol-PCR) was the reference or definitive test for bTb infection; e.g., cattle were considered to be bTb infected if positive on either test. Individual animal **apparent prevalence** (AP) for each test was also calculated as the proportion of tested animals that were test positive.

Forty-three of 494 cattle were considered bTb infected according to the Isol-PCR reference test, yielding an apparent prevalence of 8.70%. Although the CFT correctly identified 40 of these 43 cattle (93.02% sensitivity), it also resulted in a high proportion of false positives, reflected in the apparent prevalence of 15.18% (75 test-positive cattle). The majority of these false positives were correctly classified through CCT testing of CFT-positive cattle. The serial testing procedure correctly identified 38 of 43 bTb-infected cattle (88.37% sensitivity), and apparent prevalence was reduced to 9.11% (45 test-positive cattle). The performance of this serial testing strategy is summarized in Figure 4.3.

Although the sensitivity of the CFTCCT$_{SER}$ serial testing strategy was high, two of the seven herds (29%) would have had at least one positive animal left in the herd if a test and removal program had been used. In other words, the tests are more suited to the detection of infected herds than the detection of infected cattle. This suggests that when positive herds are identified, selective culling of skin test reactors is a less acceptable disease control strategy than is complete depopulation.

Serial testing should not be confused with **paired sampling**, in which the same test is performed on sequentially collected samples to detect changes in test results over time. Either decreases or increases in measured results may be sought. For example, paired sampling may be used to reduce the likelihood of false positive results due to time-related phenomena peculiar to particular patients. Examples are colostral antibody or vaccination titers that can be distinguished from immune responses to actual infection by their tendency to drop off over time. During an outbreak investigation paired sampling may be performed to identify a potential causative agent. In this case, an increased antibody titer to a specific pathogen in paired sera collected during and following a disease outbreak provides presumptive evidence for its involvement in the outbreak.

▼

> The net effect of parallel testing is to ask the patient to prove that it is healthy, whereas the net effect of serial testing is to ask the patient to prove that it is truly affected by the condition being sought.

▲

4.3.3   Herd retest

Herd retest is a modification of serial testing in which test-negative rather than test-positive animals are retested with the same test, usually at regular intervals. *The net effect is to ask the herd to prove that it is free of the condition being sought.*

Although test-negative animals are retested, herd retest does not increase the sensitivity of the testing strategy at the level of the individual because (1) the same test is used and (2) retesting occurs after a fairly long interval. Thus, a false negative may not be detected or, at best, would not be detected until some time later. However, herd retest should increase the sensitivity of the testing strategy *at the herd level* because it increases the likelihood of detecting an agent on premises that, for whatever reason (sampling, incubating infection, reintroduction of the agent), eluded detection earlier.

Herd retest forms the basis of test and removal programs designed to eradicate disease on any scale. The USDA's swine Pseudorabies Eradication Program is designed to detect infected herds and maintain continued surveillance in disease-free herds. Voluntary guidelines also exist for the eradication of such diverse diseases as bovine anaplasmosis and feline leukemia virus from their respective populations. In some cases, the option exists to cull animals or treat them to remove infection, as in the case of bovine anaplasmosis.

It is important to note that as the prevalence of disease in a population decreases, the specificity of the test procedure used to identify infected individuals becomes increasingly important. For example, application of a test that is only 80% specific in a herd that is free of infection will yield 20% test-positive individuals, all of which would be false positives. In a test and removal program these animals would be needlessly sent to slaughter, much to the embarrassment of animal health officials if follow-up definitive testing is performed postmortem.

4.3.4   Assumption of independence of multiple test results

Ideally, when multiple tests are used in parallel or in series, each test should measure a unique indicator of the health status of the individual. Body temperature, pulse, and respiratory rates are, by and large, independent measures. Immunologic tests also measure unique attributes of the individual when they depend on differences in the nature of the immune response, such as cellular vs. humoral immunity, IgM vs. IgG antibody, or differences in titer. If the assumption that the tests are completely independent is wrong, calculation of the probability of disease from several tests would tend to overestimate the value of the multiple testing strategy.

4.4 Working with differential lists

4.4.1 Rule-ins and rule-outs: the choice of sensitive or specific tests

The choice of a particular diagnostic test, or the interpretation of a test result, should be made within the context of the clinical situation. A negative result on a highly sensitive test, i.e., one that is usually positive in the presence of disease, is frequently used to rule out a disease on a differential list during the early stages of a diagnostic workup. Tests of high sensitivity are also useful when there is an important penalty for failure to detect a particular disease, e.g., when the cost of a false negative result exceeds that of a false positive.

Sensitivity should not be the sole criterion for choosing a test, however. As discussed earlier, use of a test of high sensitivity but low specificity in a disease eradication program may result in the removal from the herd of an unacceptable number of animals with false positive results. A positive result on a highly specific test, i.e., one that is rarely positive in the absence of disease, is useful to confirm (or rule in) a diagnosis that has been suggested by other data. Tests of high specificity are especially useful when a false positive diagnosis can result in physical, emotional, or financial loss to the patient or owner.

Two simple acronyms to facilitate remembering the above relationships are **SnNout** and **SpPin**. In expanded form, SnNout states that negative results on tests of high sensitivity are best for ruling out a target disorder. SpPin states that positive results on tests of high specificity are best for ruling in a target disorder (Sackett et al., 1991).

When we simply wish to choose the test with the best overall performance (fewest diagnostic errors), test accuracy provides the best criteria. Even though the accuracy of a diagnostic test varies with the likelihood of the target disorder in the individual(s) being tested, the range of variability is less than positive or negative predictive values. Test accuracy provides a simple answer to the question: *What proportion of test results are likely to be correct?*

4.5 Screening for disease

4.5.1 Definitions

When apparently healthy individuals or groups of individuals are systematically tested for the purpose of detecting certain characteristics or health problems, the process is referred to as **screening**. When screening tests are applied to large, unselected populations, this testing strategy is referred to as **mass screening**. Mass screening is sometimes employed in state and federal disease control or eradication programs, such as state bovine tuberculosis eradication programs. Abnormal test results may be followed up with confirmatory diagnosis, then treatment or destruction of affected individuals. In other scenarios, only a statistically representative sample of the herd or flock is sampled with the objective of identifying affected populations rather than individuals. This strategy has been employed in herd testing for swine pseudorabies. Sampling of groups of individuals may also be accomplished by pooling of samples, as in testing of milk samples from bulk tanks for excessive bacterial counts or violative antibiotic residues.

Identification of an affected population may be followed with **case finding**. Case finding is a strategic form of screening targeted at individuals or groups suspected to be at high risk of infection or disease because of association with known infected or diseased individuals or groups, or through other forms of exposure. Case finding may be part of a trace-back investigation of herds suspected of being sources of infected individuals involved in a disease outbreak. Case finding may also be employed during a food-borne disease outbreak investigation to identify as many affected individuals as possible.

The ongoing systematic and continuous collection, analysis, and interpretation of health data for the purpose of monitoring the spatial and temporal patterns of one or more diseases and their associated risk factors is referred to as **epidemiologic surveillance (surveillance)** or **monitoring**. An example is the systematic reporting and recording of cases of notifiable animal diseases by veterinary diagnostic laboratories. Surveillance data contribute to our understanding of the natural history of disease and are useful in the planning, implementation, and evaluation of disease control measures. Surveillance data provide the scientific basis for political, social, or economic decision making.

4.5.2   Test criteria

Several criteria are used to evaluate the suitability of a diagnostic test for screening apparently normal populations. First, the test should be sensitive and specific. Because the prevalence of the condition being tested for will usually be low, the positive predictive value of the screening test will also be relatively low, regardless of its specificity. This effect can be diminished by restricting testing to high-risk groups. In addition to its performance characteristics, the test must be inexpensive, very safe, and acceptable to both clients and practitioners.

4.6   Increasing the predictive value of diagnostic tests

Considering the relationship between prevalence and predictive value of a test, it is obviously to the clinician's advantage to apply diagnostic tests to patients with an increased likelihood of having the target disorder sought. As a rule, tests are not ordered until the patient has undergone a thorough history and physical examination. Being a member of a high-risk group increases the positive predictive value of diagnostic tests. Consequently, clinicians should be aware of risk factors for specific diseases and the corresponding confirmatory diagnostic tests.

The referral process, such as that which contributes to the case load of veterinary teaching hospitals, increases the likelihood of finding significant disease. Consequently, more aggressive use of diagnostic tests might be justified in these settings vs. the typical walk-in community practice. The same tests, performed on a routine basis on all patients, would have a lower predictive value because of the lower prevalence of disease.

▼

Being a member of a high-risk group increases the positive predictive value of diagnostic tests. Consequently, clinicians should be aware of risk factors for specific diseases and the corresponding confirmatory diagnostic tests.

▲

Table 4.5 Criteria for Abnormal Physicochemical and Microscopic Findings in Canine Urine

Physicochemical	Microscopic
pH > 7.5	>10 RBC/hpf[a]
Protein trace	>5 WBC/hpf[b]
Glucose trace	>2 hyaline casts/lpf
Ketones trace	>1 granular cast/lpf
Occult blood trace	>1 waxy cast/lpf
Bilirubin > 2+	Microorganisms
	Parasitic ova/microfilariae
	Hyperplastic or neoplastic epithelial cells
	Unusual crystals[c]

[a] hpf = high-power (magnification) field (×450).

[b] lpf = low-power (magnification) field (×100).

[c] Unremarkable crystals include triple phosphate, amorphous phosphate, calcium carbonate, and bilirubin.

Source: Fettman, M.J., *J. Am. Vet. Med. Assoc.*, 190, 892–896, 1987. With permission.

Example 4.3

Historically, routine urinalysis has consisted of a parallel testing strategy combining macroscopic or physicochemical analysis and microscopic examination of the urine sediment (Table 4.5). Although microscopic examination increases laboratory technician time and expense to the client, its use has been justified on the basis of high false negative rates when physicochemical tests alone are used. Fettman (1987) explored the use of a risk-based testing strategy that reserved microscopic analysis for patients that were negative on physicochemical analysis but deemed at high risk for genitourinary disease.

The initial signs, clinical problems, and results of urinalyses of 1000 consecutive canine patients examined at a veterinary medical teaching hospital were reviewed. Criteria for classification of high-risk patients included patient history, physical signs, and clinical problems consistent with diseases in which genitourinary disease might be highly suspect (Table 4.6). Physicochemical examination alone would have incorrectly classified 64 of 562 individuals as normal (micropositive/macronegative), resulting in a negative predictive value (D–/T–) of 88.6%. By performing follow-up microscopic urinalysis on 136 of the 562 macronegative individuals classified as being at high risk for genitourinary disease (Table 4.6), an additional 51 micropositive individuals would have been detected. As a result, only 13 of 426 macronegative individuals that tested negative would have been incorrectly classified, raising the negative predictive value of this multiple test strategy to 97.5%. This increase in negative predictive value was achieved despite the fact that 426 low-risk patients were not retested microscopically, thus resulting in considerable potential savings in laboratory technician time and client costs. These savings would have to be balanced against the cost of failing to detect a patient with genitourinary disease.

Table 4.6 False Negative Rates (Micropositive/Macronegative) for Physicochemical Tests of Canine Urine Specimens by Risk Group

Diseases and Signs	False Negative Rate (%)
Signs Associated with Predisposition to Genitourinary Disease	
Diarrhea[a]	60.0[g]
Perineal abnormalities[a,b]	45.5[g]
Genitourinary abnormalities[a,c]	40.5[g]
Serum biochemical abnormalities due to renal failure[d]	37.5[h]
Neurologic deficits[e,f]	35.3[g]
Lower vertebral disk abnormalities and hindlimb lameness[f]	29.2[g]
Signs not Associated with Predisposition to Genitourinary Disease	
Nasal neoplasia	15.8
Congestive heart disease	11.1
Neoplastic or inflammatory oral disease	10.5
Neoplastic or inflammatory lung disease	10.0
Skin neoplasia	7.1
No illness	3.5

[a] Clinical problems potentially associated with ascending genitourinary inflammatory disease.

[b] Perianal neoplasia or inflammatory disease, perineal hernia.

[c] Dysuria, stranguria, pollakiuria, polyuria.

[d] High values for urea nitrogen, creatinine, or phosphorus.

[e] Caudal lower motor neuron or upper motor neuron deficits only associated with caudal muscular dysfunction.

[f] Clinical problems potentially associated with impaired micturition.

[g] $p < 0.05$.

[h] $p = 0.08$.

Source: Fettman, M.J., *J. Am. Vet. Med. Assoc.*, 190, 892–896, 1987. With permission.

4.7   Communication of diagnostic test results

Uncertainty is an inherent part of medical practice, and the interpretation and reporting of diagnostic test results are no exception. In most cases, there is a chance that the conclusion drawn from a test result is incorrect. It is important, therefore, not only to accurately communicate test results with colleagues and clients, but also to express the level of certainty of the associated diagnosis. Diagnostic certainty is usually conveyed using terms such as *likely, probable, consistent with*, or *suggestive* (Christopher and Hotz, 2004). Although such terms are qualitative and imprecise expressions of probability, they may be preferable when people are uncomfortable with probabilities, or where numbers or percentages imply a level of precision that is unwarranted by the available information. Ultimately, whether words or numbers are used to express probability, they should communicate the intended information effectively and be clearly understood by and have value for the clinician or client.

Example 4.4

Clinical pathologists use descriptive terms or modifiers to express the probability or likelihood of a cytologic diagnosis. Words are imprecise in meaning, however, and may be used and interpreted differently by pathologists and clinicians. Christopher and Hotz (2004) surveyed 202 board-certified clinical pathologists to (1) assess the frequency of use of 18 modifiers (terms) used to express diagnostic certainty, (2) determine the probability of a positive diagnosis implied by the modifiers, (3) identify preferred modifiers for different levels of probability, (4) ascertain the importance of factors that affect expression of diagnostic certainty, and (5) evaluate differences based on gender, employment, and experience. The survey response rate was 47.5% (n = 96) and primarily included clinical pathologists at veterinary colleges (n = 58) and diagnostic laboratories (n = 31). There was high variability in the numerical percentage assigned to each of the 18 modifiers (Figure 4.4). Ninety of 96 (96.8%) respondents preferred words to numbers or percentages for expressing probability in cytology reports, and 10 terms expressing 7 probability levels ranging from 1 to 100% were preferred by 50% of respondents (Table 4.7). The authors conclude that because of wide discrepancy in the implied likelihood of a diagnosis using words, defined terminology and controlled vocabulary may be useful in improving communication and the quality of data in cytology reporting. Vagueness inherent in the use of words to express diagnostic uncertainty is not necessarily bad, as it depends on the nature of the situation (as when tests are used for screening) and the quality of the information base.

4.8   Summary

In light of the uncertainties of diagnostic testing, it would be helpful to know the likelihood of disease in an individual given a positive or negative test result. A number of techniques can be used to estimate this parameter, known as the posttest probability of disease. These include the predictive values calculated directly from a two-by-two table, and formulas based on Bayes' theorem or the likelihood ratio. The latter require that the pretest probability of disease be estimated. The likelihood ratio method is especially useful for estimating disease probability directly from the magnitude of a test result.

Multiple tests can be performed, or test results interpreted, in three different ways: parallel, serial, and herd retest. In parallel testing, two or more different tests are run on a patient or herd, usually at the same time. A positive diagnosis requires that only one of the test results be positive. The net effect is to increase test sensitivity and negative predictive value, thereby increasing the probability that a disease will be detected. However, specificity and positive predictive value are lowered. In serial testing, two or more different tests are run on a patient or herd, but all test results must be positive for a positive diagnosis to be made. Serial testing maximizes specificity and positive predictive value, but lowers sensitivity and negative predictive value, thus increasing the probability that a disease will be missed. Herd retest is commonly used in disease control and eradication programs. It is a modification of serial testing in which test-negative rather than test-positive animals are retested with the same test, usually at regular intervals. The net effect is to ask the herd to prove that it is free of the condition being sought by calling negative only those animals that are negative on all tests. Consequently, sensitivity (at the herd level) is increased. Use of tests of low specificity in disease eradication programs based on herd retesting may lead to excessive herd depopulation.

Probability Expression

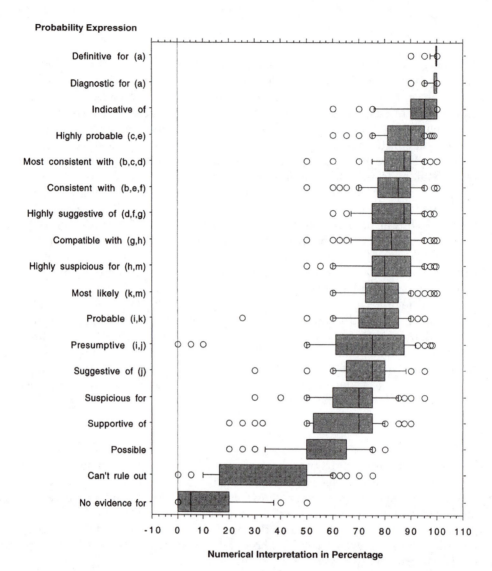

Figure 4.4 Numerical percentages attributed to 18 expressions of probability used to express uncertainty about a positive diagnosis. Boxes indicate the 25th to 75th percentile and median values; lines extend to the 10th and 90th percentile values; circles indicate outlying values. Expressions with the same letters in parentheses are not significantly different on the basis of analysis of variance of transformed probabilities. (From Christopher, M.M. and Hotz, C.S., *Vet. Clin. Pathol.*, 33, 84–95, 2004. With permission.)

The choice of a particular diagnostic test, or the interpretation of a test result, should be made within the context of the clinical situation. Two simple acronyms to facilitate remembering the above relationships are SnNout and SpPin. In expanded form, SnNout states that negative results on tests of high sensitivity are best for ruling out a target disorder. SpPin states that positive results on tests of high specificity are best for ruling in a target disorder. When we simply wish to choose the test with the best overall performance (fewest diagnostic errors), test accuracy provides the best criteria.

When apparently healthy individuals or groups of individuals are systematically tested for the purpose of detecting certain characteristics or health problems, the process

Table 4.7 Summary of Preferred Modifiers for Expressing the Probability of a Positive Diagnosis at Defined Percentage Levels

Modifier	100%	95%	75%	50%	25%	5%	0%
(No modifier)	24	3	0	0	0	0	2
Diagnostic for	37	3	0	0	0	0	0
Highly suggestive of	0	14	6	0	0	0	0
Most consistent with	1	13	4	2	0	0	0
Consistent with	5	14	9	2	0	0	0
Probable	0	12	23	4	1	0	0
Suggestive of	0	0	19	14	2	0	0
Possible	0	0	1	44	27	5	1
Can't rule out	0	0	0	6	21	30	2
Unlikely	0	0	0	0	6	10	0
No evidence for	0	0	0	0	1	11	42
Other	20	33	31	20	20	21	29
Do not express this level of probability	4	0	0	0	1	2	1
Number of different terms used	11	18	16	15	21	21	26
Total number of responses	91	92	93	92	78	77	76

Source: Christopher, M.M. and Hotz, C.S., Cytologic diagnosis: expression of probability by clinical pathologists, *Vet Clin Pathol*, 33, 84-95, 2004. With permission.

is referred to as screening. Case finding is a strategic form of screening targeted at individuals or groups suspected to be at high risk of infection or disease because of association with known infected or diseased individuals or groups, or through other forms of exposure. Sometimes only a statistically representative sample of the herd or flock is sampled, and the objective is to identify affected populations rather than individuals. The ongoing systematic and continuous collection, analysis, and interpretation of health data for the purpose of monitoring the spatial and temporal patterns of one or more diseases and their associated risk factors is referred to as epidemiologic surveillance (surveillance) or monitoring.

The positive predictive value of tests can be improved by restricting testing to individuals at greatest risk of having the condition of interest. This can be accomplished through a referral process, by restricting testing to demographic groups (by age, sex, breed, etc.) known to be at greater risk of having the condition, and by carefully conducting a screening history and physical examination before ordering additional diagnostic tests.

chapter 5

Measuring the commonness of disease

5.1   Introduction

Until now we have focused on the diagnosis of disease. We now turn our attention to measuring the frequency of disease events. Comparison of disease frequency in different groups forms the basis for assessing the risk of contracting a disease, its cause, prognosis, and response to treatment — the subjects of the next four chapters. Frequencies thus play a pivotal role in veterinary medical decision making.

5.2   Expressing the frequency of clinical events

5.2.1   Proportions, rates, and ratios

The frequency of clinical events is usually expressed as a proportion, with cases as the numerator and **population at risk** as the denominator. These proportions are commonly referred to as **rates**, although the latter term is more appropriately reserved for those proportions that include a time component, e.g., that express the occurrence of new events in a population over a defined time interval. The reason for this distinction will be discussed further below when prevalence and incidence rates are compared.

A **rate** is not the same thing as a **ratio**. In the case of a rate, the numerator is included in the denominator, while in a ratio, the numerator and denominator are mutually exclusive. In other words,

$$\text{rate} = \frac{a}{a+b} \qquad \text{ratio} = \frac{a}{b}$$

and in the special case for disease,

$$\text{rate} = \frac{\text{affected}}{\text{affected} + \text{unaffected}} \qquad \text{ratio} = \frac{\text{affected}}{\text{unaffected}}$$

An example of a rate is the proportion of students enrolled in U.S. veterinary colleges that are male or female. An example of a ratio is the comparison of the frequency of male to female veterinary students, or vice versa. This chapter focuses on rates. Ratios will be used in the following chapter to estimate risks of clinical events.

Example 5.1

During the 1985–1986 academic year, the proportion (a rate) of female students (50.8%) enrolled in U.S. veterinary medical colleges surpassed that of males (49.2%) for the first time. The ratio of female to male students was 1.034 to 1 (AVMA, 1986).

▼

A rate is not the same thing as a ratio. In the case of a rate, the numerator is included in the denominator, while in a ratio, the numerator and denominator are mutually exclusive.

▲

Veterinarians regularly use a number of rates. Some are **vital statistics rates**, which provide indirect evidence of the health status of a population. Other rates may be classified as **morbidity rates**, i.e., direct measures of the commonness of disease. Among the latter, the three most commonly used are prevalence, incidence, and attack rate. Several of the more commonly used vital statistics and morbidity rates are listed in Table 5.1.

5.2.2 *Prevalence, incidence, and attack rate*

Prevalence is the proportion of sampled individuals that possess a condition of interest at a given point in time. It is measured by a single examination of each individual of the group. Prevalence is a static measure in which the time unit is short (1 day or a few days). It can be likened to a snapshot of the population and includes both old and new cases. It is a measure of the likelihood of being a case at a given point in time.

In some cases, a distinction is made between animal-level and herd prevalence. **Animal-level prevalence** expresses the proportion of animals (the population at risk) that possess the condition of interest. When these animals reside within the same herd, this is referred to as **within-herd prevalence**. In contrast, **herd prevalence** expresses the proportion of herds in which one or more animals possess the condition of interest. Herd prevalence is useful when describing the spatial distribution of disease. As factors determining the level of within-herd prevalence are usually distinct from those determining herd prevalence, there may be a marked discrepancy between the two figures in any given region.

Example 5.2

Johne's disease (paratuberculosis) is a chronic contagious enteritis of ruminants characterized by persistent and progressive diarrhea, weight loss, debilitation, and eventually death. The disease is caused by *Mycobacterium avium* subsp. *paratuberculosis* and has a worldwide distribution. Table 5.2 lists the prevalence of *M. avium* subsp. *paratuberculosis* infection in cattle in selected U.S. states. The data were based on culture of ileocecal lymph nodes obtained from cattle culled at 76 slaughterhouses in 32 states and Puerto Rico during 1983 and 1984 (Merkal et al., 1987). The prevalence was 1.6% overall, with 2.9% in dairy culls and 0.8% in beef culls. The prevalence for female and male animals did not appear to differ significantly. We have no information on when the infections were acquired or the duration of infection. The rate thus represents the likelihood of being a case, rather than becoming a case. Standard error is defined as the

Table 5.1 Commonly Used Vital Statistics and Morbidity Rates in Veterinary Medicine

Rate and Its Calculation	Remarks
Vital Statistics	
Crude live birth rate: $$\frac{\text{No. of live births}}{\text{Average population}} \times 10^x$$	Useful as a measure of population increment due to natural causes
General fertility rate: $$\frac{\text{No. of live births}}{\text{Average no. of females of reproductive age}} \times 10^x$$	Frequently used as an index of overall herd reproductive performance
Crude death rate: $$\frac{\text{No. of deaths}}{\text{Average population}} \times 10^x$$	Useful as a measure of population loss due to natural causes
Morbidity/Mortality Rates	
Attack rate: $$\frac{\text{No. of affected individuals during an outbreak}}{\text{Population at risk at beginning of the outbreak}} \times 10^x$$	Useful for identifying risk factors for a specific disease; restricted to outbreak investigation
Incidence rate: $$\frac{\text{No. of new cases of a disease over a time interval}}{\text{Average population at risk during the time interval}} \times 10^x$$	A dynamic measure of risk of acquiring disease over a given period; useful for monitoring the course of an epidemic; used in cohort studies to measure effect of suspected or known risk factors
Prevalence: $$\frac{\text{No. of existing cases of a disease at a point in time}}{\text{Population at risk at the same point in time}} \times 10^x$$	A static measure of the risk of having a particular disease at a given point in time; used in case control studies to measure effect of suspected or known risk factors
Case fatality rate: $$\frac{\text{No. of deaths from a specified cause}}{\text{Total no. of cases of the same disease}} \times 10^x$$	Useful for determining prognosis for a specific disease

Note: Although any time period could be used, for convenience all indices refer to a defined population of animals observed for 1 year, unless otherwise stated.

Adapted from Armstead, W.W., in *Veterinary Medicine and Human Health*, 3rd ed., Schwabe, C.W., Ed., Williams & Wilkins, Baltimore, 1984, chap. 17.

standard deviation of the mean and is a measure of the variability of the reported prevalence values. See Chapter 2 for further information on the standard deviation. The derivation of standard error for this example is discussed in detail in Chapter 9 in Section 9.3.1.4.

The preceding animal-level prevalence data do not provide any insight into the prevalence of mycobacterial infection among and within individual beef or dairy herds. This kind of information was generated during a 1997 USDA-APHIS National Animal Health

Table 5.2 Prevalence, Listed by State, of *Mycobacterium paratuberculosis* Isolated from the Ileocecal Lymph Node in Culled Cattle

State[a]	No. Submitted	No. Infected Lymph Nodes	Prevalence (%)	Standard Error[c] (%)
Alabama	106	1	0.9	0.9
Arkansas	102	1	1.0	1.0
California	531	8	1.5	0.5
Colorado	111	1	0.9	0.9
Georgia	104	0	0.0	1.2
Illinois	171	2	1.2	0.8
Kansas	394	0	0.0	0.6
Kentucky	129	1	0.8	0.8
Maine	101	1	1.0	1.0
Michigan	118	2	1.7	1.2
Minnesota	238	13	5.5[b]	1.5
Mississippi	116	2	1.7	1.2
Missouri	449	4	0.9	0.4
Nebraska	249	3	1.2	0.7
New York	365	5	1.4	0.6
Ohio	214	6	2.8	1.1
Oklahoma	415	1	0.2	0.2
Oregon	141	4	2.8	1.4
Pennsylvania	307	21	6.8[b]	1.4
Tennessee	197	4	2.0	1.0
Texas	1215	9	0.7[b]	0.3
Virginia	193	3	1.6	0.9
Washington	236	2	0.9	0.6
Wisconsin	562	13	2.3	0.6
All others	776	12	1.6	0.4

[a] Only states from which at least 100 specimens were received are shown separately.

[b] States with prevalences that differed significantly from the overall mean, based on a Z-test with a level of significance of $p < 0.01$.

[c] Standard error is equal to the SD of the mean.

Source: Merkal, R.S. et al., *J. Am. Vet. Med. Assoc.*, 190, 676–680, 1987. With permission.

Monitoring System (NAHMS) comprehensive study of the health and management of the cow-calf segment of the beef industry. Dargatz et al. (2001) analyzed data from 10,371 beef cows from 380 herds in 21 states that had been tested for antibody to *M. avium* subsp. *paratuberculosis* using a commercial enzyme-linked immunosorbent assay (ELISA). Although only 40 (0.4%) of the individual cow samples yielded positive results, 30 herds had 1 or more animals for which results of the ELISA were positive, yielding a herd prevalence of 7.9%. The authors concluded that the prevalence of antibodies to *M. avium* subsp. *paratuberculosis* among beef cows in the U.S. is low and that seropositive herds were widely distributed geographically.

Although prevalence is a snapshot of the disease status of a population, series of prevalence measurements can be combined to obtain a picture of the occurrence of disease over time. This approach is particularly useful for depicting disease trends.

Example 5.3

Guptill et al. (2003) studied time trends and risk factors for diabetes mellitus in dogs using records from the Veterinary Medical Database (VMDB), a hospital-

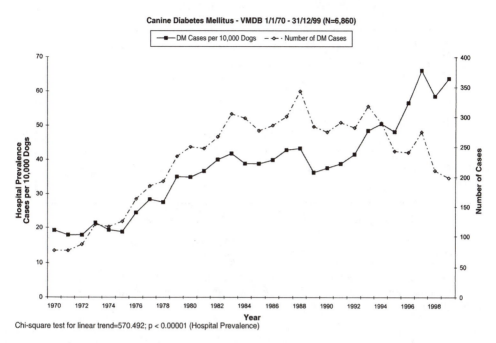

Figure 5.1 Hospital prevalence of canine diabetes mellitus (DM), VMDB, 1970–1999. Prevalence of DM increased over the study period. The number of institutions for which data are recorded is lower from 1995 to 1999, resulting in lower numbers of cases per year in these years. (From Guptill, L. et al., *Vet. J.*, 165, 240–247, 2003. With permission.)

based animal disease surveillance system that has been in existence since 1964. Electronic records of 6860 dogs diagnosed with diabetes mellitus between 1970 and 1999 were evaluated. The prevalence of diabetes mellitus in dogs presented to veterinary teaching hospitals increased from 19 cases per 10,000 admissions per year in 1970 to 64 cases per 10,000 in 1999 (Figure 5.1), while the case fatality rate decreased from 37 to 5% over the same period (Figure 5.2). Although diabetes mellitus diagnoses are reported over a period of time, this is still a measure of disease prevalence because we do not know what proportion of normal dogs developed diabetes mellitus each year, but only when the condition was first diagnosed. Although we cannot calculate the actual incidence, the trend in disease prevalence does suggest that the incidence of diabetes mellitus has increased over the 30-year study period. The authors suggest that changes in the genetic makeup or dietary practices over the years may be responsible for the apparent increase in canine diabetes mellitus. The case fatality rate is an incidence rate because it represents the number of new events (deaths) in the population at risk (diabetes mellitus cases) each year. The authors suggest that the decline in the case fatality rate may be due to the willingness of both owners and veterinarians to undertake long-term management of diabetic dogs. The importance of considering the size of the population at risk when interpreting trends in diagnoses can be appreciated in Figure 5.1. The decline in the number of diabetes mellitus cases after 1993 is due to a decline in reported hospital visits overall. The proportion of diabetes mellitus cases among reported visits actually increased during this period. The misleading effect of such **dangling numerators** will be discussed later in this chapter.

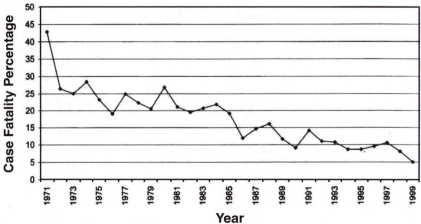

Chi-square test for linear trend=30.585; p <0.00001; includes died and euthanased

Figure 5.2 Case fatality percentage for canine diabetes mellitus (DM), VMDB, 1970–1999. The case fatality percentage for dogs with DM decreased steadily between 1970 and 1999. (From Guptill, L. et al., *Vet. J.*, 165, 240–247, 2003. With permission.)

------------------------------▼------------------------------

Prevalence represents the likelihood of being a case, whereas incidence represents the likelihood of becoming a case.

------------------------------▲------------------------------

Incidence is the proportion of individuals in a susceptible population that develop a condition of interest over a defined period. Although birth rates, death rates, and similar vital statistics are based on new events, incidence is commonly understood to refer to disease events. Incidence takes into account new cases only, i.e., cases that have their onset during the specified period. It is therefore a measure of the risk of becoming a case over a defined period. An example would be the incidence of postoperative surgical site infections for different kinds of surgeries performed in a veterinary teaching hospital. The population at risk would be animals undergoing surgery during a specified period. Surgeries might be further classified by site, duration, etc., for comparative purposes.

Ideally, the population at risk is a cohort of all susceptible individuals at the beginning of the follow-up period. A **cohort** is a group of individuals who have something in common when they are first assembled, and who are then observed for a period to see what happens to them. Often, because of the difficulty of conserving the original composition of a cohort over follow-up periods of long duration, the denominator is expressed as the average population at risk during that period (Figure 5.3).

Example 5.4

Straw et al. (1985) studied the effect of a number of management factors on productivity in a swine feedlot. One of the outcomes monitored was the daily death rate, which was calculated by dividing the number of deaths occurring each day (new cases) by the number of swine present in the feedlot at that time (population at risk). When adjusted for length of stay in the feedlot, it was found that the average incidence of death among pigs that failed to reach

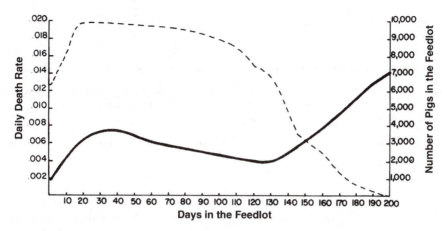

Figure 5.3 Comparison of daily death rate (solid line) vs. length of stay (dashed line) of swine in a feedlot. (From Straw, B.E. et al., *J. Am. Vet. Med. Assoc.*, 186, 986–988, 1985. With permission.)

market weight within 150 days of entry into the feedlot (0.0104) was nearly twice that of pigs that reached market weight before 150 days (0.0054) (Figure 5.3). Although the specific cause(s) was not identified, the authors recommended that all animals be marketed by 150 days after entry into the feedlot, regardless of weight. The two lines cross at the 150-day mark. Note that a change in either of the y-axis (ordinal) scales would result in a shift of the crossover point and perhaps a different recommendation.

Attack rate is a term that is often used to specify the proportion of a defined population affected during an outbreak. In its simplest form, the attack rate is equal to the total number of cases during the outbreak period divided by the number of individuals initially exposed, i.e., those present at the beginning of the outbreak. Since the attack rate is based only on new cases of the disease, it is comparable to incidence. Attack rate tables are particularly useful for evaluating the relative contribution of various risk factors to the onset or course of an epidemic or a food-borne disease outbreak. Measurement of risk is discussed in greater detail in Chapter 6.

5.3   Measuring the frequency of clinical events

5.3.1   Prevalence

Prevalence is measured by surveying a population, some of whose members are diseased and the remainder healthy, at a particular point in time. The proportion that are diseased constitute the prevalence of the disease. Such snapshots of the population are referred to as **cross-sectional studies**.

Prevalence can be estimated through examination of a group of animals at a single point in time (**point prevalence**), a single examination of each of a series of animals seen over a period (**period prevalence**), or a combination of the two. For example, determination of the proportion of swine afflicted with pneumonia during a slaughter check represents the proportion of cases in a population at a single point in time, or point prevalence. The proportion of different types of neoplasia among all equine neoplasms diagnosed in an animal disease diagnostic laboratory over a 5-year period represents the cumulative results of individual diagnoses over time, or period prevalence. Both are expressions of prevalence since we do not know when disease first appeared or how long it has lasted.

Neither provides information on the risk of becoming a case (incidence), only on the risk of being a case (prevalence).

▼

> Prevalence studies can be based on the examination of a group of animals at a single point in time, on a single examination of each of a series of animals seen over a period, or a combination of the two.

▲

5.3.2   Incidence

Incidence is measured by recording the appearances of a condition of interest over time in a population initially free of the condition. This study design, called a **longitudinal** or **prospective study**, is discussed in detail in Chapter 6. Whereas time is assumed to be instantaneous in cross-sectional studies, it is a key component in the measurement and expression of incidence.

Incidence is commonly measured in one of two ways. In the first, a **defined group** of susceptible individuals, known as a **cohort**, is followed over time and each occurrence of the event of interest is recorded as it occurs. This approach is frequently used to determine the prognosis, with or without treatment, for a group of individuals known to be affected with a particular disease.

Incidence can also be measured by recording the number of new events occurring in an ever-changing population whose members are at risk for varying periods of time (as the pigs in Figure 5.3). This approach is useful for determining the effect of a risk factor on the subsequent incidence of disease in a dynamic population. In this case, the denominator of the incidence rate must be adjusted to account for the variable period that each animal is exposed to the risk factor. Sometimes the average number of animals present over the specified time interval is used as the denominator. A more accurate approach is to use **animal time at risk** rather than number of animals in the denominator. The resulting incidence rate is then referred to as an **incidence density**, and reflects the number of new events, or cases, per total number of animal days, weeks, months, or years at risk. The following example illustrates the difference in the way prevalence and incidence are calculated using bovine mastitis as an example.

Example 5.5

Erskine et al. (1988) estimated the incidence and prevalence of mastitis in 18 dairy herds, 12 with low herd mean somatic cell counts (SCC 150,000 cells/ml) and 6 with high (>700,000 cells/ml) SCC. Mean incidence of clinical mastitis in low SCC herds was 4.24 infections/100 cows/month. The highest recorded incidence of clinical mastitis was in July and August. The prevalence of intra-mammary infection attributable to all major pathogens in the same herds was <4% of all quarters.

Figure 5.4 draws on these findings to depict the onset of clinical mastitis (■) and persistence of intramammary infection (—) in a hypothetical sample of 100 dairy cows from a low SCC herd over a 4-month period. It is assumed that recovery from an episode of mastitis does not confer immunity to subsequent intramammary infection and disease. Consequently, the population at risk re-mains constant. In this example, monthly incidence of mastitis ranged from 3

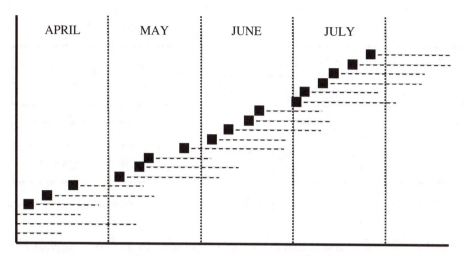

Figure 5.4 Occurrence of mastitis in 20 dairy cows from a hypothetical population of 100 over a 4-month period. ■, onset of clinical mastitis; —, duration of detectable intramammary infection with pathogenic bacteria.

to 6 new infections/100 cows/month. Mean monthly incidence can by calculated by summing all new cases over the 4-month period (n = 17) and dividing by 4, yielding 4.25 new infections/100 cows/month. The mean duration of intramammary infection was approximately 28 days. Three additional cows had actually contracted mastitis prior to April, but their infections were still detectable at the beginning of the 4-month period depicted in Figure 5.4. On any given day the prevalence of mastitis ranged from 3 to 5 detectable infections/100 cows. The significance of the difference between incidence and prevalence can be appreciated by considering that although 17 new cases of clinical mastitis occurred over this 4-month period, cross-sectional sampling would have detected only 3 to 5% of the herd infections at any given time.

In the preceding example it was assumed that the dairy herd population was stable, e.g., no animals entered or left the herd during the observation period. The following example describes how incidence can be estimated in a constantly changing population with variable periods of follow-up. This is often the case when conducting patient-based research in a clinical setting.

Example 5.6

Case control studies had shown that cryptorchid dogs are at greater risk of developing certain kinds of testicular neoplasia than their normal counterparts. However, because of the study design, the actual incidence of testicular neoplasia in exposed (cryptorchid) and unexposed (normal) male dogs could not be estimated. In an attempt to estimate actual incidence rates, a 4-year prospective study of the risk of developing canine testicular neoplasia incorporated cryptorchid (risk group) and matched controls into the study as they were identified by veterinary practitioners (Reif et al., 1979). Once dogs developed testicular neoplasia or were castrated for other reasons, they were considered to be no longer at risk, and their remaining months in the study were not counted. The average follow-up period for all dogs was 2 years, and ranged

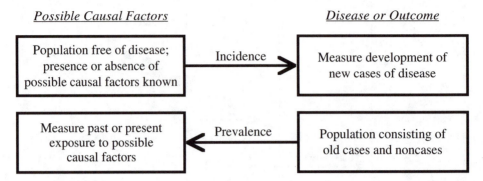

Figure 5.5 Temporal relationship between possible causal factors and disease; approaches based on incidence vs. prevalence.

from 1 to 4 years for individual dogs. Since dogs were in the study for variable periods of time, incidence was calculated on the basis of dog years of observation. Dog years (the denominator) were estimated by dividing the total months of observation for all dogs in the risk group by 12, the number of months in a year.

5.4   Factors affecting the interpretation of incidence and prevalence

5.4.1   Temporal sequence

Prevalence studies can be used to obtain a static picture of a situation at a fixed point in time, e.g., a snapshot of the population. Examples are provided in Chapters 3 and 4, in which prevalence data were used to evaluate the performance of diagnostic tests. Other examples are the routine surveillance activities of animal disease control programs, diagnostic laboratories, and veterinary teaching hospitals.

   Prevalence studies can also be used to examine the possible causal relationship (association) between suspected risk factors and the health status of a population. Unlike incidence studies, this relationship was not studied over time. Thus, we can only infer which came first, the putative cause or the outcome of interest. These relationships are further depicted in Figure 5.5.

> An important limitation of prevalence studies of cause is that one must infer the sequence of events.

5.4.2   Disease duration

The population included in the numerator of an incidence rate may differ from that in a prevalence rate. In an incidence study new cases are recorded as they occur over time. In a prevalence study it is difficult to distinguish new from old cases. Furthermore, if a disease is of short duration or fatal, some cases may be missed because they are no longer detectable at the time the prevalence study is conducted.

> Prevalence of a disease in a population may be higher or lower than incidence, depending on the average duration of the disease.

The prevalence of a disease in a population may be higher or lower than incidence, depending on the average duration of the disease. Diseases that are rapidly fatal, such as rabies, or of short duration, such as bovine mastitis, might have a higher incidence than prevalence. Chronic diseases, such as some parasitic infections, might be readily detected for long periods and would be more likely to appear in a prevalence study.

Example 5.7

The Animal Disposition Reporting System (ADRS), maintained by the USDA's Food Safety and Inspection Service (FSIS), contains slaughter totals and disposition summaries for federally inspected livestock and poultry slaughter establishments. Each animal carcass is inspected for diseases and other conditions that, if present, may result in the animal being condemned as unfit for human consumption. If a carcass is condemned, the reason for condemnation, also referred to as the disposition, is recorded in the ADRS database. Because of the way in which data are gathered, the ADRS database is biased in favor of diseases of long duration. For this reason, the USDA initiated the National Animal Health Monitoring System in 1983 to collect, analyze, and disseminate data on animal health, management, and productivity across the U.S. The NAHMS program uses federal, state, and university veterinary medical officers to conduct periodic national studies or targeted epidemiologic research on current animal health issues. NAHMS personnel visit sampling units, or premises, where they collect incidence data through personal interviews, evaluation of herd health records, and direct observations of the livestock or poultry (King, 1985). This approach provides better estimates of incidence than inspection-based surveillance systems.

5.4.3 Relationship among incidence, prevalence, and duration of disease

Since prevalence is the likelihood of being a case at any particular time, anything that increases the duration of disease will increase prevalence. Stated mathematically, prevalence can be estimated by multiplying incidence times the duration of disease (prevalence = incidence × average duration of disease). The equation can be rearranged to calculate any one of the parameters of interest.

Example 5.8

Let us return to the example by Erskine et al. (1988), depicted in Figure 5.4. The prevalence of intramammary infection was approximately 4%. If the duration of detectable infection is typically 1 month (0.083 years), then the annual incidence of mastitis would be 4%/0.083 years, or 48% of susceptibles per year. In other words, 48% of the herd will contract mastitis over the year, but at any given point in time only 4% of cows are affected. The accuracy of this estimate of incidence depends in large part on the accuracy of our estimate of the duration of the disease and the extent to which recovered animals are reinfected. If certain cows are more prone to mastitis, then incidence in the herd as a whole would be less.

5.4.4 True vs. apparent prevalence

Chapters 3 and 4 discussed how results derived from tests of less than 100% sensitivity and specificity may not indicate the **true prevalence** of disease. These tests measure the

apparent prevalence of disease in a population, as distinguished from true prevalence, which is usually estimated through use of an appropriate gold standard. If estimates of the sensitivity and specificity of a diagnostic test are available, it is possible to use them to estimate true prevalence from apparent prevalence.This estimate would be useful during the course of a disease eradication program, where the actual level of disease still present in the test population must be known as accurately as possible. The formula for estimating true prevalence from apparent prevalence is

$$\text{True Prevalence} = \frac{\text{Apparent Prevalence} + \text{Specificity} - 100\%}{\text{Sensitivity} + \text{Specificity} - 100\%}$$

Example 5.9

Collins et al. (1993) conducted a random cross-sectional survey of Wisconsin dairy herds to determine the geographic distribution and prevalence of paratuberculosis, and to identify herd management factors associated with higher prevalence rates. An ELISA test with a sensitivity of 50.9% and specificity of 94.9% was used. Overall, 7.29% of the cattle had positive test results. According to the equation,

$$\text{True Prevalence} = \frac{7.29\% + 94.9\% - 100\%}{50.9\% + 94.9\% - 100\%} = 4.78\%$$

In this case, the true prevalence (4.78%) is a third less than the apparent prevalence (7.29%). This equation will not tell us whether a given test result is correct or not, but it does provide a better estimate of the true prevalence of disease.

5.4.5   Case definition

In many instances it is difficult to define a set of disease signs, referred to as the **case definition**, that will include all true cases of the disease and exclude similar, but unrelated, conditions. For example, in Chapter 3 (Table 3.2) a list of clinicopathologic findings associated with chronic renal disease in cats was presented. The percentage of cats exhibiting any one finding ranged from 2.7 to 96.9%. As the number of signs required to diagnose chronic renal disease increases, the definition becomes more and more restrictive and includes a progressively smaller number of cases.

5.4.6   Dangling numerators

Expressing the frequency of disease as a rate or proportion, using appropriate denominators rather than in terms of absolute numbers, e.g., **dangling numerators**, permits comparisons of disease frequency in comparable populations. Comparing numbers of cases (numerator data) without taking into consideration the population at risk (denominator data) does not tell us anything about the risk of becoming (incidence) or of being (prevalence) a case.

Example 5.10

Cryptosporidium sp. is a protozoan pathogen that can causes diarrhea in calves, lambs, goats, deer, immunocompromised and immunocompetent humans, and

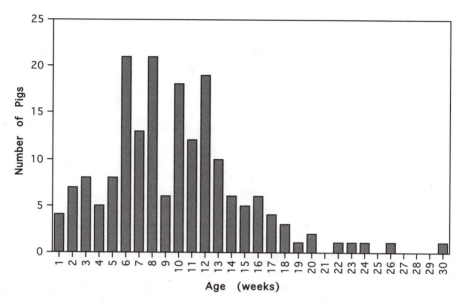

Figure 5.6 Age distribution of 184 pigs with enteric infection with *Cryptosporidium* sp. (From Sanford, S.E., *J. Am. Vet. Med. Assoc.*, 190, 695–698, 1987. With permission.)

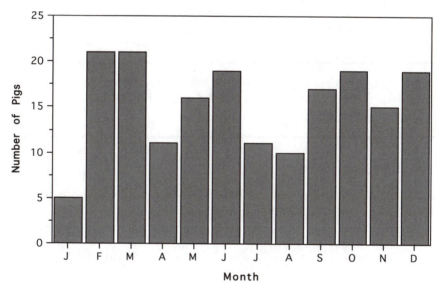

Figure 5.7 Monthly frequency of submissions for 184 pigs infected with *Cryptosporidium* sp. (From Sanford, S.E., *J. Am. Vet. Med. Assoc.*, 190, 695–698, 1987. With permission.)

other domestic and wild animals. Sanford (1987) reviewed the records of all 3491 live pigs submitted to a veterinary diagnostic laboratory over a 5-year period to obtain information on the characteristics of infected pigs. A total of 184 infected pigs from 133 farms were identified. He reported that the frequency of cryptosporidial infection was greatest in pigs 6 to 12 weeks old and that there was no seasonal pattern of infection. A perusal of the data from which these conclusions were drawn (Figure 5.6 and Figure 5.7) reveals that these conclusions were based on the number rather than the proportion of submissions with cryptosporidial infection, i.e., dangling numerators. It is not clear whether the observed outcomes were real or whether the numerator data are merely a reflection of overall submission patterns. Had proportions been used, then the populations at risk would have been comparable.

5.4.7   Population at risk

Incidence rates and prevalence must be interpreted in the context of the population at risk. If the population at risk differs significantly from one's own patients, then extrapolations may be meaningless. For example, because of the frequency of referral cases and usage patterns of veterinary services, the population of animals presented to the typical veterinary teaching hospital (VTH) is not representative of the population as a whole. This does not mean that the VTH patient population cannot serve as a denominator. If we wish to know the frequency with which findings occur among individuals with particular diseases (sensitivity data), then patients must be the denominator. On the other hand, if we wish to know the prevalence of the condition in the general population, then we would have to change our sampling strategy.

It is seldom feasible to sample the entire population at risk. Typically, a representative sample is selected by a random procedure in which all individuals have an equal chance of being included in the study. Sampling techniques and statistics are discussed further in Chapter 9. Comparison of disease rates among different groups is fundamental to determining the presence, cause, source, or probable mode of transmission of a disease. When comparing rates, care should be taken to ensure that populations used as denominators are truly comparable.

▼

> Comparing numbers of cases without taking into consideration the population at risk does not tell us anything about the risk of becoming (incidence) or of being (prevalence) a case.

▲

5.4.8   Crude vs. adjusted rates

Rates such as incidence, prevalence, and attack rate are considered **crude rates** when they are expressed in the standard format:

$$\frac{\text{Total number of affected individuals}}{\text{Total population}} \times \text{Multiplier}$$

It should be recognized that the crude rate summarizes the effects of two factors:

1. **Specific rate**: The probability of the event occurring in each subgroup (or stratum) of a population (such as subgroups based on age, breed, or sex)
2. **Subgroup distribution**: The characteristics or distribution of the subgroups in the population under consideration

Because a crude rate is a composite figure, it is necessary to disentangle these two factors before meaningful comparisons can be made between population groups. **Adjusted rates** compensate for subgroup effects by converting their distribution to that of a **standard population**.

Table 5.3 Death Rates of Calves by Age on Two Farms According
to Antibiotic Use

Age Group	Farm A Antibiotics Given to Calves[a]		Farm B Antibiotics Not Given to Calves	
	Population at Risk	Death Rate	Population at Risk	Death Rate
0–14 days	105	10.5	118	7.6
15–60 days	307	4.2	40	2.5
All ages	412	5.8	158	6.3

[a] Antibiotics were being used therapeutically rather than prophylactically.

Source of age-specific death rates: Oxender, W.D. et al., *J. Am. Vet. Med. Assoc.*, 162, 458–460, 1973.

Age is one of the most important characteristics governing the distribution of disease. Before morbidity or mortality rates in two populations can be compared, account must be taken of differences in age composition (Morton et al., 1990). Consider the data in Table 5.3. A paradox is seen. Age-specific death rates were higher for calves in both age groups on Farm A, where antibiotics were given. Yet, the overall death rate was higher on Farm B, where antibiotics were not given to calves. The apparent advantage of antibiotic use in calves is the result of the difference in age distribution of calves in the two comparison groups (Farms A and B). As a matter of record, the original findings showed that overall mortality for live births was 7.6% among calves given antibiotics vs. 5.2% among those not given antibiotics; i.e., antibiotics were being used therapeutically rather than prophylactically. Mortality figures were based on cohorts of calves followed from birth through 60 days of age (Oxender et al., 1973).

The effect of differences in age distribution among subgroups of calves in the preceding example is an example of **confounding**. In this case, age is referred to as a **confounding factor** because it confounds or blurs the comparison of interest. When differences in the distribution of one or more host characteristics, such as age, occur among the groups we wish to compare, **adjusted rates** should be used (Morton and Hebel, 1979).

▼

Because a crude disease rate is a composite figure reflecting two factors, namely, specific disease rates and population compositions, it is necessary to disentangle the two factors before meaningful comparisons can be made between population groups.

▲

5.5 *Adjusted rates: the direct method*

One method that can be used to adjust rates is referred to as the **direct method** (Kleinbaum and Kleinbaum, 1976). To understand what is meant by an adjusted rate, it must first be recognized that a crude rate may be expressed as the weighted sum of **specific rates**. Each component of the sum (crude rate) has the following form:

Proportion of the population in each subgroup × Subgroup-specific rate

The basic idea in computing direct rates for comparison of populations is to compute what the hypothetical crude rates would be for the populations if the confounding factor

Table 5.4 Direct Adjustment of Death Rates among Calves on Two Farms According to Antibiotic Use

Age Group	Standard Population at Risk	Farm A Antibiotics Given to Calves		Farm B Antibiotics Not Given to Calves	
		Death Rate per 100	Expected Deaths	Death Rate per 100	Expected Deaths
0–14 days	223	10.5	23.4	7.6	16.9
15–60 days	347	4.2	14.6	2.5	8.7
Totals	570		38		25.6
Direct rate (per 100) for Farm A	$\dfrac{38}{570}$ = 6.7		Direct rate (per 100) for Farm B	$\dfrac{25.6}{570}$ = 4.5	

Source of age-specific death rates: Oxender, W.D. et al., *J. Am. Vet. Med. Assoc.*, 162, 458–460, 1973.

were similarly distributed among their respective subgroups. In other words, we force a comparison of populations based on a *common* distribution of the confounding factor.

To compute directly adjusted rates, we need only two basic pieces of information: (1) the subgroup-specific rates for each subgroup and (2) a standard population. The **standard population** is that common distribution whose primary purpose is to serve as a reference group or substitute for the different distributions of the populations being compared.

5.5.1 Age-adjusted rates

Age is one of the most common confounding factors that is adjusted for. In the following example we calculate and compare age-adjusted rates using the data on calf mortality from Table 5.3. We arbitrarily define the standard population to be the sum of calves from the two farms in each age group. The method for calculating age-adjusted death rates involves three steps and is presented in Table 5.4:

1. Estimate the number of expected deaths for each age group by multiplying the standard population at risk by the observed death rate for each age-specific group.
2. Estimate the total number of expected deaths by adding expected deaths over all age-specific groups.
3. Estimate the direct rate by dividing the total expected deaths by the total standard population.

Comparing the age-adjusted death rates for the two farms, we see that the risk of death is greater for Farm A than it is for Farm B. This finding is consistent with the conclusion derived by comparing age-specific death rates for the two farms. This means that antibiotics were not a contributing factor in the deaths of calves on Farm A. Rather, antibiotics were used *in response to* the higher death rate and other disease problems on the farm.

5.5.2 Rate adjustment for other factors

A variety of other confounding factors may bias the comparison of groups. Two of the most common in veterinary medicine are breed and sex. Furthermore, age/breed- and age/sex-specific and adjusted rates can be computed and compared as was done previously for age alone. Cause-specific disease and death rates may be stated for the entire population or for any age, breed, or sex subgroup.

Example 5.11

Responses of atopic dogs to intradermal challenge with 60 allergens were determined and compared for four regions of the U.S.: northern Florida (n = 53), southern Florida (n = 67), Illinois (n = 130), and North Carolina (n = 28) (Schick and Fadok, 1986). Responses to allergens were compared among the first three regions to determine their relative prevalence or frequency and whether significant ($p < 0.05$) differences existed, using chi-square analysis. The number of patients seen in North Carolina (n = 28) was deemed too small for statistical analysis. Sex and breed prevalence of atopic dogs in northern and southern Florida were analyzed (chi-square) for significant ($p < 0.05$) differences from the general hospital population at the University of Florida VMTH.

Sex and breed predispositions to atopy were detected. Females were found to have an increased tendency ($p < 0.05$) to develop clinical signs of atopy. West Highland white terriers, cairn terriers, English and Irish setters, Dalmatians, Lhasa apsos, and golden and Labrador retrievers were predisposed to develop atopy. Poodles had a significantly ($p < 0.05$) lower prevalence of atopy. Regional differences in responses to allergens were also found. Twenty-seven allergens incited significantly greater responses in dogs from northern Florida and 28 allergens in dogs from southern Florida, when compared with dogs from Illinois. Of Florida dogs with atopy, 79% had a positive response for flea antigen, compared with only 9% of dogs from Illinois. On the basis of these findings, the authors concluded that region-specific allergens should be used for diagnosis and hyposensitization treatment.

Though these findings are interesting and may be clinically important, a nagging question is whether the results could be explained by the age–breed–sex composition of comparison groups. If age is a factor, could the breed and sex predisposition to atopy be the result of the age distribution of respective comparison groups? Likewise, could different age, breed, or sex distributions in Illinois and Florida dogs explain the increased prevalence of atopy in Florida dogs? Use of adjusted rates would have strengthened the validity of this study.

Example 5.12

PigCHAMP is a computerized record-keeping system for swine herds. It provides a valuable management and diagnostic tool for swine producers and veterinarians. One of the outputs of the program, the Farm Comparison Report, compares a series of performance monitors, expressed as crude rates, for up to 12 farms. A number of these performance monitors, such as preweaning mortality, are parity specific; i.e., their values are known to be influenced by parity, e.g., number of litters the sow has produced (Stein and Duffy, 1988). Preweaning mortality rates exceeding 15% (action threshold) suggest that a problem exists that should be rectified. However, unless preweaning mortality rates are adjusted for parity, one may erroneously ascribe unacceptable mortality rates to disease rather than the age distribution of the sow herd.

In Table 5.5 actual crude preweaning mortality rates for two Illinois farms, Farm A (16.7% mortality) and Farm B (13.1% mortality), are adjusted by the direct method. Since preweaning mortality is calculated based on litters that are

Table 5.5 Direct Adjustment of Preweaning Mortality Rates on Two Illinois Swine Farms According to Parity of the Sow[a]

		Farm A		Farm B	
Parity	Standard Population at Risk	Preweaning Mortality (%) (p)	Expected Deaths (E)	Preweaning Mortality (%) (p)	Expected Deaths (E)
1	133	13.6	18.1	13.2	17.6
2	130	13.7	17.8	9.7	12.6
3	120	2.5	3.0	9.8	11.8
4	105	10.4	10.9	15.0	15.8
5	80	20.0	16.0	16.5	13.2
6	45	21.6	9.7	16.6	7.4
7	30	19.7	5.9	21.0	6.3
8	39	37.5	14.6	11.5	4.5
Totals	682		96.0		89.2

Direct rate (per 100) for Farm A	$\dfrac{96.0}{682} = 14.1\%$	Direct rate (per 100) for Farm B	$\dfrac{89.2}{682} = 13.1\%$

[a] Crude preweaning mortality rate for Farm A was 16.7% and for Farm B was 13.1%.

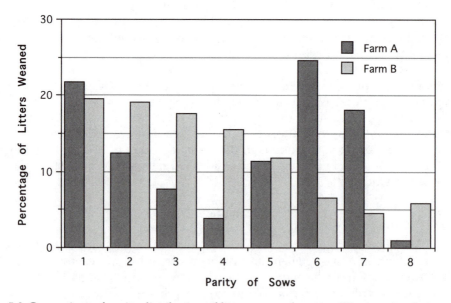

Figure 5.8 Comparison of parity distribution of litters weaned on two Illinois swine farms.

weaned or nursed off in the report period, the crude rates are adjusted for number of litters weaned for each parity group. The standard population chosen was that of Farm B, whose preweaning mortality was below the action threshold.

After rate adjustment we see that preweaning mortality for both farms is below the action threshold. A comparison of parity-specific mortality rates does not suggest overall difference between the two farms. The reason that the crude rates differed was due to a greater proportion of higher-parity sows on Farm A (Figure 5.8), which generally have higher preweaning mortality values.

5.5.3 The choice of a standard population

The choice of a standard population is relatively unimportant if the specific rates in one group are consistently lower than or equal to those in the other group. On the other hand, if disease rates, for example, favor younger animals in one group and older animals in another, then either group can be made to appear to have lower age-adjusted mortality rates, depending on the age distribution of the standard population. If a standard population is chosen so that it contains a large proportion of young animals, the group having the lower rates in young animals will have the lower standardized mortality. If a standard population contains a large proportion of older animals, the herd having lower age-specific rates among older animals will have a low age-adjusted mortality rate. In these instances, rate adjustment or standardization may not provide more information beyond that obtained by simple comparison of specific rates (Schwabe et al., 1977).

5.5.4 When to adjust rates

Rates are adjusted in order to remove the effect of a factor that may confound a comparison. However, it is always necessary to first look at the overall crude rates, because they represent the actual events. An adjusted rate gives an accurate comparison, but does not reveal the underlying raw data, which are shown by the crude rate (Morton and Hebel, 1979).

Although the presence of a (1) confounding factor is the primary condition for rate adjustment, three additional conditions must be met to justify adjusting rates:

(2) A comparison is to be made (not a single population).
(3) The event or characteristic of interest is defined for purpose of analysis as a rate or proportion.
(4) The comparison involves overall rates (not specific rates).

Populations that appear comparable at first glance may in fact be found to differ in important ways if complete census data are examined. Adjustment of rates by age, sex, or other relevant demographic factors may reveal differences that might otherwise be lost in the population as a whole.

5.5.5 The uses of incidence and prevalence

Incidence provides a measure of the likelihood of something happening. This could be the likelihood of contracting or recovering from disease, or the duration of a disease-free state following treatment. Incidence is therefore the preferred statistic for expressing risk or predicting the future course of disease.

Prevalence is a measure of the status of a population at a given point in time. Because of its relationship to the predictive value of diagnostic tests, prevalence should be considered when choosing a test and interpreting its results. It is also useful in evaluating the importance of a risk factor at the population level. A factor that is associated with a high risk of disease may not be important if it is present in only a fraction of the population.

Incidence and prevalence are especially useful when used to make comparisons. Incidence and prevalence measurements are fundamental to identifying the cause during outbreak investigations.

5.6   Summary

Measurement of the frequency of clinical events is fundamental to assessing the risk of contracting a disease, its cause, prognosis, and response to treatment. The frequency of clinical events is usually expressed as a proportion, with cases as the numerator and population at risk as the denominator. These proportions are commonly referred to as rates, although the latter term is more appropriately reserved for those proportions that include a time component. A rate is not the same thing as a ratio. In the case of a rate, the numerator is included in the denominator, while in a ratio, the numerator and denominator are mutually exclusive.

Veterinarians routinely deal with a number of rates. Some are vital statistics that can be used to provide indirect evidence of the health status of a population. Others may be classified as morbidity rates, i.e., direct measures of the commonness of disease. Among the latter, the three most commonly used are prevalence, incidence, and attack rate.

Prevalence is the proportion of sampled individuals that possess a condition of interest at a given point in time. It can be likened to a snapshot of the population and includes both old and new cases. It is a measure of the likelihood of being a case at a given point in time. Incidence is the proportion of individuals in a susceptible population that develop a condition of interest over a defined period. Incidence takes into account new cases only, i.e., cases that have their onset during the period under study. It is therefore a measure of the risk of becoming a case over a defined period. Attack rate is a general term used to express the proportion of a defined population affected during an outbreak. It is equal to the total number of cases during the outbreak period divided by the number of individuals initially exposed, i.e., those present at the beginning of the outbreak. Since the attack rate is based only on new cases of the disease, it is comparable to incidence. Prevalence is determined through cross-sectional studies, whereas incidence and attack rates are determined through longitudinal or prospective studies.

Sources of bias in prevalence studies include interpretation of the temporal sequence of suspected cause–effect relationships, inclusion of old as well as new cases, and true vs. apparent prevalence. The interpretation of incidence and prevalence rates also depends on the degree to which cases and the population at risk are comparable to the populations that we are interested in. When making comparisons, rate adjustment is used to remove the effect of confounding factors, such as age, breed, and sex distribution, upon overall crude rates. The direct method of rate adjustment forces a comparison of populations based on a common distribution of the confounding factors.

chapter 6

Risk assessment and prevention

6.1 Risk factors and their identification

An understanding of the concept of risk is fundamental to an understanding of the subsequent chapters on prognosis, treatment, and cause. The reason is twofold. First, all analyses rely on similar approaches to organizing and interpreting the data. Second, the statistical approach to proving that relationships exist is similar. The previous chapter focused on rates and proportions. In this chapter we will also use ratios to study associations between risk factors and outcomes.

Factors that are associated with an increased likelihood of an event occurring (such as disease) are called **risk factors**. Exposure can take place at a point in time, as when an individual comes in contact with an infectious agent or receives a drug, or may also be ongoing, like the risk of mosquito exposure for heartworm infection or cryptorchidism for testicular neoplasia.

Risk factors for many animal diseases are poorly defined or unknown and only come to light through the systematic study of naturally or spontaneously occurring cases. Clinical studies in which the researcher gathers data by simply observing events as they happen, without playing an active part in what takes place, are called **observational studies**. They are contrasted with **experimental studies**, in which the researcher determines which individuals are exposed or not exposed to the factor being investigated. Although experimental studies are more scientifically rigorous, observational studies are the only feasible way of studying most questions of risk.

Observational studies are subject to many more potential biases than are experiments. Observational study designs must minimize unwanted differences between exposure groups in order to mimic, as closely as possible, an experiment.

▼

Observational studies are subject to many more potential biases than are experiments.

▲

6.2 Factors that interfere with the assessment of risk

Many risks are obvious enough that their impact on animal health can easily be documented. Exposure to pathogenic organisms and their vectors, and acute toxins or environmental stresses associated with weather extremes or transportation are recognized as major risk factors for disease. For many diseases, however, the risks are not as readily discernible, and individual clinicians are seldom in a position to assess their possible importance. Some of the reasons for this follow:

1. **Long latency**: For many conditions the time between exposure and development of an outcome is too long to be perceived by a practitioner. Examples are environmental hazards such as pollutants or nutritional deficiencies, and sequelae of certain infectious diseases that may not appear until long after recovery from the initial disease, such as Lyme arthritis.

2. **High prevalence of risk factors or disease**: If a disease is relatively common among all members of a population, and some of the risk factors for it are already known, it becomes difficult to distinguish a new risk factor from the others. The effects of chronic or widespread risk factors on animal health and production may be easily misinterpreted as the norm until they are compared with unexposed animals.

3. **Low incidence of disease**: Diseases of low incidence do not provide enough cases to prompt a practitioner to suspect that a cause–effect relationship may exist. For example, it has been claimed that 20% of a small animal practitioner's time is spent diagnosing or treating canine genetic diseases (Padgett, 1985). The risk of occurrence of genetic diseases in any particular individual, however, is usually very low. The genetic heterogeneity of outbred animals and possible polygenic nature of inherited disorders contribute to a relatively low incidence of any particular genetic defect in the population as a whole. Research into genetic diseases is slow and requires large numbers of individuals to prove an association.

4. **Small risk from exposure**: As the amount of risk conferred by a factor decreases, a larger number of subjects will be required to confirm the relationship.

5. **Multiple causes**: Many diseases exist as complexes. Examples are shipping fever, neonatal mortality, and the postpartum dysgalactia syndrome (PPDS) in sows. For these diseases no single cause can be identified. Rather, a combination of factors acting synergistically appears to be responsible for the disease syndrome.

Example 6.1

Ruble and Hird (1993) examined 1679 6- to 18-week-old dogs for congenital abnormalities over a 2-year period. Fifteen percent had at least one congenital defect, and 1.5% had multiple congenital abnormalities. Defects observed, in descending order, were patellar luxation (7.2%), palpebral abnormalities (3%), cryptorchidism (2.6%), inguinal hernia (1.3%), faciodental malformations (1.3%), cardiac abnormalities characterized by murmurs (0.7%), and umbilical hernia (0.6%). Although practitioners are likely to encounter many cases of congenital abnormalities among their patients, detection of any breed associations would require systematic examination and record keeping of a large number of such cases.

6.3 *Uses of risk*

1. **Prediction**: Risk is useful for estimating the likely future incidence of disease among comparable individuals. While risk for groups of individuals can be predicted rather well in this way, it is not possible to be precise about risk to any one individual in the group.

2. **Diagnosis**: The presence of a risk factor in an individual increases the likelihood that an associated disease is present and the positive predictive value of diagnostic tests for that disease. If the association between a risk factor and disease is strong, the absence of the risk factor can be used to rule out the disease. Thus, knowledge of risk factors and their associated diseases is useful for screening patients and generating a differential list.

3. **Cause**: Risk factors are frequently identified because they exhibit a statistically significant association with a disease. In some cases, this association is causal. In others, the risk factor is merely an innocent bystander, confounded with a causal factor. Because of confounding, an association may not necessarily be a cause.

4. **Prevention**: If a risk factor is also a cause of disease, its removal can be used to prevent disease, even if the disease mechanism is unknown. For example, before bacteria were identified, a 19th-century physician by the name of John Snow found an increased rate of cholera among people drinking water supplied by a particular company in London. He stopped a local cholera epidemic by cutting off that supply of contaminated water (Schwabe et al., 1977). He was unaware, however, of the specific cause of the disease. The concept of cause and its relationship to prevention is discussed further in Chapter 10.

▼

If the association between a risk factor and disease is strong, the absence of the risk factor can be used to rule out the disease.

▲

6.4 Comparison of risks

Several study designs and analytical techniques can be used to explore the association between presumed risk factors and outcomes. The choice of analytical technique depends, in part, on the study design employed. Regardless of the approach, results are usually expressed in terms of (1) the strength of association between the risk factor and outcome and (2) the statistical significance of this association. In the following sections we will discuss how these parameters are estimated.

6.4.1 Univariate analysis

Univariate (or univariable) analysis is the simplest approach to exploring the association between a potential risk factor (**variable**) and an outcome of interest. A **two-by-two table**, illustrated in Figure 6.1, is often used to describe and analyze this relationship. The study design can be longitudinal or cross-sectional, but the layout of the table is the same. What differs is the way in which the magnitude of risk is calculated. Longitudinal studies permit disease incidence in exposed and unexposed groups to be calculated, and magnitude of risk is expressed as **relative risk**. On the other hand, cross-sectional studies provide no information on the incidence of disease, but do allow us to compare how common a risk factor is among diseased (cases) and nondiseased individuals. The resulting statistic, the **odds ratio**, provides the same information as relative risk.

The derivation of these two estimates of risk is summarized in Figure 6.1 and discussed in greater detail in subsequent sections on study design.

6.4.2 Multivariate analysis

Cross-sectional studies are especially useful for testing the possible causal association between a number of potential risk factors, or variables, and an outcome of interest. The analysis can be performed by constructing a two-by-two table for each of the variables, one at a time. However, it is entirely possible that two or more variables that appear to be associated with the outcome in a simple two-by-two analysis are also related to each other, such as herd size and type of housing system, or that the magnitude of risk varies

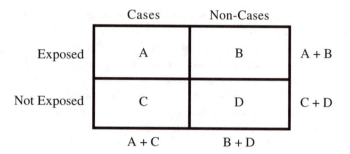

$$\text{Relative Risk} = \frac{A/(A+B)}{C/(C+D)} \qquad \text{Odds Ratio} = \frac{\dfrac{A/(A+C)}{C/(A+C)}}{\dfrac{B/(B+D)}{D/(B+D)}} = \frac{A/C}{B/D} = \frac{AD}{BC}$$

Figure 6.1 Two-by-two table comparing how the strength of the association between exposure and outcome is estimated from cohort vs. case control studies.

with subgroups within the population being evaluated. This is known as **confounding** and makes it difficult to determine the actual contribution of suspected risk factors to disease. In these cases, two basic approaches are available to the investigator to disentangle relationships between individual variables and outcome.

6.4.2.1   Mantel–Haenszel stratified analysis

When the number of variables is small, a series of two-by-two analyses can be performed with each subgroup, or stratum, within the population. By stratifying on a variable, we eliminate the effect of confounding by that variable. The contribution of each subgroup to the whole is weighted on the basis of its relative abundance within the population, much like direct rate adjustment (Chapter 5). This is known as a Mantel–Haenszel stratified analysis and yields an adjusted measure of risk. Further discussion of the application and limitations of Mantel–Haenszel stratified analysis appears later in this chapter.

6.4.2.2   Multivariate logistic regression analysis

Multivariate (or multivariable) logistic regression (MLR) is used to assess the contribution of each of a number of variables to a dichotomous outcome (such as presence or absence of disease) while controlling for confounding. Multiple logistic regression is especially useful if there is more than one major predictor variable (risk factor) for an outcome, such as the contribution of a number of management factors to calf mortality. Rather than performing a series of stratified two-by-two tables (Mantel–Haenszel stratified analysis) for each subgroup, MLR is performed by constructing and solving a logistic regression equation in which the relative contribution of each risk factor is represented as an exponent. The resulting equation provides information on the magnitude and statistical significance of each variable's contribution to the outcome of interest. Often a univiariate analysis of each potential risk factor is performed first to identify those to be included in MLR analysis. Confounding variables that are found to be suitable for inclusion in the model from univariate analysis usually drop out of the final MLR model because they are found to be statistically insignificant. Thus, MLR is often used to reduce the number of risk factors to those that are most likely to be associated with the outcome of interest.

Table 6.1 Cohorts and Their Uses

Characteristic in Common	To Assess Effect of	Example
Age	Age (duration of exposure)	Effect of duration of cryptorchidism on incidence of testicular neoplasia (Reif et al., 1979; Chapter 5)
Date of birth	Calendar time	Effect of improved radiation safety procedures on incidence of lymphatic and hematopoietic tumors in veterinary practitioners (Blair and Hayes, 1982; Chapter 6)
Exposure	Etiologic agent	Effect of infection with feline leukemia virus upon mortality from selected diseases (Hardy et al., 1976; Chapter 7)
Disease	Prognosis	Prognosis for untreated feline dilated cardiomyopathy (Pion et al., 1992; Chapter 8)
Treatment	Therapeutic intervention	Prognosis for taurine-treated feline dilated cardiomyopathy (Pion et al., 1992; Chapter 8)

In the following sections we will examine more closely the study designs and analytical methods employed to identify and test the strength of association of potential risk factors for disease outcomes.

6.5   Cohort studies of risk

6.5.1   True cohort study designs

Cohort studies, also known as longitudinal or prospective studies, involve the assembly of a group of individuals (the **cohort**) that have something in common and following them over time to detect occurrences of the outcome of interest. The duration of a cohort study should be consistent with the natural history of the disease being studied. If the study is terminated too early, many cases may not yet have become detectable or run their course. Ideally, all members of the cohort study should be followed for the entire follow-up period. The study group may be assembled in the present (concurrent cohort) or from past records (historical cohort) based on any of a number of criteria. Some examples of how cohorts are used in clinical research are listed in Table 6.1. Examples of concurrent and historical cohort studies follow. An example of the use of both historical and concurrent cohorts in a clinical trial appears in Chapter 8 (Figure 8.2).

6.5.1.1   Concurrent cohort studies

In a **concurrent cohort study** the study group is assembled in the present and followed into the future. This study design usually requires periodic examination of members of the cohort to record new occurrences of the event of interest.

Example 6.2

Let us return to our earlier discussion of the effect of low serum gamma globulin levels in newborn calves on subsequent survival (see Table 2.6). The data have been rearranged in Table 6.2 in a format that facilitates the comparison of risk. Since the four groups of calves were assembled at one time, each group may be treated as a cohort and the outcome (survival or removal from the cohort) as incidence. Notice that the "Loss" column is now referred to as "Incidence" and that two additional parameters, designated **relative risk** and **attributable risk**, have been calculated. These are discussed in the following sections.

Table 6.2 A Concurrent Cohort Study of Risk in Neonatal Calves with Various Levels of Serum Gamma Globulin

Gamma Globulin (%)	Cohort Size	Deaths or Culls	Incidence (%)	Relative Risk[a]	Attributable Risk[a]
1.1–6.2	73	12	16.44	12.16	15.09
6.3–12.0	73	3	4.11	3.04	2.76
12.1–19.3	73	2	2.74	2.03	1.39
19.4–46.7	74	1	1.35	1.00	0.00
Totals	293	18	6.14		

[a] Compared with the high gamma globulin group.

Adapted from data in Table 2.6.

Table 6.3 A Historical Cohort Study of the Risks Associated with Being a Veterinarian (Based on Cause of Death in 5016 White Men, 1947–1977)

Cause of Death	Mortality in Veterinarians (%)	Mortality in General Population (%)	Relative Risk	Attributable Risk (%)
All cancers (including the following)	16.59	16.39	1.01	0.20
Brain and CNS	0.56	0.34	1.63	0.22
Skin	0.48	0.30	1.61	0.18
Lymphatic and hemopoietic	2.23	1.50	1.49	0.73
Colon	2.21	1.65	1.34	0.57
Stomach	0.94	1.44	0.65	−0.51
Lung	2.29	3.71	0.62	−1.42
Suicide	2.73	1.60	1.70	1.13
Motor vehicle accidents	3.15	2.19	1.44	0.96
Circulatory disease	50.36	48.57	1.04	1.79
Respiratory disease	3.27	5.17	0.63	−1.90
All others	23.90	26.08	0.92	−2.18
Total	100.00	100.00		

Source of data: Blair, A. and Hayes, H.M., Jr., *Int. J. Epidemiol.*, 11, 391–397, 1982. With permission.

6.5.1.2   Historical cohort studies

In a **historical cohort study** the study group is assembled from past records and followed into the future, usually up to the present. The term *retrospective cohort* is also used to describe a historical cohort. The term *cohort* is used because every individual has an equal chance of being included in the study, e.g., sampling based on exposure. The term *retrospective* is used because evidence of exposure is based on past records or recall.

Example 6.3

Causes of death among 5016 white male veterinarians identified from obituary listings in the *Journal of the American Veterinary Medical Association* were compared with a distribution based on the general U.S. population, matched by 5-year age and calendar period (age-adjusted mortality; Table 6.3). Proportions of deaths were significantly elevated for cancers of the lymphatic and hematopoietic system, colon, brain, and skin. Fewer deaths were observed than expected for cancers of the stomach and lung. Sunlight exposure was suspected

Table 6.4 A Survival Cohort Study of the Benefits of Chemotherapy for Advanced Mammary Adenocarcinoma in Cats

Patient	Breed	Age (yr)	OVH[a] (yr)	Duration of Signs (mo)	No. of Recurrences	Metastases to Thorax	Survival Time (d)
1	DSH	9	1	14	2	No	NA
2	DSH	13	11	72	2	No	NA
3	Persian	11	7	3	0	Yes	NA
4	Siamese	13	11	24	3	Yes	4
5	Siamese	9	5	10	1	Yes	45
6	Siamese	11	9	24	2	Unknown	47
7	DSH	8	NA	8	0	Yes	67
8	Siamese	12	Intact	5	2	Yes	106
9	DSH	13	2	17	1	Yes	149
10	DSH	12	Intact	6	1	No	170
11	DSH	11	NA	9	2	Yes	180
12	DSH	14	Intact	16	1	No	182
13	Siamese	7	6	6	2	Yes	283
14	DSH	11	10	12	3	Yes	344

Note: DSH = domestic shorthair; NA = not available.

[a] Years since ovariohysterectomy.

Source: Jeglum, K.A. et al., *J. Am. Vet. Med. Assoc.*, 187, 157–160, 1985. With permission.

for the excess of skin cancer among veterinarians whose practices were not limited exclusively to small animals. Ionizing radiation exposure was suspected for the excess of leukemia among veterinarians practicing during years when diagnostic radiology became widely used. Mortality was also high for motor vehicle accidents and suicides, but low for diseases of the respiratory system (Blair and Hayes, 1982).

▼

Cohort studies, also known as prospective studies, involve the assembly of a group of individuals that have something in common and following them over time to detect occurrences of the outcome of interest.

▲

6.5.2 Survival cohorts

Concurrent and historical cohorts are sometimes referred to as **true cohorts**, since they are studied from the point at which they are first exposed to a risk factor or at the onset of disease. Sometimes this is not possible and the cohort must include individuals at any stage of their disease. This assembly of individuals is referred to as a **survival cohort**. The name does not imply that survival is being studied, but rather that each individual has survived, or is available for study, after a given period of exposure or disease.

Example 6.4

Table 6.4 summarizes the results of a study in which a chemotherapeutic regimen for treating advanced feline mammary adenocarcinoma was evaluated. This is a classic survival cohort in that the only thing the patients have in common is the particular type of tumor. The extent of tumor development

Table 6.5 Advantages and Disadvantages of Cohort Studies

Advantages	Disadvantages
The only way of establishing incidence (e.g., absolute risk) directly	Inefficient and expensive because many more subjects are included than experience the event of interest. Therefore, inappropriate for diseases of low incidence
Follow the same logic as the clinical question: If the subjects are exposed, do they get the disease?	Can assess the effects of exposure to relatively few factors (i.e., those recorded at the outset)
Can assess the relationship between exposure and many possible outcomes (diseases)	Results not available for a long time

Source: Fletcher, R.H. et al., *Clinical Epidemiology: The Essentials,* 3rd ed., Lippincott Williams & Wilkins, Baltimore, 1996. With permission.

among the patients when they were included in the study is highly variable. Aside from being in different stages of the disease, additional variables such as breed, age, and ovariohysterectomy exist within the group. Survival time was measured from the start of chemotherapy to death (Jeglum et al., 1985).

▼

Regardless of the way in which a cohort study is conducted, if all individuals are identical at the time they enter into a study, and the only variable is the time over which they will be followed, then a true cohort study exists.

▲

6.5.3   Limitations of cohort studies

Some of the advantages and disadvantages of cohort studies are compared in Table 6.5. Since they are conducted in the present, concurrent cohort studies permit the collection of any data required for the specific purposes of the study. In contrast, data for historical cohort studies are often limited to what was recorded in medical or herd records. Vital information may be difficult or impossible to obtain. Historical cohorts are useful when it would take so long for an event to occur that the experiment would be jeopardized. For example, the study examining the risks associated with being a veterinarian (Table 6.3) could conceivably extend beyond the lifetime of the investigators if it were conducted as a concurrent cohort study.

Regardless of the way in which a cohort study is conducted, if all individuals are identical at the time they enter into a study, and the only variable is the time over which they will be followed, then a true cohort study exists. If there is reason to believe that differences exist among individuals that may influence the outcome of the study, then a biased view of risk may result. An example is the survival cohort study of chemotherapy for advanced mammary adenocarcinoma in cats (Table 6.4).

One of the major difficulties in cohort studies is assembly of all members of the cohort at the same time. As described in Chapter 5 (canine testicular neoplasia in cryptorchid dogs; Reif et al., 1979), individuals exposed to a risk factor may not all be available at the same point in time. This affects their follow-up period, and outcome must be expressed as incidence density. Even if all individuals can be assembled at the same point in time, additional difficulties may affect the validity of cohort studies. If the outcome is infrequent, a large number of subjects must enter and remain in the study for a long time before results are available.

Cohort studies also lack the controls inherent in laboratory experiments. Additional factors such as diet, housing, management, and exposure to other animals are difficult to control and may influence the outcome of cohort studies. Diseases of low incidence present a special problem. The number of animals that must be assembled to ensure that a sufficient number of cases will arise may make a cohort study impractical. An alternate approach, the **cross-sectional study**, is discussed later in this chapter.

6.5.4   Comparing risks in cohort studies

Incidence is the basic expression of risk. It is the number of new events (usually disease) arising in a defined population over a given period. Incidence is especially useful for evaluating the relationship between presumed risk factors and disease. Several measures, called **measures of effect**, can be estimated from incidence data.

6.5.4.1   Relative risk

Relative risk (RR), or **risk ratio**, is calculated by dividing incidence in individuals exposed to a risk factor by incidence in nonexposed individuals. Relative risk can range from zero to infinity. If no additional risk is associated with exposure, then both incidences should be equal and the ratio would be equal to 1. Relative risk is an index of the strength of the association between a risk factor and disease, but tells us nothing about the absolute magnitude of that risk. For this we must calculate the attributable risk.

6.5.4.2   Attributable risk

Attributable risk, also known as **risk difference**, is calculated by subtracting incidence among those not exposed to a risk factor from incidence among exposed individuals. Since subtraction removes background incidence, attributable risk is the additional incidence of disease attributable to the risk factor itself. Considered another way, it is the disease incidence that would not occur had the risk factor not been present.

The difference between relative risk and attributable risk can be appreciated if we consider that a 10-fold reduction in incidence among both exposed and unexposed would result in a 10-fold reduction in attributable risk, but would have no effect on relative risk.

6.5.4.3   Population attributable risk

Relative and attributable risks provide information on the contribution of risk factors to the overall rates of disease in exposed individuals. However, neither tells us how much a risk factor contributes to the overall rate of disease in the population or herd. This information would be useful in deciding which risk factors are important and which are trivial in the overall incidence of a particular disease in a population, or which risks are associated with the greatest economic loss.

Population attributable risk is estimated by multiplying the attributable risk for a particular risk factor by the prevalence of that risk factor in the population. It provides a measure of how much a risk factor contributes to disease incidence at the population level. A relatively weak risk factor that is quite prevalent could contribute more to overall disease incidence than a stronger risk factor that is rarely present.

6.5.4.4   Population attributable fraction

We may also wish to know what fraction of disease occurrence in a population is associated with a particular risk factor. This is called the **population attributable fraction** and is estimated by dividing the population attributable risk by the total incidence of disease in the population. The population attributable fraction permits us to predict the proportion

Table 6.6 Measures of Effect in Studies of Risk of Disease

Expression	Clinical Question	Calculation[a]
Relative risk (risk ratio)	How many times more likely are exposed individuals to become diseased relative to unexposed?	$RR = IE \div Ie$
Attributable risk (risk difference)	What is the incidence of disease attributable to exposure?	$AR = IE - Ie$
Population attributable risk	What is the incidence of disease in a population associated with the occurrence of a risk factor?	$ARp = AR \times P$
Population attributable fraction	What fraction of disease in a population is attributable to exposure to a risk factor?	$AFp = ARp \div RT$

[a] Where IE = incidence in exposed individuals; Ie = incidence in nonexposed individuals; P = prevalence of exposure to a risk factor; and RT = total incidence of disease in a population.

Source: Fletcher, R.H. et al., *Clinical Epidemiology: The Essentials,* 3rd ed., Lippincott Williams & Wilkins, Baltimore, 1996. With permission.

of cases of a particular disease that will be eliminated through control of a particular risk factor. If all cases are associated with the risk factor being measured, then the population attributable fraction would be 1.00, or 100%.

Table 6.6 compares the various measures of effect for the risk of disease, while the following example describes how the indices can be used to describe the risks associated with low gamma globulin levels in neonatal calves.

Example 6.5

As discussed in Chapter 2, one way of defining abnormality is by association with disease. To illustrate how this association might be evaluated using the measures of effect approach, let us return to the study summarized in Table 6.2 evaluating the impact of low serum gamma globulin levels on calf survival. For this analysis, the lowest serum gamma globulin group is considered as the exposed (at-risk) group, while members of the other three groups are pooled as controls. This approach is appropriate since the former group suffered by far the greatest calf losses, either through death or culling. The longitudinal study design and data distribution are depicted in Figure 6.2. A univariate analysis is depicted in Table 6.7 and the resulting values incorporated into the calculation of measures of effect in Table 6.8.

From the results in Table 6.8 we can conclude the following:

1. Calves with low serum gamma globulin levels are approximately six times more likely to be culled or die than their normal counterparts (relative risk).
2. Low serum gamma globulin levels are associated with an additional 13.71% incidence of culls and deaths among exposed calves (attributed risk).
3. Low serum gamma globulin levels are associated with an additional 3.42% incidence of culls and deaths among all calves (i.e., the herd, population attributable risk).
4. Low serum gamma globulin levels are associated with approximately 56% of calf losses among all calves (population attributable fraction).

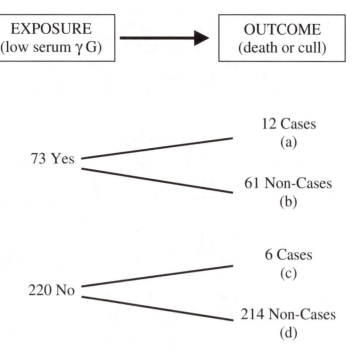

Figure 6.2 Study design employed to evaluate the effect of low serum gamma globulin upon calf survival. This is a longitudinal study design employing concurrent cohorts. The data are derived from Table 6.2. Low serum gamma globulin = 1.1% to 6.2%.

Table 6.7 Two-by-Two Table Analysis of Data from Figure 6.2

	Cases	Noncases	Total
Exposed (to low gamma globulin levels)	(a) 12	(b) 61	73
Not exposed (to low gamma globulin levels)	(c) 6	(d) 214	220
Total	18	275	293

Incidence in exposed = 16.44%
Incidence in unexposed = 2.73%
Relative risk = 6.03 (2.35 – 15.49)

6.6 Case control studies of risk

The prospective approach to the estimation of risk, prognosis, and treatment outcomes relies on assembly of a large number of individuals, some of whom are exposed to a factor or an intervention, and some who are not. This approach makes for good science, but does not make the best use of the unique resource most readily available to the practitioner, i.e., the clinical cases. Furthermore, the frequency of many diseases of veterinary concern is relatively low. A statistically significant cohort study of risk factors may require us to follow extremely large numbers of animals over long periods. This could make prospective studies of risk and prognostic factors, and treatments for these diseases, impossible.

Table 6.8 Calculation of Measures of Effect:
Suboptimal Gamma Globulin Levels in Calves

Simple Risks
Incidence of calf losses among low gamma globulin group = 16.44%
Incidence of calf losses among remaining calves = 2.73%
Prevalence of low gamma globulin levels in all calves = 24.91%
Incidence of calf losses = 6.14%

Compared Risks
Relative risk = 16.44 ÷ 2.73 = 6.03%
Attributable risk = 16.44 − 2.73 = 13.71%
Population attributable risk = 13.71 × 24.91 = 3.42%
Population attributable fraction = 3.42 ÷ 6.14 = 55.61%

Rather than forming cohorts with the desired characteristics (risk factors) and then waiting an unpredictable amount of time for something to happen, would it not make more sense to start with diseased individuals and look backward to compare the proportion of cases that were exposed to the factor(s) of interest with a comparable group of noncases? This approach, known as a **case control study**, is a cross-sectional study design fundamental to studies of uncommon diseases, and in outbreak investigations where the practitioner must rule out a number of possible risk factors. The approach also lends itself to clinical studies of risk and prognosis using medical records.

6.6.1 Advantages of case control studies

Case control studies lend themselves to clinical research since they take advantage of a resource that practitioners have in abundance — cases. Since case control studies start with cases, comparisons are not constrained by diseases of low frequency or long latency. For example, in order to gather information about the risk factors for tuberculosis in 100 swine at a representative U.S. incidence of approximately 0.02% (Dey and Parham, 1993), a cohort of at least 500,000 animals would have to be formed and followed from birth to slaughter. Obviously, the expense and logistic difficulties of such a study design would render it unrealistic. In contrast, it would be more feasible and relatively inexpensive to assemble 100 or more cases of swine tuberculosis from USDA-FSIS surveillance records, find similar groups of animals without the disease, and compare frequencies of hypothesized risk factors.

Another advantage of case control studies is that large numbers of possible risk or causal factors for a disease syndrome of unknown etiology can be explored. Whereas cohort studies are designed to examine the role of a limited number of causal factors, the number of causal factors that a case control study can consider is much greater, provided, of course, that data on the frequency of the suspected causal factors can be obtained from the medical records or through interviewing techniques. The case control design lends itself to fishing expeditions.

▼

Advantages of case control studies are: (1) cases can be identified unconstrained by the natural frequency of disease, (2) studies are unaffected by latency of disease, and (3) large numbers of possible risk or causal factors can be explored.

▲

6.6.2   Comparing risks in case control studies

In the cohort approach sampling is based on exposure, whereas in the case control approach sampling is based on outcome. Both cohort and case control designs measure frequency, but in cohort studies the frequency of different outcomes is measured, whereas in case control studies the frequency of the presumed causal factors is measured. As opposed to the cohort study, evidence of exposure in case control studies usually relies on memory and the availability and completeness of medical or herd records. It is the past, not the present, that is important, and therein lies the potential for bias in case control studies (Fletcher et al., 1982).

▼

In the cohort approach sampling is based on exposure, whereas in the case control approach sampling is based on outcome.

▲

6.6.3   The odds ratio

Since the case control study begins with the selection of cases, we have no data on the size of the population at risk, and consequently the incidence of disease. Mathematically, adding cases or controls to a two-by-two table would alter the value obtained for incidence, which does not make biological sense. It is therefore not possible to calculate relative risk in the usual way. However, it is possible to obtain an estimate of relative risk in another way. The **odds ratio (OR)**, defined as the odds that a case is exposed divided by the odds that a control is exposed, provides a measure of risk for case control studies that is conceptually and mathematically similar to the relative risk (Figure 6.1). The meaning of the odds ratio is analogous to the relative risk obtained in cohort studies; e.g., the higher the odds ratio, the stronger the association between exposure and disease.

▼

The meaning of the odds ratio is analogous to the relative risk obtained in cohort studies, e.g.; the higher the odds ratio, the stronger the association between exposure and disease.

▲

Example 6.6

A marked increase in the number of early fetal losses (EFLs) (fetal loss prior to 60 days of gestation) was reported to University of Kentucky extension veterinarians in the spring of 2001 (Dwyer et al., 2003). No infectious cause for the abortions could be identified. A case control study was conducted to identify farm, pasture, and demographic factors that might be associated with increased EFLs. Questionnaires were administered to managers of 97 case farms and 36 noncase (control) farms that met the inclusion criteria for the study. Among the variables investigated was the presence of high concentrations of Eastern tent caterpillars (i.e., blankets of caterpillars on fences, waterers, or other surfaces) on case vs. control farms. The case control study design and data distribution are depicted in Figure 6.3 and the corresponding univariate analysis in Table 6.9. The high odds ratio (OR = 7.11) and 95% confidence

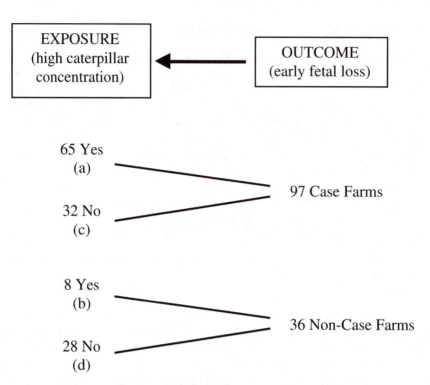

Figure 6.3 Case control study evaluating the effect of high concentrations of Eastern tent caterpillars upon the likelihood of a farm having excessive numbers of early fetal losses in broodmares. (Source of data: Dwyer, R.M. et al., *J. Am.Vet. Med. Assoc.*, 222, 613–619, 2003. With permission.)

Table 6.9 Two-by-Two Table Analysis of Data from Figure 6.3

	Case Farms	Noncase Farms	Total
Exposed (high caterpillar concentration)	(a) 65	(b) 8	73
Not exposed (to low gamma globulin levels)	(c) 32	(d) 28	60
Total	97	36	133

Odds that a case was exposed = 2.031
Odds that a noncase was exposed = 0.286
Odds ratio (95% CI) = 7.11[a] (2.71 – 19.25)

[a] OR differs from that reported in the original article, which was adjusted through logistic regression.

interval for the OR suggest that limiting exposure to Eastern tent caterpillars may help decrease the risk of excessive proportions of early fetal losses. This investigation will be discussed in greater detail in Chapter 12. See Chapter 9 for a discussion of confidence intervals.

6.6.4 Bias in case control studies

There are three major sources of bias in case control studies: (1) the selection of groups, (2) measurement of exposure, and (3) presumed temporal relationships.

6.6.4.1 Bias in selecting groups

Case control studies are designed to test whether there is a significant difference between cases and controls with regard to exposure to a suspected risk factor. It is essential, therefore, that the selection process ensures that both groups have an equal likelihood of being detected as cases if they develop the condition of interest. This will facilitate the detection of risk factors that are significantly associated with disease. Bias in selection of groups can be reduced by (1) matching cases with one or more controls for factors already known to be related to disease and (2) choosing more than one control group, preferably from a different geographic location.

6.6.4.2 Bias in measuring exposure

Measurement bias may occur when the presence of the outcome affects the owner's recollection of the exposure (recall bias), or the measurement or recording of the exposure. These sources of bias may be reduced by (1) using alternative sources for the same information and (2) concealing the specific purpose of the study from interviewers and interviewees.

6.6.4.3 Presumed temporal relationships

Although case control studies are often considered to be longitudinal, the fact remains that sampling is cross-sectional, i.e., occurs at one point in time. Unless presumed risk or causal factors are innate characteristics of the individual (as breed or sex), it may be difficult to document the temporal relationship between the risk factors being examined and the outcome of interest.

6.7 Prevalence surveys of risk

A **prevalence survey** is a cross-sectional design that bears some similarities to both cohort and case control approaches. As in the cohort study, the prevalence survey begins with a **defined population**. However, rather than measuring an outcome, the investigator divides the population into cases and noncases and then measures the prevalence of the putative risk factor in each group, as in the case control approach.

6.7.1 Comparing risks in prevalence surveys

In a prevalence survey we can be certain that cases and noncases came from the same population, but the exposure history must be reconstructed from interviews or medical records. Additionally, the cases include only those detected, or prevalent, during the examination. Because the sampling strategy is essentially random, the resulting relative risk or odds ratio estimates would remain relatively unchanged if additional individuals were added to the study. However, since incidence is not being measured, it is preferable to use the odds ratio to express risk in prevalence surveys. An exception is a prevalence survey conducted during the course of an outbreak investigation. In this case, incidence (attack rate) is actually being measured and it is possible to define the temporal sequence between exposure and disease. Examples are food-borne disease and other similar outbreaks that occur over a defined, and relatively short, period. In these cases, attack rates are calculated, so relative risk can be used.

Table 6.10 Proportion of Diagnoses of Congenital Portosystemic Shunts in a Selection of Canine Breeds Accessed from the Veterinary Medical Database (VMDB) from January 1, 1980 to February 28, 2002

Breed	No. of Affected Dogs (%)	Reference Hospital Population	Odds Ratio	Adjusted Confidence Interval[a]
Havanese	6 (3.2%)	187	64.9	8.9–234.3
Yorkshire terrier	483 (2.9%)	16,538	58.7	42.9–80.2
Maltese	100 (1.6%)	6231	32	20.2–49.8
Dandie Dinmont terrier	4 (1.6%)	251	31.7	2.3–140.1
Pug	75 (1.3%)	5681	26.2	15.7–42.5
Mixed	169 (0.05%)	331,234	1.0	NA

Note: NA = not applicable (comparison group).

[a] 99.9995% confidence interval adjusted for 106 comparisons with mixed-breed dogs.

Source: Tobias, K.M. and Rohrbach, B.W., *J. Am. Vet. Med. Assoc.*, 223, 1636–1639, 2003. With permission.

Prevalence surveys are especially common in clinical research using medical records. Typically, the records are scanned for all cases of the condition of interest over some time interval. The prevalence of one or more suspected risk factors (age, breed, sex, etc.) among cases is then compared with prevalence for the remaining clinic population, or a defined, low-risk subpopulation, over the same period (e.g., the noncases). The strength of association of each suspected factor is expressed as an odds ratio and its statistical significance tested with the **chi-square test**.

Example 6.7

The most common circulatory anomaly of the liver in dogs is the portosystemic shunt (PSS), a connection between the portal vessels and systemic circulation that diverts blood flow, in varying degrees, from the liver. The PSS may be acquired, due to portal hypertension, or appear congenitally (congenital portosystemic shunt (CPSS)). Knowing which canine breeds are at greater risk of CPSS can help the veterinarian diagnose the condition and counsel owners on breeding dogs with a family history of CPSS. Tobias and Rohrbach (2003) used data recorded in the Veterinary Medical Database (VMDB) to calculate the proportion of diagnoses of CPSS for all dogs and each breed over the 22.2-year period from January 1, 1980 to February 28, 2002. Odds ratios and adjusted confidence intervals were calculated for breeds with at least 100 accessions by comparing odds of each breed with a diagnosis of CPSS with those for mixed-breed dogs. Thirty-three breeds were significantly more likely to have a diagnosis of CPSS than mixed-breed dogs. The greatest proportions of diagnoses were found in Havanese, Yorkshire terriers, Maltese, Dandie Dinmont terriers, and pugs (Table 6.10). The prevalence survey study design and data distribution for Yorkshire terriers are depicted in Figure 6.4 and the corresponding univariate analysis in Table 6.11. The authors concluded that the elevated odds ratios among specific breeds support the hypothesis of a genetic predisposition for CPSS. Clients and veterinarians should consider appropriate diagnostic tests for dogs with clinical signs and those used for breeding from breeds with increased risk of CPSS.

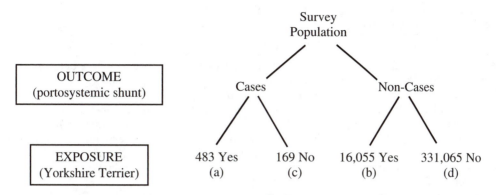

Figure 6.4 Prevalence survey evaluating the risk of congential portosystemic shunts in Yorkshire terrier breeds. (Source of data: Tobias, K.M. and Rohrbach, B.W., *J. Am. Vet. Med. Assoc.*, 223, 1636–1639, 2003. With permission.)

Table 6.11 Two-by-Two Table Analysis of Data from Table 6.10

	Cases	Noncases	Total
Exposed (Yorkshire terrier)	(a) 483	(b) 16,055	16,538
Not exposed (mixed breed)	(c) 169	(d) 331,065	331,234
Total	652	347,120	347,772

Odds that a case was exposed = 2.858
Odds that a noncase was exposed = 0.048
Odds ratio = 58.93[a] (49.25 – 70.54)

[a] OR differs from that reported in the original article, which was adjusted for 106 individual comparisons.

6.7.2   Limitations of prevalence surveys

Prevalence surveys are especially useful in situations where we wish to determine which of a number of potential risk factors is associated with an outcome, as during disease outbreak investigations. Prevalence surveys are less useful for examining the role of a specific causal factor, because cases and controls are not purposely matched to control for bias. Whatever matching of cases and controls that does occur in a prevalence survey is merely a fortuitous result of their being drawn from the same population. Another problem with prevalence surveys (and cross-sectional surveys in general) is that it may not be possible to distinguish between a risk factor and a prognostic factor for a condition. In other words, a factor that does not affect disease incidence but is related to survival of the cases will be associated with disease prevalence in a cross-sectional study.

Characteristics of cohort, case control, and prevalence survey designs are compared in Table 6.12.

Table 6.12 Comparison of Characteristics of Cohort, Case Control, and Prevalence Survey Study Designs

Cohort	Case Control	Prevalence Survey
Begins with a defined population at risk	Population at risk generally undefined	Begins with a defined population
Cases not selected but ascertained by continuous surveillance	Cases selected by investigator from an available pool of patients	Cases not selected but ascertained by a single examination of the population
Comparison group not exposed to risk factor but similar to at-risk group in other regards	Controls selected by investigator to resemble cases	Noncases include those free of disease at the single examination
Exposure measured before the development of disease	Exposure measured, reconstructed, or recollected after development of disease	Exposure measured, reconstructed, or recollected after development of disease
Risk or incidence of disease and relative risk measured	Risk or incidence of disease cannot be measured directly; relative risk of exposure can be estimated by odds ratio	Risk or incidence of disease cannot be measured directly; relative risk of exposure can be estimated by odds ratio

Source: Fletcher, R.H. et al., *Clinical Epidemiology: The Essentials*, 3rd ed., Lippincott Williams & Wilkins, Baltimore, 1996. With permission.

6.8   Biological plausibility and cross-sectional study designs

A distinguishing feature of both case control and prevalence survey designs, which contributes to their fallibility, is that subjects possess the outcome of interest at the time that the clinical findings or causal factors are measured. In some cases, temporal relationships between presumed causes and their effects are obvious, such as breed or sex predisposition to particular disease outcomes. In others, the cause–effect relationship is not so clear. In these cases, the validity of the presumed temporal relationships must be based on our understanding of the mechanisms of disease, e.g., **biological plausibility**. In fact, this illustrates the mutual dependency of epidemiologic and mechanistic (or basic) research. Epidemiologic studies cannot prove with certainty that a cause–effect relationship exists, but only that an association exists. Research on mechanisms of disease provides the biological basis for believing that associations are, in fact, causal. Likewise, information derived from research on mechanisms of disease cannot assume that a particular phenomenon behaves in nature as it does in the laboratory. For this, epidemiologic studies must be conducted.

Example 6.8

Blood samples were collected from 53 dairy cows with uterine prolapse (cases) and from 53 cows with normal parturition matched by dairy for various management programs (controls). Cows with uterine prolapse had significantly lower ($p < 0.01$) total serum calcium content than did controls, suggesting a cause–effect relationship. Since treatment of prolapse and blood collection were done shortly after the prolapse had occurred, the authors believed that there was little likelihood of hypocalcemia developing after the prolapse and before the time of sampling. Hypothesized mechanisms (biological plausibility) for the association between hypocalcemia and uterine prolapse were (1) prolonged recumbency and tenesmus due to hypocalcemia, thus predisposing to uterine prolapse, (2) reduced uterine tone due to hypocalcemia, and (3) delayed involution of the cervix due to hypocalcemia (Risco et al., 1984).

6.9 Summary

An understanding of the concept of risk is fundamental to an understanding of such diverse clinical issues as prognosis, treatment, and cause. Factors that are associated with an increased likelihood of an event occurring (such as disease) are called risk factors. Exposure to risk factors may occur instantaneously or may be ongoing (chronic).

Several study designs and analytical techniques can be used to explore the association between presumed risk factors and outcomes. Univariate analyses consider one variable at a time without adjusting for the possible contribution of, or associations among, other potential risk factors. Multivariate analysis provides a means to adjust for such associations among variables, generally referred to as confounding. Regardless of the approach, results are usually expressed in terms of (1) the strength of association between the risk factor and outcome and (2) the statistical significance of this association.

Risk may be estimated through the use of cohort (prospective or longitudinal) or cross-sectional (case control or prevalence survey) study designs. In a true cohort study, a group of individuals that have something in common (the cohort) is assembled and followed over time to detect occurrences of the outcome of interest. True cohort studies can be conducted in two ways. In a concurrent cohort study, the cohort is assembled in the present and followed into the future. In a historical cohort study, the study group is assembled from past records and followed into their future, usually up to the present. A survival cohort is the name given to a group of individuals who are assembled at various times in the course of their illness, rather than at the beginning. The name does not imply that survival is being studied, but rather that each individual has survived, or is available for study, after a given period of exposure or disease. If there is reason to believe that differences exist among individuals that may influence the outcome of the study, then a biased view of risk may result.

To compare risks in cohort studies, several measures of the association between exposure and disease, called measures of effect, are commonly used. Relative risk, or risk ratio, is the ratio of incidence in exposed individuals to incidence in nonexposed individuals. If no additional risk is associated with exposure to a suspected risk factor, then both incidences should be equal and the ratio would be equal to 1. Relative risk is an index of the strength of the association between exposure and disease, and is frequently used in studies of disease etiology. Attributable risk, also known as risk difference, is equal to the incidence of disease in exposed individuals minus the incidence in nonexposed individuals. It represents the additional incidence of disease among individuals attributable to a risk factor. Two other expressions, population attributable risk and population attributable fraction, convey the impact of a risk factor by considering its prevalence in the population.

Cohort studies are often impractical due to the relative infrequency of many diseases. An alternative approach is the cross-sectional study, which looks backward to compare the proportion of cases and noncases that were exposed to the factor(s) of interest. In a case control study, each case is matched with one or more noncases on factors that are not under study but that could confound the results. In a prevalence survey, cases and controls emerge naturally from within a defined population. The odds ratio, defined as the odds that a case was exposed to a particular risk factor divided by the odds that a noncase was exposed, provides a measure of risk for cross-sectional studies that is conceptually and mathematically similar to the relative risk. The stronger the association between exposure and disease, the higher the odds ratio. There are three major sources of bias in cross-sectional studies: (1) the selection of groups, (2) measurement of exposure, and (3) presumed temporal relationships.

chapter 7

Measuring and communicating prognoses

7.1 Expressing prognoses

Prognosis is a prediction of the expected outcome of disease with or without treatment. Prognosis is expressed as the probability or likelihood that something will occur in the future. The significance of this probability depends on your point of view. Clinical experience may indicate that the likelihood of improvement following a given treatment regimen is 75%, but from the patient's perspective it is either 0 or 100%. Practitioners should avoid statements that can be misconstrued as a contract — a definite statement about an outcome. Clients must be appraised of the probabilities of unfavorable, as well as favorable, outcomes. The objective is to avoid expressing prognosis with vagueness when it is unnecessary, and with certainty when it is misleading. Breach of contract and malpractice are bases for lawsuits, but therapeutic reassurance — the desire to appear positive while making an explanation or obtaining informed consent — is not (Hannah, 1985).

When communicating a prognosis, the practitioner should strive to supply facts and figures that really help the client make a decision. Specifically, a prognosis should include (1) the variability in course relative to treatment options, (2) a time reference, (3) risk of treatment-related death (or other untoward reaction), (4) cost, and (5) the nature of the benefit attainable (Crow, 1985).

There are few animal diseases that are documented with this kind of clinically useful information. Instead, evaluations of disease frequently document improvement in tissue morphology, changes in blood chemistries, or physiologic adjustments. Although this information may be useful in understanding the origins and mechanisms of disease, it may lack clinical relevance. Wherever possible, prognoses should be assessed in ways that can be perceived by the patient and its owner.

▼

Clinical experience may indicate that the likelihood of improvement following a given treatment regimen is 75%, but from the patient's perspective it is either 0 or 100%.

▲

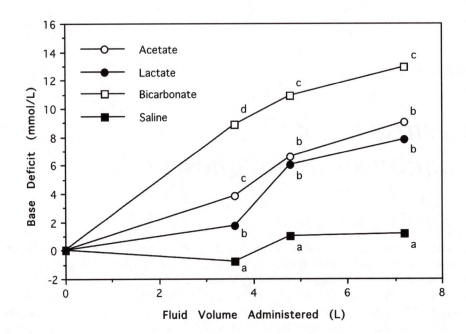

Figure 7.1 Base deficit of 36 dehydrated diarrheic calves (9 calves per group) that received different alkalinizing compounds (50 mmol/l) during extracellular fluid replacement therapy. At a given volume of fluid, means with different letters are significantly different ($p < 0.01$). The initial base deficit was 18.2 ± 1.3 mmol/l. (From Kasari, T.R. and Naylor, J.M., *J. Am. Vet. Med. Assoc.*, 187, 392–397, 1985. With permission.)

Example 7.1

Metabolic changes associated with diarrhea in neonatal calves include a number of blood biochemical changes. Several investigators have indicated that acidosis and hyperkalemia are major causes of death in many of these diarrheic calves. Kasari and Naylor (1985) evaluated the relative merits of treating acidosis in dehydrated, diarrheic calves using sodium bicarbonate, sodium L-lactate, sodium acetate, and saline (sodium chloride) concomitant with parenteral fluid therapy. Thirty-six calves with spontaneously occurring diarrhea and dehydration were randomly assigned to four double-blind experimental fluid groups (nine calves per group) designated saline control, lactate, acetate, and bicarbonate groups. Acid–base values and selected hematologic and biochemical values were determined from venous blood samples collected from each calf immediately before and after administration of fluid therapy. Dramatic improvements in base deficit relative to controls were measured in calves receiving lactate, acetate, and bicarbonate solutions. The magnitude of the response was also related to volume of fluid administered (Figure 7.1). However, the degree of clinical response of calves to rehydration therapy was directly related to the volume of fluid administered, regardless of the fluid used (Figure 7.2). Despite this, the authors concluded that rehydration of a calf without attention to correcting acidosis via alkalinizing compounds should be avoided.

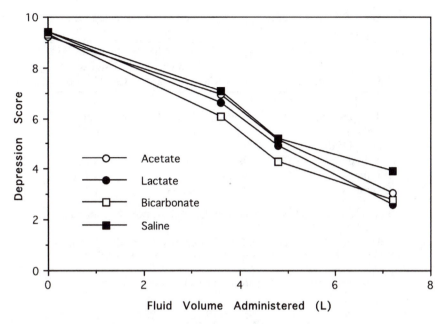

Figure 7.2 Influence of extracellular fluid replacement therapy on depression scores in dehydrated calves. Statistically significant differences were not found between groups, as determined by analysis of variance. (From Kasari, T.R. and Naylor, J.M., *J. Am. Vet. Med. Assoc.*, 187, 392–397, 1985. With permission.)

▼

Wherever possible, prognoses should be assessed in ways that can be perceived by the patient and its owner.

▲

7.2   Natural history vs. clinical course

The **natural history of a disease** describes its evolution without medical intervention. Because of the availability of veterinary services, it is often difficult to obtain information on the natural history of a disease. Once disease is recognized, it is likely to be treated. The **clinical course** of a disease describes its progression once it has come under medical care.

The true natural history of unselected cases of a disease, and the course of those that are recognized, can be quite different. The recognized cases may be a biased sample of all manifestations of the disease that may be particularly symptomatic or may have come to attention because the patients had other symptoms that were not related to the disease. Reports of prognosis from veterinary teaching hospitals and other referral centers may not be representative of cases seen in the typical private practice. Reported cases are often those that had been referred because they were doing poorly.

▼

Reports of prognosis from veterinary teaching hospitals and other referral centers may not be representative of cases seen in the typical private practice.

▲

Table 7.1 Mortality among FeLV-Infected and Uninfected Cats from the Time at Which Infection Was Acquired

Cause of Death	Incidence in FeLV-Infected Cats[a] (n = 46)	Incidence in Uninfected Cats[b] (n = 512)
FeLV diseases		
Lymphosarcoma	15.2%	0.6%
Others[c]	13.0%	0.2%
Non-FeLV diseases		
Feline infectious peritonitis	6.5%	1.2%
Others	17.4%	14.1%
Overall	52.2%	16.1%

[a] Based on 2-year follow-up. Source of data: Hardy, W.D., Jr. et al., *Nature*, 263, 326–328, 1976.

[b] Based on 3.5-year follow-up. Source of data: McClelland, A.J. et al., in *Feline Leukemia Virus*, Hardy, W.D., Jr. et al., Eds., Elsevier, New York, 1980, pp. 121–126.

[c] Nonregenerative anemias, panleukopenia-like syndrome.

Example 7.2

A study of the prognosis for feline leukemia virus (FeLV) infection in a cohort of cats with newly acquired infection provided a rare opportunity to study the natural history of the disease (Hardy et al., 1976). Fifty-five clinically normal cats that acquired FeLV infection from household contacts over a 3-month period were followed over time. Over the 2-year follow-up period nine cats were euthanized. Fifty-two percent of the remaining 46 FeLV-infected cats died: 13 (28%) from lymphosarcoma and other FeLV-caused diseases and 11 (24%) from other diseases. Based on data from unmatched controls (McClelland et al., 1980), fewer than 16% of FeLV-free cats would be expected to die over the same period, and fewer than 1% from lymphosarcoma or FeLV-caused diseases (Table 7.1).

7.3   *Prognosis as a rate*

It is convenient to summarize the course of disease as a rate. Rates commonly used for this purpose are shown in Table 7.2. All are expressions of incidence, e.g., events arising in a cohort of patients over time. Two variables that must be considered in the interpretation of rates are assignment of "zero time" and interval of follow-up.

Most reports of prognosis are really based on a survival cohort of patients. Zero time may be assigned at any point in the course of disease, such as onset of signs, diagnosis, or treatment. Consequently, the computed rates will reflect the way in which zero time is assigned. Cases should be followed for a sufficient period for all events to occur. Any period of follow-up that falls short will lower observed rates relative to true ones.

Example 7.3

The results of natural disease development over a 3.5-year period in initially healthy, FeLV-infected and uninfected cats is summarized in Table 7.3 (McClelland et al., 1980). The feline cohort in this study differs from that in Table 7.1

Table 7.2 Rates Commonly Used to Describe a Prognosis

Rate	Definition
Survival	Percent of patients surviving a defined period of time from some point in the course of their disease
Case fatality	Percent of patients with a disease who die of it
Response	Percent of patients showing some evidence of improvement following an intervention
Remission	Percent of patients entering a phase in which disease is no longer detectable
Recurrence	Percent of patients who experience a return of disease after a disease-free interval

Source: Fletcher, R.H. et al., *Clinical Epidemiology: The Essentials*, Williams & Wilkins, Baltimore, 1982. With permission.

Table 7.3 Mortality over 3.5-Year Follow-Up among FeLV-Infected and Uninfected Cats from the Time at Which Infection Was Diagnosed

Cause of Death	Incidence in FeLV-Infected Cats (n = 96)	Incidence in Uninfected Cats (n = 512)	Relative Risk	Attributable Risk
FeLV diseases				
Lymphosarcoma	27.1%	0.6%	45.2	26.5%
Others[a]	7.3%	0.2%	36.5	7.1%
Non-FeLV diseases				
Feline infectious peritonitis	5.2%	1.2%	4.3	4.0%
Others	43.7%	14.1%	3.01	29.6%
Overall	83.3%	16.1%	5.21	67.2%

[a] Nonregenerative anemias, panleukopenia-like syndrome.

Source of data: McClelland, A.J. et al., in *Feline Leukemia Virus*, Hardy, W.D., Jr. et al., Eds., Elsevier, New York, 1980, pp. 121–126.

in that the duration of infection at the start of this study is not known (i.e., it is a survival cohort). Thus, the interval of follow-up is from time of diagnosis, rather than time of infection. In Table 7.3 the original data have been used to calculate relative and attributable risks. The cause of death has been partitioned into FeLV-related and -unrelated diseases. Despite the difference in study design, yearly mortality for FeLV-infected cats in Table 7.1 (26.1%) and Table 7.3 (23.8%) is very similar. Yearly mortality for uninfected cats in the same studies was only 4.6%.

Rates, such as those in Table 7.2, are a relatively simple way of expressing prognosis. However, similar overall rates may cover up important differences in prognosis over the course of a disease. Additional information can be extracted from the same data if it is analyzed over time.

7.4 Survival analysis

When interpreting a prognosis, we would like to know the likelihood, on average, that patients with a given condition will experience an outcome at any point in time. When prognosis is expressed as a summary rate, it does not contain this information. However,

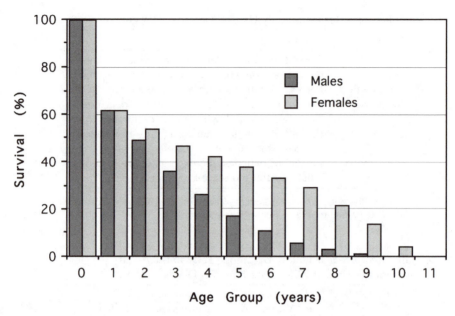

Figure 7.3 Survival of white-tailed deer. (Source of data: Spain, J.D., *BASIC Microcomputer Models in Biology*, Addison-Wesley, Reading, MA, 1982, p. 114.)

a method called **survival analysis** provides information about average time to event for any point in the course of disease. The plotted data are referred to as a **survival curve**.

▼

Similar overall rates may cover up important differences in prognosis over the course of a disease.

▲

7.4.1   *Survival of a cohort*

The most direct way of learning about survival is to assemble a cohort of patients with the condition of interest and periodically count the number remaining throughout the course of their illness. Life expectancy, the expected survival of presumably normal individuals, is a form of prognosis. Indeed, the term *terminal* is not unique to diseases — life itself follows a terminal course, which begins at birth. Knowledge of the expected survival of normal individuals provides a baseline for comparison with their diseased counterparts.

7.4.1.1   *Steady-state population models*

When populations are in a **steady state**, i.e., constant rates of birth and death with no migration in or out of the population over the life span of the individuals, the age frequency distribution can be used to estimate the survival of a cohort of the population. This is depicted graphically in Figure 7.3, where survival curves for white-tailed deer have been derived from a **population model** of a Michigan herd (Spain, 1982). The additional insight provided by survival curves is apparent when we compare the survival of male vs. female deer. The survival rates for male and female deer are identical through 1 year of age, but they diverge markedly thereafter. The reduced survival in the male population over 1 year of age is due primarily to hunting pressure.

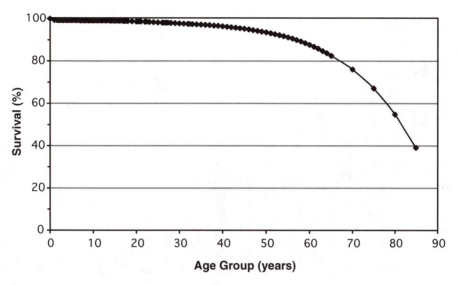

Figure 7.4 Survival curve for the U.S. population for 2001. (Source of data: U.S. Census Bureau, Expectation of life and expected deaths by race, sex, and age: 2001, in *Statistical Abstract of the United States*, 2004–2005 ed., U.S. Department of Commerce.)

7.4.1.2   Vital statistics data

Many populations are not in a steady state. For example, we are all familiar with the ups and downs of the birth rate in the U.S. population and have heard many accounts of the effect of the baby boomers and their offspring on the demand for teachers, goods and services, and the housing market. Changes in the birth and death rate over time are reflected in statistics on the age frequency distribution of the U.S. population. However, the death rate for any particular year can be used to estimate a surviorship curve for the human population. Since a rate is used, rather than absolute numbers of deaths (dangling numerators), the resulting survival data are unaffected by the number of individuals in each age class. Figure 7.4 depicts a human survival curve based on the age class death rates of the 2001 U.S. population (U.S. Census Bureau, 2004–2005).

Unfortunately, comparable vital statistics data are not routinely collected for animal populations. The closest that we can come is the distribution of age at death. The following example was taken from diagnostic laboratory data that were used to estimate the longevity of different breeds of dogs (Bronson, 1982). There are a number of biases inherent in these data. The survival analysis that follows hinges on two assumptions: (1) the age distribution of dogs presented for necropsy is representative of all dogs dying in the area, and (2) the population is in a steady state. Figure 7.5 is based on the assumption that a dog that died in a given age interval would have been alive during all preceding intervals (Lebeau, 1953), an assumption inherent to the Reed and Muench method of estimating the 50% lethal dose. Despite the likely effect of bias on the resulting survival curve, it is apparent that the pattern of canine survival is markedly different from that of human beings. This should emphasize the inaccuracy of estimating the canine–human age equivalence solely on maximum life span. For example, dividing 90 by 15 = 6 years, suggesting that 1 year of a dog's life is equal to 6 years in the life of a human. Actually, after 1 year only about 70% of dogs are alive vs. about 99% of humans at 6 human years. Lebeau (1953) estimated that the ratio of human to canine age decreased from 20:1 at a canine age of 6 months to 4.76:1 at a canine age of 21 years. A more recent study of 1290 canine patients seen by 19 California practices yielded similar results (Reichenbach, 1989).

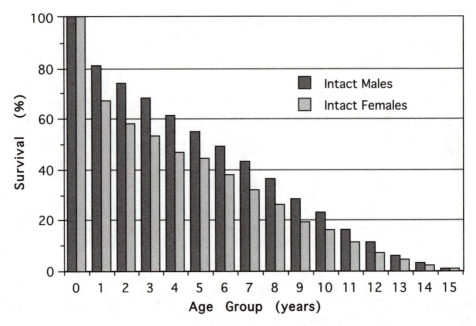

Figure 7.5 Canine survival curve for intact males and females. (Source of data: Bronson, R.T., *Am. J. Vet. Res.*, 43, 2057–2059, 1982.)

7.4.1.3   *Clinical trials*

Clinical trials frequently describe the prognosis for diseased patients with or without treatment. The results may be expressed as rates, as mentioned previously, or depicted as survival curves. Frequently, sufficient information is available for construction of survival curves, but it is "hidden away" in the text of the report.

Example 7.4

In Chapter 6, data were presented from a survival cohort of cats with advanced mammary adenocarcinoma in which the chemotherapeutic cycle was repeated every 21 days until death (see Table 6.4). If we exclude the three cats for which no follow-up data were available, we are left with a cohort of 11 cats from which a survival curve can be constructed. It is important to note that all 11 cats were followed until the outcome (death) occurred. The original data are analyzed in Table 7.4, along with the resulting survival curve (Figure 7.6).

Note that the results can be expressed over fixed time intervals (as in this case) or time to event (death). The former was chosen to simulate the results of a monthly checkup of patients; however, the latter would actually have provided a more accurate representation of the data. The number of individuals on which values for each interval are based is indicated above the interval. The median survival was 149 days, which means that half of the patients survived for this period. The mean (average) survival time was 143 days. The median is a better expression of prognosis since the mean value is influenced by extreme values.

7.4.2   *Life table analysis*

Maintaining the integrity of a cohort is often difficult in clinical practice because (1) patients ordinarily become available for a study over a period of time, thus resulting in variable

Table 7.4 Analysis of Data from a Cohort of Cats Undergoing Chemotherapy for Advanced Mammary Adenocarcinoma Where All Were Observed until Death (Complete Follow-Up)

Original Data		Survival of the Cohort			
Patient	Survival Time (d)	Time Interval (d inclusive)	Deaths	Remaining No.	Percent
4	4	0	0	11	100
5	45	30	1	10	91
6	47	60	2	8	73
7	67	90	1	7	64
8	106	120	1	6	55
9	149	150	1	5	45
10	170	180	2	3	27
11	180	210	1	2	18
12	182	240	0	2	18
13	283	270	0	2	18
14	344	300	1	1	9
		330	0	1	9
		360	1	0	0
		Total	11		

Note: Survival times from Table 6.4. Mean = 143; median = 149.
Source of data: Jeglum, K.A. et al., *J. Am. Vet. Med. Assoc.*, 187, 157–160, 1985.

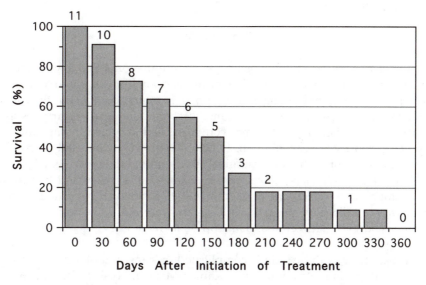

Figure 7.6 Survival curve for a cohort of 11 cats following chemotherapy for advanced mammary adenocarcinoma. Numbers above bars correspond to the number of cats remaining in the cohort. (Source of data: Jeglum, K.A. et al., *J. Am. Vet. Med. Assoc.*, 187, 157–160, 1985.)

time of follow-up, and (2) patients may drop out of the study before the end of the follow-up period. **Life table analysis** can be used to more efficiently utilize follow-up data, regardless of the time at which an individual enters or leaves a study. There are two principal techniques for carrying out a life table analysis: the **actuarial method** and the **Kaplan-Meier** (or **product-limit**) method (Kramer, 1988). In both techniques patient data

Table 7.5 Original Data from Follow-Up Study
of Cats Treated Surgically for Hemangiosarcoma

Group	Time to Event (weeks)
Still alive at last follow-up	18, 19, 40, 77, 90, 112
Died during follow-up	6, 13, 15, 20, 27, 32, 35, 75, 86

Source of data: Scavelli, T.D. et al., *J. Am. Vet. Med. Assoc.*, 187, 817–819, 1985.

are used only up to the point of their last follow-up. Thereafter, they are dropped, or **censored**, from the population at risk. The major difference between the two techniques lies in the way time intervals are defined: the Kaplan-Meier method groups analyses into **time-to-event intervals** rather than the fixed chronological intervals used in the actuarial method. The Kaplan-Meier method is the method most commonly used in clinical epidemiology and is discussed further below. The actuarial method has been used extensively by the insurance industry.

In the Kaplan-Meier method, each time interval is defined by the occurrence of the outcome of interest (the event). In many studies this is the death of the patient. The probability of surviving over each time interval is calculated by dividing the number of patients surviving by the number at risk of dying over that interval. Individuals who have already died, dropped out of the study, or have not been followed up to that point are not included in the population at risk for that interval. The probability of surviving to any point in time since the beginning of the study (zero time) is obtained by multiplying the probability of surviving over the preceding time interval by the probability of surviving up to the beginning of that interval. The mechanics of these calculations are illustrated in the following example.

Example 7.5

Hemangiosarcoma, also known as hemangioendothelioma and angiosarcoma, is a malignant neoplasm originating in the endothelium of blood vessels. It develops commonly in the dog, but reports of hemangiosarcoma in the cat are rare. During retrospective analysis of medical records in a veterinary hospital, 31 cases of feline hemangiosarcoma were identified in which therapeutic surgery was performed (Scavelli et al., 1985). Owners were contacted for follow-up information from which postsurgical survival time data were obtained for 20 of the 31 cats. Of these, three were euthanized at surgery and two in the first postoperative week. Nine of the remaining 15 cats died over the 112-week postoperative follow-up period, while 6 cats were still alive from 18 to 112 weeks postsurgery. The original data appear in Table 7.5.

Survival analysis of these data is complicated by **censored observations**, e.g., five cats with incomplete follow-up. A Kaplan-Meier analysis of the data, which adjusts for the censored observations, is depicted in Table 7.6. The population at risk over each interval is adjusted for previous deaths and loss to follow-up. Thus, even though surviving cats were not followed for the same period, each contributed to the analysis for the period that it remained in the study. The resulting survival curve appears in Figure 7.7.

Life table analysis can be used to describe outcomes of disease besides death, e.g., recurrence of tumor, remission duration, rejection of graft or reinfection, and to identify

Table 7.6 Kaplan-Meier Analysis of Data from Table 7.5
on Feline Hemangiosarcoma

Interval (weeks)	No. of Events		At Risk	Survival	
	Censored	Death		Interval (%)	Overall (%)
0	0	0	15	—	100
6	0	1	15	93	93
13	0	1	14	93	87
15	0	1	13	92	80
20	2	1	10	90	72
27	0	1	9	89	64
32	0	1	8	88	56
35	0	1	7	86	48
75	1	1	5	80	38
86	1	1	3	67	26
90	0	0	2	100	26
112	1	0	1	100	26

Source of data: Scavelli, T.D. et al., *J. Am. Vet. Med. Assoc.*, 187, 817–819, 1985.

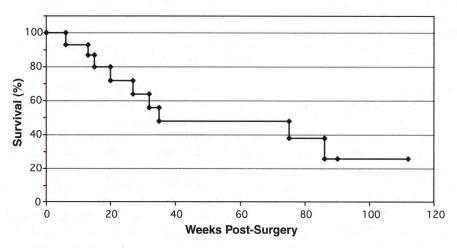

Figure 7.7 Kaplan-Meier graph of postoperative survival of 15 cats being treated for hemangiosarcoma. (Source of data: Table 7.6.)

prognostic factors for these outcomes. In fact, the frequency of any event can be studied by means of life tables, so long as the outcome is dichotomous (i.e., either/or) and can occur only once during the follow-up period. The following example illustrates the use of life table analysis to evaluate the prognostic value of the TNM tumor classification system in dogs afflicted with malignant mammary tumors.

Example 7.6

Next to skin tumors, mammary tumors are the second most commonly occurring neoplasm in dogs. Various factors such as complicated histologic types, site distribution, onset time, and biological behavior make it difficult to make a prognosis for affected patients. In an attempt to identify prognostic indicators,

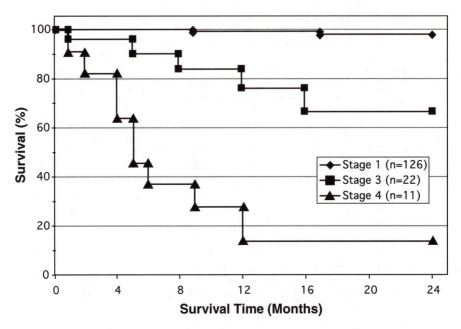

Figure 7.8 Kaplan-Meier graph depicting survival of untreated dogs with malignant mammary tumors according to TNM classification. Stage 1 — T1, N0, M0; Stage 3 — any T, any N, M0; Stage 4 — any T, any N, M1. There were an insufficient number of stage 2 cases (n = 3) for meaningful analysis. As the grade of staging increased, the prognosis was significantly poorer ($p < 0.01$). (Source of data: Yamagami, T. et al., *J. Vet. Med. Sci.*, 58, 1079–1083, 1996. With permission.)

Yamagami et al. (1996) evaluated 2-year follow-up data on randomly selected canine patients with histologically confirmed malignant mammary tumors. Cases that died from causes unrelated to mammary tumors or that underwent anticancer chemotherapy were excluded from the study. A number of potential prognostic factors for patient survival were evaluated, including clinical staging based on the **TNM classification system** (T = maximum diameter of the primary tumor; N = extent of regional lymph node involvement; M = presence or absence of distant metastases). Kaplan-Meier survival analysis was employed to compare 2-year cumulative survival for each prognostic factor. The relationship between TNM classification stage and prognosis is depicted in Figure 7.8. The survival curve clearly shows that as the grade of staging increased, the prognosis was significantly poorer ($p < 0.01$). The TNM **clinical staging** system thus appears to provide clinically useful information on the prognosis for untreated cases of canine malignant mammary tumors.

7.4.3   Interpreting survival curves

Several points must be considered when interpreting survival curves. First, since the data include censored observations, the percentage of individuals at each data point may not be equivalent to the actual number of individuals remaining in the study. This can be appreciated if Figure 7.6 and Figure 7.7 are compared. The former is based on follow-up of a cohort of individuals with no censored observations. Consequently, the number of individuals remaining at any point on the curve can be estimated by multiplying the percent survival at this point by the number of individuals initially present. In contrast, if we multiply 26% survival by the 15 cats initially present in Figure 7.7, we obtain 4 cats.

Table 7.7 Numeric Equivalents for 16 Literal Prognoses Based
on the Response of 47 Large and Small Animal Practitioners

		Numeric Designation of Probability of Recovery[a]		
Prognostic Term or Phrase	No. of Responses	Mean	±SD	Range
Terminal	45	0.11	0.38	0–2
Incurable	43	0.21	0.51	0–2
Horrible	41	0.80	0.84	0–3
Grave	47	0.96	0.86	0–3
Dismal	41	1.22	0.88	0–3
Very poor	46	1.96	0.99	0–5
Poor	47	2.64	1.01	0–5
Unfavorable	46	2.78	1.47	0–5
Guarded	46	3.83	1.73	1–8
Not so good	42	3.93	1.54	2–9
Fair	47	5.79	1.59	2–10
Not too bad	42	7.10	1.51	6–10
Favorable	46	8.07	0.83	6–10
Good	47	8.32	0.78	6–10
Very good	46	8.96	0.70	7–10
Excellent	47	9.83	0.38	9–10

[a] Recovery was defined as absence of disease-related signs for at least 1 year after appropriate treatment/management.
Source: Crow, S.E., *J. Am. Vet. Med. Assoc.*, 187, 700–703, 1985. With permission.

Actually, the 26% survival figure is based on only one cat, as the others were not available for the entire 112-week follow-up period.

Second, the number of individuals at risk declines as we move from left to right along the survival curve. Consequently, our estimates of the probability of survival depend on what happens to fewer and fewer individuals. A single event toward the end of the follow-up period will have a much greater impact than at the beginning. As a result, we can have less confidence in our estimates of survival toward the end of the survival curve.

Finally, the survival curve reflects the effect of a survival rate upon a steadily decreasing population at risk. This accounts for the steadily decreasing slope of the survival curve over the follow-up period. Although the percentage survival appears to improve over time, the survival rate may actually remain unchanged. This is similar to a radioactive decay curve whose shape reflects the steady decay of a radionuclide over time.

7.5 Communication of prognoses

The use of qualitative terms to express chances of success or failure is inherently ambiguous. Furthermore, veterinarians frequently do not agree regarding the prognosis for many common illnesses. Unfortunately for veterinary clinicians, there is no definitive source of prognostic information about diseases of domestic animals.

Example 7.7

Table 7.7 summarizes the responses of 47 large and small animal practitioners at a university teaching hospital who were asked to designate numeric equivalents for each of 16 literal terms, on a scale of 0 to 10. The number 0 was assigned to no probability of recovery, and each increment of 1 represented a

Table 7.8 Numeric Designation for Probability of Recovery from 22 Common Illnesses of Small Animals

Prognostic Term or Phrase	No. of Responses	Numeric Designation of Probability of Recovery[a]		
		Mean	±SD	Range
Fleabite dermatitis	20	7.80	2.89	0–10
Otitis externa	20	7.40	3.12	1–10
Hypoadrenocorticism	20	7.25	2.43	2–10
Epilepsy	20	6.30	2.96	0–10
Intervertebral disk disease	19	6.22	2.94	0–9
Diabetes mellitus	19	5.79	2.90	1–9
Hyperadrenocorticism	19	5.68	2.96	2–8
Atopic dermatitis	19	5.21	3.44	0–10
Exocrine pancreatic insufficiency	20	5.20	3.40	0–10
Chronic bronchitis	18	5.06	3.15	0–10
Collapsing trachea	19	4.89	3.13	0–9
Mammary carcinoma	19	4.63	2.77	1–10
Glaucoma	19	4.53	3.13	0–10
Mitral insufficiency with congestive failure	19	4.21	2.57	0–8
Granulomatous colitis	19	3.89	2.54	0–8
Chronic active hepatitis	19	3.00	2.29	0–7
Nasal aspergillosis	18	3.00	2.54	0–9
Distemper	20	2.85	2.78	0–8
Lymphosarcoma	20	2.75	2.36	0–7
Cardiomyopathy	18	2.33	1.91	0–6
Chronic progressive renal disease	18	2.05	1.67	0–5
Osteosarcoma	21	1.52	1.63	0–6

[a] Recovery was defined as absence of disease-related signs for at least 1 year after appropriate treatment/management.

Source: Crow, S.E., *J. Am. Vet. Med. Assoc.*, 187, 700–703, 1985. With permission.

10% probability of recovery. Recovery was defined as absence of disease-related signs for at least 1 year after appropriate treatment/management (Crow, 1985). Small animal practitioners were also asked to apply the same numeric scale to 22 common illnesses of dogs and cats, for the purpose of evaluating the disorders with respect to an animal's chances for recovery. The results are summarized in Table 7.8.

Because of the considerable overlap of terms in Table 7.7, the author suggested that veterinarians use the prognostic terms listed in Table 7.9 to express prognoses.

7.6 Summary

Prognosis is a prediction of the expected outcome of disease with or without treatment. A prognosis should include (1) variability in course relative to treatment options, (2) a time reference, (3) risk of treatment-related death (or other untoward reaction), (4) cost, and (5) the nature of the benefit attainable.

The natural history of a disease describes its evolution without medical intervention. The clinical course of a disease describes its progression once it has come under medical care. The true natural history of unselected cases of a disease, and the course of those that are recognized, can be quite different. Reports of prognosis from veterinary teaching

Table 7.9 Qualitative Terms for Clinical Outcomes

Prognosis	Probability of Recovery (%)
Excellent	90–100
Good	70–89
Fair	40–69
Poor	10–39
Grave	0–9

Source: Crow, S.E., *J. Am. Vet. Med. Assoc.*, 187, 700–703, 1985. With permission.

hospitals and other referral centers may not be representative of cases seen in the typical private practice. Reported cases are often those that had been referred because they were doing badly.

It is convenient to summarize the course of disease as a rate. All rates used for this purpose are expressions of incidence, e.g., events arising in a cohort of patients over time. Two variables that must be considered in the interpretation of rates are assignment of zero time and interval of follow-up.

Survival analysis can be used to estimate the average time to event for any time in the course of disease. The plotted data are referred to as a survival curve. The most direct way of learning about survival is to assemble a cohort of patients with the condition of interest and periodically assess their status throughout the course of their illness.

Maintaining the integrity of a cohort is often difficult in clinical practice because (1) patients frequently drop out of the study before the end of the follow-up period, and (2) patients ordinarily become available for a study over a period of time, leading to variable duration of follow-up. Data on patients with incomplete follow-up are referred to as censored observations. Life table analysis can be used to more efficiently use follow-up data, regardless of the time at which an individual enters or leaves a study. With the life table method, the probability of surviving during each time interval is calculated and is used to estimate overall survival through the end of each time interval.

The life table approach can be used to describe other outcomes of disease besides death, such as recurrence of tumor, remission duration, graft rejection, or reinfection, and to identify prognostic factors for these outcomes.

Several points must be considered when interpreting survival curves. First, since the data include censored observations, the percentage of individuals at each data point may not be equivalent to the actual number of individuals remaining in the study. Second, the number of individuals at risk declines as one progresses along the survival curve, which reduces the precision of survival estimates. Finally, the decreasing slope (or tail) of a survival curve over the follow-up period may simply be the effect of a relatively constant survival rate upon a steadily decreasing population at risk.

The use of qualitative terms to express chances of success or failure is inherently ambiguous. Furthermore, veterinarians frequently do not agree on the prognosis for many common illnesses. There is a clear need for quantitative prognostic information about diseases of domestic animals.

chapter 8

Design and evaluation of clinical trials

8.1 Introduction

Throughout this text a distinction has been made between epidemiologic studies of naturally occurring disease and laboratory studies of experimentally induced disease. Within the field of clinical epidemiology, the evaluation of treatment effects (the clinical trial) comes as close to a laboratory experiment as any activity that we have discussed. In evaluating clinical trials, the practitioner must consider not only whether the data support the authors' conclusions, but also whether the study design was appropriate for the question being asked. In this chapter we first examine factors that can influence the outcome of clinical trials and then apply criteria to selected case studies.

▼

> Treatments should be adopted "not because they ought to work, but because they do work."

▲

Therapeutic hypotheses may come from an understanding of the mechanisms of disease, clinical observations, or epidemiologic studies of populations. Regardless of their source, new treatment regimens must be tested. In other words, treatments should be adopted "not because they ought to work, but because they do work" (Anonymous, 1980).

8.2 Efficacy, effectiveness, and compliance

Efficacy is a measure of how well a treatment works among those who receive it. **Effectiveness**, on the other hand, is a measure of how well a treatment works among those to whom it is offered. **Compliance** is a measure of the proportion of patients (or their owners) that adhere to the prescribed treatment regimen. Thus, an efficacious treatment could be ineffective due to poor compliance. This relationship can be summarized as effectiveness = efficacy × compliance. **Intention to treat (ITT) analysis** considers the outcome for all subjects entered into a trial, whether or not they had actually received the intervention and completed the study. ITT analyses may prevent overestimation of treatment efficacy in case of substantial withdrawal of study subjects, as in response to adverse drug effects (Olivry and Mueller, 2003).

127

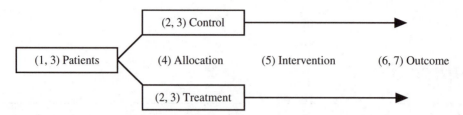

Figure 8.1 Design and potential sources of bias (Table 8.1) in clinical trials. (From Fletcher, R.H. et al., *Clinical Epidemiology: The Essentials*, Williams & Wilkins, Baltimore, 1982. With permission.)

8.3   Clinical trials: structure and evaluation

Practitioners initiate an observational study of treatment every time they treat a patient. However, because of the many potential sources of bias during routine patient care, a more formal approach to evaluating treatment outcomes is usually required. The **clinical trial** is a cohort study specifically designed to facilitate the detection and measurement of treatment effects, free of extraneous variables. Because of the experimental nature of clinical trials, they are sometimes referred to as **intervention or experimental studies**.

The design and potential sources of bias in a clinical trial are depicted in Figure 8.1. The first step should be a determination of the minimum number of subjects required to achieve the desired level of **statistical power**. Too few subjects and random variation in outcome may obscure the effects of a beneficial treatment. Study subjects are allocated to either treatment or control groups. Both are treated identically, with the exception that the treatment group receives an intervention that is believed to be beneficial. The control group usually receives a **placebo**, an intervention designed to simulate the act of treatment but lacking its beneficial component(s). Any differences that emerge between the two groups over time are attributed to the treatment. Virtually any parameter can be used to measure and express the outcome of a clinical trial. In veterinary medicine, the outcome may be expressed in terms of the health benefit to the patient, or as productivity or economic benefits.

▼

The clinical trial is a cohort study specifically designed to facilitate the measurement of treatment effects, free of extraneous variables.

▲

There a two measures of validity for clinical trials: internal and external (Fletcher et al., 1996). **Internal validity** is the extent to which conclusions drawn from a study are correct for the sample of patients being studied. **External validity** (*generalizability*) is the degree to which results of a study can be generalized to the population at large from which the sample was drawn, e.g., the **target population**. The first requirement for external validity is internal validity; e.g., invalid conclusions from a clinical trial will also be invalid when applied to the broader population of patients. However, a study may produce valid results but still lack external validity because study subjects are not representative of the general patient population. Examples might be clinical trials whose patient composition does not accurately reflect the gender or age distribution, or clinical severity of patients at large. External validity can be maximized by selecting study subjects that are as similar as possible to the patient population to which the results are to be generalized.

Many factors can affect the internal validity of cohort studies of risk, prognosis, and treatment. These generally originate from one of the following sources:

Table 8.1 Factors That May Influence the Outcome and Relevance of Clinical Trials

1. Is the case definition explicit, exclusive, and uniform?
2. Is a comparison group explicitly identified?
3. Are both treated and control patients selected from the same time and place?
4. Are patients allocated to treatment and control groups without bias?
5. Is the intended intervention, and only that intervention, experienced by all of the patients in the treated group and not in the control group?
6. Is the outcome assessed without regard to treatment status?
7. Is the method used to determine the significance of the observed results defined explicitly? Can we be certain that the observed results could not have occurred by chance alone?

Source: Fletcher, R.H. et al., *Clinical Epidemiology: The Essentials*, Williams & Wilkins, Baltimore, 1982. With permission.

1. **Assembly bias**: Assembly (or selection) bias occurs when the criteria for inclusion of patients in a study do not ensure uniformity of individuals. Patients may differ in ways that are not under study but that can affect the outcome.
2. **Migration bias**: Migration bias occurs when patients that leave a study (censored observations) are systematically different from those that remain.
3. **Measurement bias**: Measurement bias occurs when uniform standards for measurement of clinical events cannot be maintained over time.

An additional form of bias, **confounding bias**, occurs when two factors are associated with each other, or "travel together," and the effect of one is confused with or distorted by the effect of the other (Fletcher et al., 1996). Confounding bias is usually dealt with during data analysis, after the study is over.

The criteria outlined in Table 8.1 have proven useful for reducing bias in cohort studies. The points at which they influence the outcome of a clinical trial are indicated in Figure 8.1 and discussed in greater detail below.

▼

Many factors can affect the outcome of cohort studies of risk, prognosis, and treatment. These generally originate from assembly, migration, measurement, or confounding bias.

▲

8.3.1   Case definition

The first step in a clinical trial is selection of patients who meet the **case definition**. This is not as easy as it might first appear. It may be difficult to define a set of disease signs that will include all true cases of a disease and exclude similar, but unrelated conditions. Few cases will show the complete range of disease signs and symptoms; thus, minimal criteria for a diagnosis often have to be established. As the number of signs and symptoms required to meet the case definition increases, the definition becomes more and more restrictive and includes a progressively smaller number of cases. Furthermore, the criteria used for the case definition should be uniformly applied when multiple clinics are involved.

8.3.2   Uncontrolled clinical trials

In **uncontrolled clinical trials** the effects of treatment are assessed by comparing patients' clinical courses before and after treatment, without reference to an untreated comparison group, to see whether an intervention changes the established course of disease in individual patients. The difficulty in interpreting the results of an uncontrolled trial relates to the predictability of the course of disease.

For some conditions, the prognosis without treatment is so predictable that an untreated control group is either unnecessary or unethical. In most cases, however, the clinical course is not so predictable. Some diseases normally improve after an initial attack. If a treatment is given at this time, it may be mistakenly credited with the favorable outcome. Clients tend to seek care for their animals when signs are at their worst. Patients sometimes begin to recover after seeing the veterinarian because of the natural course of events (natural history of the disease), regardless of what was done. Severe diseases that normally are not self-limiting may nonetheless undergo spontaneous remission. In these cases, improvement in the patient's condition would mistakenly be attributed to the treatment if it had been initiated when signs were most evident.

Example 8.1

Canine ehrlichiosis is a tick-borne rickettsial disease of dogs characterized by fever, pancytopenia, particularly thrombocytopenia, hemorrhage, and persistent infection (Smith, 1977). During the initial, acute phase of the disease, clinical signs (nasolacrimal discharge, crusting of the nares, leukopenia) resemble those of several other infectious diseases, particularly canine distemper. Routine hemograms are consistent with this diagnosis. Consequently, veterinarians are seldom prompted to prepare Giemsa-stained buffy coat smears and look for the occasional *Ehrlichia*-infected monocyte, which is pathognomonic for the disease. The natural history of the disease is such that most dogs undergo an uneventful recovery from the acute phase of the disease, regardless of treatment. Consequently, uncontrolled clinical trials of any therapeutic regimen for the disease, correctly diagnosed or not, are likely to be favorable if initiated during the acute phase of infection. More severe complications usually develop months later, during the chronic phase of canine ehrlichiosis.

8.3.3 *Comparisons across time and place*

Diagnosis and treatment strategies change over time. Similarly, the nature of patients, clinical expertise, and medical procedures differ among clinical settings. Thus, the time and place in which conditions are diagnosed and treated can affect the expected prognosis. Clinical trials in which treatment and comparison groups are selected at the same time (concurrent controls) and place are less likely to be biased. However, a historical comparison group may be the only alternative when it is ethically inappropriate to withhold a promising new treatment from client-owned animals.

Example 8.2

Until recently **dilated cardiomyopathy (DCM) in cats** was considered a progressive, irreversible condition with a grave prognosis, despite medical intervention. The incidence in cats has dropped dramatically since the discovery in 1985 that taurine deficiency was responsible for most cases. Pion et al. (1992) observed rapid reversal of signs following taurine supplementation of affected cats, and designed a clinical trial to evaluate the long-term benefits of administering taurine to cats with DCM. A concurrent cohort of 37 taurine-treated DCM cats (treatment group) was compared with a historical cohort of 33 DCM

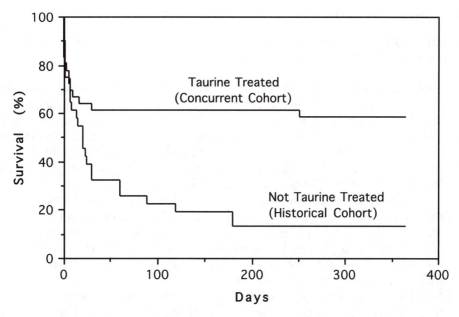

Figure 8.2 Effect of taurine supplementation upon survival of cats from the time of diagnosis of dilated cardiomyopathy. Fifty-eight percent of 36 taurine-treated cats (concurrent cohort) survived a year or more vs. only 14% of 31 untreated cats (historical cohort). (Source of data: Pion, P.D. et al., *J. Am. Vet. Med. Assoc.*, 201, 275–284, 1992. With permission.)

cats (control group) who had been treated with conventional therapy, before the role of taurine was suspected. The latter group was assembled from medical records by identifying cats with an echocardiographically confirmed diagnosis of DCM. Treatment and survival time data were obtained from the medical records, and verified and supplemented through follow-up telephone interviews with clients. According to treatment records, most control cats had received digoxin and furosemide. Cats in the treatment group with evidence of congestive heart failure were treated symptomatically with a combination of digoxin, diuretics, angiotensin-converting enzyme inhibitors, and pleurocentesis. All treatment group cats received oral taurine supplementation initially. Medications other than taurine were discontinued in the treatment group as clinical improvement became evident. Taurine supplementation was discontinued once echocardiographic improvement occurred, and plasma levels were maintained through feeding of commercial cat food containing additional taurine.

The survival curves for the two groups (Figure 8.2) diverged markedly within a few weeks after the initiation of taurine supplementation of treatment group cats. Twenty-one (58%) of 36 taurine-treated cats with a known outcome survived for at least 1 year vs. only 4 (14%) of 31 untreated cats with a known outcome. Although the differences in the survival curves of the groups were statistically significant, differences in the nature of supportive medications given the two groups confounded the interpretation of the results. Based on historical data, the authors discarded the possibility that medications other than taurine were responsible for the improved survival. They also pointed out that it would have been ethically inappropriate to withhold taurine supplementation from a concurrent control group of client-owned animals once the beneficial effects of taurine became apparent.

8.3.4   Allocating treatment

When concurrent controls are used, assignment of study subjects to treatment or comparison groups can be done in several ways.

1. **Nonrandom allocation**: If the clinician or owner decides how a case is to be treated, then allocation is considered to be nonrandom. This approach is prone to systematic differences among treatment groups. Many factors, such as severity of illness, concurrent diseases, local preferences, owner cooperation, etc., can affect treatment decisions. As a result, it is difficult to distinguish treatment effects from other prognostic factors when nonrandom allocation to treatment groups is used.
2. **Random allocation**: The best way to study unique effects of a clinical intervention is through randomized controlled trials in which patients are randomly allocated to treatment and comparison groups. The purpose of randomization is to achieve an equal distribution of all factors related to prognosis among treatment and control groups. If the number of patients is small, the investigator can compare the distribution of a number of patient characteristics among the groups to ensure that randomization has been achieved.
3. **Stratified randomization**: If certain patient characteristics are known to be related to prognosis, then patients can first be allocated to groups (strata) of similar prognosis based on this characteristic and then randomized separately within each stratum. Although stratification can be accomplished mathematically after the data are collected, prior stratification reduces the likelihood of unequal cohorts during the randomization process.

8.3.5   Remaining in assigned treatment groups

It is not uncommon for patients in treatment or comparison groups to cross over into another group or drop out of the study entirely. The way in which these deviations from protocol are handled depends on the question being asked in the clinical trial. **Explanatory trials** are designed to assess the **efficacy** of a treatment. Treatment outcomes are measured only in those patients who actually receive it, regardless of where they were originally assigned. Thus, patients who fail to adhere to the treatment plan or drop out of the study are ignored, and those who transfer into the treatment group may be included.

   Management trials seek to determine how **effective** a treatment is among those to whom it is offered. Consequently, treatment outcomes are based on the original allocation of patients, even if the clinician or owner ultimately decides not to follow treatment guidelines.

8.3.6   Assessment of outcome

The perceptions and behavior of the participants (clinical investigators and clients) in a clinical trial may be affected systematically (biased) if they know who received which treatment. This is not a problem when the outcome is unequivocal, such as life or death. However, many clinical outcomes are subject to the interpretations of the observers. The rigor with which a patient is examined and the objectivity of the observers may be influenced by prior knowledge of an animal's treatment status. Clients may be anxious to see improvement in their pets or please the clinician. Clinicians may be more thorough in their examination of one group vs. another.

   These sources of bias can be avoided by **blinding** the owners, the clinicians, or both to the treatment status of individual patients. Owners can be blinded by dispensing a placebo for control group patients. Clinicians can be blinded by use of a placebo or by not informing them of an animal's treatment status.

8.3.7 Placebo effect

A **placebo** is defined as any medical intervention that has a nonspecific, psychological, or psychophysiologic therapeutic effect, or that is used for a presumed specific therapeutic effect on a patient, symptom, or illness, but is without specific activity for the condition being treated (McMillan, 1999). It follows that the **placebo effect** is the nonspecific psychological or psychophysiologic therapeutic effect induced by a placebo. The effect may be positive or negative, e.g., favorable or unfavorable. Placebos are important both as a control in clinical trials and for understanding the mechanism of how they work.

A possible mechanism of action of a placebo in animal subjects is through the effect of human contact (visual and tactile) on animal health. In humans, expectations of a response may influence the subjective interpretation of the results of animal studies and erroneously attribute a response to either the placebo or treatment. This is really a form of **investigator bias** rather than a biologically mediated effect.

In clinical trials in which a placebo is selected as the control method, it may be useful to include a second control group in which a placebo is not administered. This would permit placebo effects to be distinguished from other causes of disease resolution.

▼

Statistical significance does not automatically equate with clinical significance.

▲

8.3.8 Statistical analysis

Many reports of clinical trials end by concluding that a treatment offered a significant improvement over existing techniques or controls. Whenever this word is used, it should be backed up by appropriate statistical analysis, and it should be stated at the outset how the results were analyzed. Statistical tests must answer one fundamental question: *How certain can we be that the observed results did not arise by chance alone?*

Statistical significance does not automatically equate with **clinical significance**. As the number of animals in each comparison group increases, the statistical significance of differences in group means also tends to increase. However, if there is considerable overlap among individuals across comparison groups, then we may not be able to accurately predict clinical outcomes for individual patients.

8.4 Subgroups

During the analysis of a clinical trial the investigators may be tempted to compare outcomes among specific subgroups of patients. If the number of patients in the clinical trial is large, then the number of individuals in each subgroup may be adequate for meaningful comparisons, provided that systematic differences among the groups being compared are adjusted for. However, as the number of subgroup comparisons increases, so does the likelihood that a statistically significant difference will be detected, even if it is not real. Validity of findings from subgroups is not a problem unique to clinical trials. Clinical studies of frequency, risk, prognosis, and cause often include the frequency of findings in various subgroups.

▼

As the number of subgroup comparisons increases, so does the likelihood that
a statistically significant difference will be detected, even if it is not real.

▲

Example 8.3

Hoskins et al. (1985) evaluated the case records for 416 heartworm-infected
dogs for complications following treatment with thiacetarsamide sodium (Ca-
parsolate). Complications occurred in 26.2% of dogs and were most frequently
seen 5 to 9 days following therapy. Frequency of selected complications ranged
from 95.4% (increased lung sounds) to 0.9% (disseminated intravascular coag-
ulopathy). There were no statistically significant differences between the age,
sex, body size, or breed of dogs that experienced complications and those that
did not. However, 56 of 65 breeds were represented by six or fewer patients
and had to be excluded from the statistical analysis.

8.5   Clinical trials in practice

Randomized controlled trials are the best available means of assessing the value of treatment. However, because of many practical difficulties with randomized controlled clinical
trials, the majority of therapeutic questions are answered by other means, particularly
uncontrolled and nonrandomized trials. The need to administer some sort of treatment is
largely responsible for the large percentage of case reports and uncontrolled clinical trials.

8.6   Summary

Within the field of clinical epidemiology, the evaluation of treatment effects (the clinical
trial) comes as close to a laboratory experiment as any activity that we have discussed.
Because of the experimental nature of clinical trials, they are sometimes referred to as
intervention or experimental studies. In evaluating clinical trials, the practitioner must
consider not only whether the data support the authors' conclusions, but also whether
the study design was appropriate for the question being asked.

   Efficacy is a measure of how well a treatment works among those who receive it.
Effectiveness, on the other hand, is a measure of how well a treatment works among those
to whom it is offered. Compliance is a measure of the proportion of patients (or their
owners) who adhere to the prescribed treatment regimen. Thus, an efficacious treatment
could be ineffective due to poor compliance. Intention to treat (ITT) analysis considers the
outcome for all subjects entered into a trial, whether or not they had actually received the
intervention and completed the study. ITT analyses may prevent overestimation of treatment efficacy in case of substantial withdrawal of study subjects, as in response to adverse
drug effects.

   The clinical trial is a cohort study specifically designed to facilitate the detection and
measurement of treatment effects, free of extraneous variables. The first step should be a
determination of the minimum number of subjects (treated and controls) required to
achieve the desired level of statistical power. Too few subjects and random variation in
outcome may obscure the effects of a beneficial treatment.

   Virtually any parameter can be used to measure and express the outcome of a clinical
trial. In veterinary medicine, the outcome is sometimes expressed in terms of productivity
or economic benefit, rather than the health status of individuals. There are two measures

of validity for clinical trials: internal and external. Internal validity is the extent to which conclusions drawn from a study are correct for the sample of patients being studied. External validity (generalizability) is the degree to which results of a study can be generalized to the population at large from which the sample was drawn, e.g., the target population.

Many factors can affect the outcome of cohort studies of risk, prognosis, and treatment. Among the most important are:

1. Is the case definition explicit, exclusive, and uniform?
2. Is a comparison group explicitly identified?
3. Are both treated and control patients selected from the same time and place?
4. Are patients allocated to treatment and control groups without bias?
5. Is the intended intervention, and only that intervention, experienced by all of the patients in the treated group, and not in the control group?
6. Is the outcome assessed without regard to treatment status?
7. Is the method used to determine the significance of the observed results defined explicitly? Can we be certain that the observed results could not have occurred by chance alone?

chapter 9

Statistical significance

Figures don't lie but liars can figure.

—Anonymous

There are three types of lies: lies, damn lies and statistics.

—Mark Twain

Torture numbers and they'll confess to anything.

—Gregg Easterbrook in *The New Republic*

9.1   Introduction

Statistical analyses, once a rarity in medical journals, are now routinely encountered in the medical literature, and veterinary journals are no exception (Shott, 1985). Almost half of the articles published in 1992 in six practice-oriented veterinary journals included statistical methods other than simple descriptive statistics (Hammer and Buffington, 1994). The authors reported that knowledge of five categories of statistical methods (analysis of variance (ANOVA), t-tests, contingency tables, nonparametric tests, and simple linear regression) would facilitate reader comprehension of 90% of the veterinary literature surveyed.

Statistical analyses often have immense practical importance since research results are frequently the basis for decisions about patient care. If the choice of treatment hinges on faulty statistics, a great deal of harm may be done. An effective treatment may be dismissed as worthless, and an ineffective treatment may be adopted. Besides treatment outcomes, statistics are used to confirm or refute the significance of risk and prognostic factors, and as a quality control component in population surveys. The likelihood of failing to detect disease in a population depends not only on the properties of diagnostic tests being used, but also on the degree to which the sample represents the population as a whole. Thus, all aspects of the practice of medicine require that statistics be used, and that they be used correctly.

Until now we have used **descriptive statistics** (measures of central tendency and dispersion) to describe clinical data. We now turn to **inferential statistics** to help us determine whether observed outcomes are real or the result of random variation.

Statistical analyses are now much easier to perform than in the past. Many statistical routines are built into handheld calculators, while others are available as microcomputer software packages. Statistical errors are not uncommon in medical research. Since most investigators rely on preprogrammed statistical packages, the most frequent statistical errors arise from analyses that are inappropriate for the type of data or study design, rather than errors of execution. In this chapter we discuss the application and interpretation of statistical tests in clinical epidemiology and the rules that guide the selection of appropriate statistical tests.

▼

Statistical analyses, once a rarity in medical journals, are now routinely encountered in the medical literature, and veterinary journals are no exception.

▲

9.2   *Hypothesis definition and testing: an overview*

In this chapter many of the details of the design and analysis of scientific research are discussed from the perspective of statistical testing. The primary purpose of statistical testing is to determine whether the observed results are real, or could have occurred by chance. Before embarking on the details, it may be useful to provide a brief overview of hypothesis testing and introduce some of the major concepts. Each will be discussed in greater detail in the pages that follow.

Any scientific investigation, epidemiologic or otherwise, begins with a research question, e.g., the objective or purpose of the study (Hulley et al., 2001). The initial research question may reflect a general concern to be restated as one or more specific research questions. For example, an initial research question might be whether exposure of pets to chemically treated lawns is harmful. More specific questions might ask what kinds of chemicals are applied and whether they increase the risk of certain kinds of cancers, such as malignant lymphoma (Hayes et al., 1991).

The next step is to formulate a research hypothesis that summarizes the elements of the study: the sample, the design, and the predictor and outcome variables. The research hypothesis should establish the basis for tests of statistical significance. This is usually done by restating the research hypothesis in the form of null and alternative hypotheses. The **null hypothesis** states that there is no association between the predictor and outcome variables. In the lawn chemical example above, this might be stated as: *There is **no difference** in the frequency of exposure to lawn chemicals between dogs that develop malignant lymphomas and those that do not.* By default, the alternative hypothesis would state that: *There is **a difference** in the frequency of exposure to lawn chemicals between dogs that develop malignant lymphomas and those that do not.* The alternative hypothesis cannot be tested directly; it is accepted by default if the test of statistical significance rejects the null hypothesis (see below).

Research hypotheses are usually stated as either directional or nondirectional. A **directional (one-sided) hypothesis** of the lawn chemical example would state that the frequency of exposure to a specific lawn chemical is greater among dogs that developed malignant lymphoma. A **nondirectional (two-sided) hypothesis** would simply state that there is an association between exposure and outcome without specifying whether exposed dogs are at greater or less risk. The practical significance of choosing between directional and nondirectional hypotheses lies in the fact that the nondirectional hypothesis is more stringent, e.g., the evidence (data) required to reject the null hypothesis must be stronger for a nondirectional hypothesis than for a directional hypothesis. Nondirectional hypotheses also

| | True Difference | |
	Present	Absent
Different (reject null hypothesis)	(a) Correct	(b) Incorrect (Type I or alpha error)
Not Different (accept null hypothesis)	(c) Incorrect (Type II or beta error)	(d) Correct

Conclusion of Statistical Test

Figure 9.1 The relationship between the statistical analysis of study results and the true difference between possible outcomes.

require a larger sample size. For these reasons, nondirectional hypothesis are generally preferred when planning sample size and analyzing the data.

When the data are analyzed, statistical tests determine the *p* **value**, the probability or likelihood of obtaining the observed or more extreme results by chance alone if the null hypothesis were true. The *p* values are expressed as **one-tailed** or **two-tailed** in accordance with whether the hypotheses being tested are directional or nondirectional, respectively. The null hypothesis is rejected in favor of the alternative hypothesis if the *p* value is less than the predetermined level of statistical significance. By convention this is usually 5%; e.g., we are willing to erroneously conclude that an association between predictor and outcome variables exists less than 5% of the time. Statistical tests thus give us an idea of the level of confidence that we can have in our results.

9.3   Interpretation of statistical analyses

Many of the rules that apply to the interpretation of statistical tests are similar to those discussed earlier in the context of diagnostic tests. In the usual situation, the outcome of clinical studies is expressed in dichotomous terms: *either a difference exists or it does not*. Since we are using samples to predict the true state of affairs in the population, there always exists a chance that we will come to the wrong conclusion. When statistical tests are applied, there are four possible conclusions — two are correct and two are incorrect (Figure 9.1).

Two of the four possibilities lead to correct conclusions — either a real difference exists (cell a) or it does not (cell d). There are also two ways of being wrong. **Alpha or type I error** (cell b) results when we conclude that outcomes are different when in fact they are not. Alpha error is analogous to the false positive result of diagnostic tests. **Beta or type II error** (cell c) occurs when we conclude that outcomes are not different when in fact they are. Beta error is analogous to the false negative result of diagnostic tests.

▼

When statistical tests are applied there are four possible conclusions — two are correct and two are incorrect.

▲

9.3.1   Concluding a difference exists

9.3.1.1   The null hypothesis

Statistical tests reported in the medical literature are usually used to disprove the null hypothesis that no difference exists between groups. If differences are detected, they are reported with the corresponding *p* value, which expresses the probability of obtaining the observed data (or more extreme data) under the assumption that the null hypothesis is true, e.g., by chance. This *p* value is sometimes referred to as P_a to distinguish it from beta error.

9.3.1.2   Statistical significance

A *p* value is usually considered to be statistically significant if it falls below 0.05; e.g., we are willing to be wrong up to 5% of the time. Since not everyone agrees with this criterion, it is preferable to specify the actual probability of an alpha error, such as $p = 0.10$, $p = 0.005$, etc.

The *p* value does not indicate the magnitude of the difference between groups, only the likelihood that a difference of that magnitude could have arisen by chance alone. If individual animal variability is such that considerable overlap occurs between groups, the difference in group means could be statistically significant but not clinically relevant. (See Figure 9.3 for an example of a statistically significant association that is not clinically significant.)

▼

The *p* value does not indicate the magnitude of the difference between groups, only the likelihood that a difference of that magnitude could have arisen by chance alone.

▲

9.3.1.3   Confidence intervals

The **confidence interval (CI)** provides a way of expressing the range over which a value is likely to occur. This value could be the difference between the means of two groups, or the theoretical range over which a measurement, such as blood pressure, might occur. Although any range can be used, the 95% confidence interval is most commonly used in the medical literature. It means that the probability of including the true value within the specified range is 0.95.

Example 9.1

Returning to the topic of risk assessment, Table 6.10 listed canine breeds at increased risk of congenital portosystemic shunt (CPSS) compared with mixed-breed dogs. Risk was expressed as the odds ratio and its 99.9995% confidence interval. The reported odds ratio is actually a mean value, and we can be 99.9995% sure that the true odds ratio falls within the reported confidence interval for each breed. In this example the confidence interval actually allows us to estimate the *p* value for each odds ratio. The null hypothesis assumes that the odds ratio is 1.00 for each breed, e.g., no increase or decrease in risk compared with mixed-breed dogs. Since 1.00 is not included in the 99.9995% confidence interval, we can reject the null hypothesis with a *p* value of <0.0005%, a highly significant result.

9.3.1.4   *Confidence interval for a rate or proportion*

Confidence intervals used in descriptive statistics often derive the mean, variance, and standard deviation from measured interval-level values. Frequency measures such as incidence and prevalence present a special problem in that they are derived from dichotomous outcomes (as presence or absence of disease) rather than measured values. The confidence interval for such proportions can be estimated by using the **binomial distribution** (Petrie and Watson, 1999). In this approach the disease prevalence value is considered to be the mean. The variance of disease prevalence equals $[p(1 - p)/n]$, where p is the proportion of diseased individuals and n is the sample size. The standard deviation of disease prevalence equals the square root of the variance. Since we are really estimating the standard deviation of the sampling distribution of a proportion (or mean), rather than the standard deviation of individual values around the mean, the derived value is called the **standard error of the proportion**.

For example, in Table 5.2 the prevalence (p) of *Mycobacterium paratuberculosis* among Illinois cattle (n = 171) was 1.2%.

$$\text{The variance of the disease prevalence} = \frac{0.012 \times .988}{171} = 0.0000693$$

The standard error of the proportion (square root of the variance) = 0.00832 or 0.8%, which is consistent with the estimate reported by the investigators. The 95% confidence interval for the prevalence of *M. paratuberculosis* would be 1.2% ± 1.96 (0.832%), or –0.4 to 2.8%. The fact that there is a chance that *M. paratuberculosis* prevalence could be less than 0%, even though the organism was isolated from ileocecal lymph nodes, results from the fact that the binomial distribution of proportions is not symmetrical around the mean, except for the special case where $p = 0.50$.

9.3.1.5   *One-tailed vs. two-tailed tests of significance*

When performing a statistical test, we may be given the option of choosing a one- or two-tailed test of significance. The p values will differ depending on which is chosen. If we are certain that differences can only occur in one direction, then a one-tailed test can be used. Examples might be whether an observed temperature rise or drop in erythrocyte count deviated significantly from normal. If a difference could occur in either direction, then a two-tailed test should be used. Two-tailed tests are more conservative; e.g., the difference required for statistical significance must be greater than that with one-tailed tests. On the other hand, one-tailed tests are more likely to detect true differences when they occur. Refer to Figure 2.9 and Figure 2.10 for a comparison of one- and two-tailed cutoffs.

9.3.2   *Concluding a difference does not exist*

9.3.2.1   *Statistical significance*

By default, p values of 0.05 imply that no difference between outcomes or treatment groups exists. Actually, p 0.05 does not mean that one factor is comparable to, equivalent with, or not different from the second factor. All that has been demonstrated is an absence of evidence of a difference (Christley and Reid, 2003). In other words, failing to reject the null hypothesis does not mean that we have proven it. There is a chance that a true difference occurred but we failed to detect it because of poor study design, inadequate numbers of individuals, or bad luck. The probability of this kind of error, known as **beta or type II error**, is expressed as $\mathbf{P_b}$.

Table 9.1 Scale for Interpretation of Kappa Statistic Values, the Chance-Corrected Probability of Agreement between Two Independent Observations or Measurements Assessing the Same Subject

Kappa Value	Strength of Agreement
0	No better than chance
0.01–0.20	Slight
0.21–0.40	Fair
0.41–0.60	Moderate
0.61–0.80	Substantial
0.81–0.99	Almost perfect
1.00	Perfect

Source: Holton, L.L et al., *J. Am. Vet. Med. Assoc.*, 212, 61–66, 1998. With permission.

9.3.2.2 Power

Power is the probability that a study will find a statistically significant difference when one exists. Power is analogous to diagnostic test sensitivity and is related to beta error by the equation

$$Power = 1 - P_b$$

P_b is the major determinant of sample size in epidemiologic research. Whereas alpha error is generally set at <5%, beta error is generally set at 20%. Thus, when viewed as a diagnostic test, statistical criteria for determining sample size are more specific than sensitive. The determination of sample size is further discussed later in this chapter.

9.3.3 Concluding an association exists

9.3.3.1 Agreement between tests

As defined in Chapter 3, **concordance** is the proportion of all test results on which two or more different tests agree. The level of agreement is frequently expressed as the **kappa (k) statistic**, defined as the proportion of potential agreement beyond chance exhibited by two or more tests. Expected agreement by chance is calculated by the method of **marginal cross-products**. The value of kappa ranges from –1.0 (perfect disagreement) through 0.0 (chance agreement only) to +1.0 (perfect agreement). The conventional interpretation of kappa values is summarized in Table 9.1 (Holton et al., 1986).

To illustrate how the kappa statistic is estimated, let us compare an enzyme-linked immunosorbent assay (ELISA) test for circulating heartworm (*Dirofilaria immitis*) antigen with the modified Knott's test for circulating microfilariae (Figure 9.2) (Courtney et al., 1990). In this study there were 341 heartworm-infected and 206 uninfected dogs. Infection status (gold standard) was determined at necropsy. Although none of the uninfected dogs harbored adult *D. immitis*, 22 had circulating microfilariae of *Dipetalonema reconditum* and one had circulating microfilariae of both *D. immitis* and *D. reconditum*.

Test concordance was 82% [(201 + 247) ÷ 547]. On the basis of column and row totals, we would expect the two tests to agree 49% of the time by chance alone, and the remaining potential agreement beyond chance would therefore be 100% – 49%, or 51%. The observed agreement beyond chance was 82% – 49%, or 33%, yielding a value for kappa of 33% ÷ 51% = 0.65. In this case (k = 0.65), there was substantial agreement between the Knott's and ELISA tests.

KNOTT'S TEST

		Positive	Negative	
		(a)	(b)	(a + b)
E	Positive	201 (110)	98	299
L				
I				
S		(c)	(d)	(c + d)
A	Negative	1	247 (156)	248
		(a + c) 202	(b + d) 345	(a + b + c + d) 547

Figure 9.2 Two-by-two table comparing concordance of Knott's and ELISA test results for *Dirofilaria immitis* infection in dogs. Numbers in parentheses are expected values based on the method of marginal cross-products. (Source of data: Courtney, C.H. et al., *J. Am. Anim. Hosp. Assoc.*, 26, 623–628, 1990.)

It should be pointed out that percent concordance and the kappa statistic do not tell us which test is correct, only the level of agreement between them. In this study, 41% (140 of 341) of heartworm infections were occult and undetectable by the Knott's test. The ELISA test detected 65% (91) of these, which accounts for most of the ELISA-positive/ Knott's-negative test results in cell b.

Observed agreement (concordance) =

$$\frac{a+d}{a+b+c+d} = \frac{(\text{observed a}) + (\text{observed d})}{a+b+c+d} = \frac{(201+247)}{547} = 82\%$$

Expected (chance) agreement for cell a =

$$\frac{(a+b)\times(a+c)}{a+b+c+d} = \frac{(299\times202)}{547} = 110$$

Expected (chance) agreement for cell d =

$$\frac{(c+d)\times(b+d)}{a+b+c+d} = \frac{(248\times345)}{547} = 156$$

Expected (chance) agreement overall =

$$\frac{(\text{expected a}) + (\text{expected d})}{a+b+c+d} = \frac{(110+156)}{547} = 49\%$$

Agreement beyond chance (kappa) =

$$\frac{\text{observed agreement} - \text{expected agreement}}{100\% - \text{expected agreement}} = \frac{82\% - 49\%}{100\% - 49\%} = \frac{33\%}{51\%} = 0.65$$

9.3.3.2   Association between two variables

Statistics are also used to describe the degree of association between variables. The **Pearson product-moment correlation coefficient**, or **Pearson r**, is a measure of the strength and direction of a linear (straight line) association between two interval-level variables (Woodward, 1999). Examples might be the relation between body weight and blood volume, or between biochemical or physiologic measures such as blood packed cell volume and hemoglobin concentration. The value of r may take any value between –1 and 1. If r is either –1 or 1, the variables have a perfect linear relationship. If r is near –1 or 1, there is a high degree of linear correlation. A positive correlation means that as one variable increases, the other also increases. A negative correlation means that as one variable increases, the other decreases. If r is equal to 0, we say the variables are uncorrelated and that there is no linear association between them.

The correlation coefficient is the square root of the **coefficient of determination**, r^2, which expresses the amount of variation in the data that is accounted for by the linear relationship between two variables and may take any value between 0 and 1. The coefficient of determination is sensitive to the variability in data. As the amount of variability, or scatter, around the fitted regression line increases, the value of r^2 decreases. An r^2 value of 1 means that all values fall on the regression line.

In some cases an association between variables may exist, but it is not strictly linear. **Spearman's correlation coefficient**, or **Spearman rho**, is the counterpart of the Pearson correlation coefficient for ordinal data (Woodward, 1999). It is a **nonparametric measure** (see below) for use with data that are either reduced to ranks or collected in the form of ranks. It provides a way to quantify by how much two variables go up (or down) together without assuming that the relationship follows a straight line. The Spearman rho, like the Pearson coefficient of correlation, yields a value from –1 to 1, and it is interpreted in the same way.

When an association between two variables is suspected, it is best to construct a **scatterplot** before deciding on an analysis strategy. A scatterplot may reveal unique patterns in the data such as outliers, clusters, nonlinear relationships (or no apparent relationship at all), and may suggest not only the most appropriate analysis strategy but the **clinical relevance** of the suspected association.

Example 9.2

Pain management is an important component of patient care. Because of the personal and subjective nature of pain, accurate and reliable assessment of animal pain is especially challenging for the veterinary practitioner. Nevertheless, a number of methods have been used to assess pain in animals. Holton et al. (1998) evaluated the association between heart rate, respiratory rate, and pupil dilation and a subjective pain score allocated using a numerical rating scale (NRS). Four groups of dogs (n = 17 to 20 per group) were included: orthopedic surgery cases, soft tissue surgery cases, dogs with nonpainful medical conditions (diabetes, cardiac disease, hyperadrenocorticism, etc.), and healthy dogs. Each dog was examined by five veterinary surgeons within a 4-hour period. The relationships between physiologic signs and NRS scores were evaluated graphically (through scatterplots) and statistically using the correlation coefficient between heart rate, respiratory rate, and the NRS score. The relationship between pupil dilation and NRS scores was evaluated using chi-square tests of association. The correlation coefficient between heart rate and NRS scores for all groups combined was small (0.168) and statistically insignificant

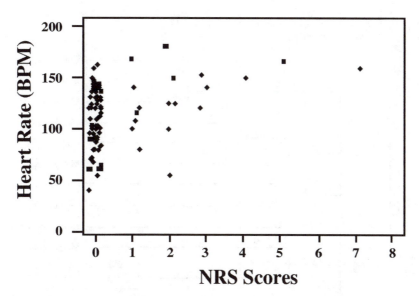

Figure 9.3 Scatterplot of heart rate (beats per minute) vs. numerical rating scale (NRS) score for 20 dogs with nonpainful medical conditions scored by five veterinary surgeons. (From Holton, L.L. et al., *J. Small Anim. Pract.*, 39, 469–474, 1998. With permission.)

($p < 0.05$). Only the medical group yielded a statistically significant correlation ($p = 0.01$) between heart rate and NRS score. However, the small correlation coefficient, 0.38, and considerable scatter of data points (Figure 9.3) indicated that the relationship was not biologically (clinically) significant; e.g., *statistical significance did not equate with clinical relevance.* This is also apparent from the high NRS scores for many dogs in the medical group, none of which were considered to be in pain by the attending clinician. There was no association between respiratory rate and NRS score, and pupil dilation achieved statistical significance only with the surgical groups. The authors concluded that heart rate and respiratory rate are not useful indicators of pain in hospitalized dogs. They also concluded that pupil dilation was unlikely to be a useful tool in the assessment of pain.

9.4 The selection of an appropriate statistical test

In most cases statistical tests are used to estimate the probability of an alpha error, e.g., the likelihood of concluding that a difference exists when, in fact, it does not. The validity of each test depends on certain assumptions about the data. If the data at hand do not satisfy these assumptions, the resulting P_a may be misleading.

In research there are many different statistical tests of significance. Research studies differ in such things as the type of data collected, the kind of measurement used, and the number of groups used. These factors decide which statistical test is appropriate for a particular study design.

For the uninitiated (most of us), the choice of an appropriate statistical test is not intuitively obvious. The tree diagram in Figure 9.4 provides guidelines for 15 of the most widely used statistical tests (Sharp, 1979). It takes into account the major requirements of each statistical test, which serve as directions for determining the appropriate test. Relevant questions for each branch of the tree follow.

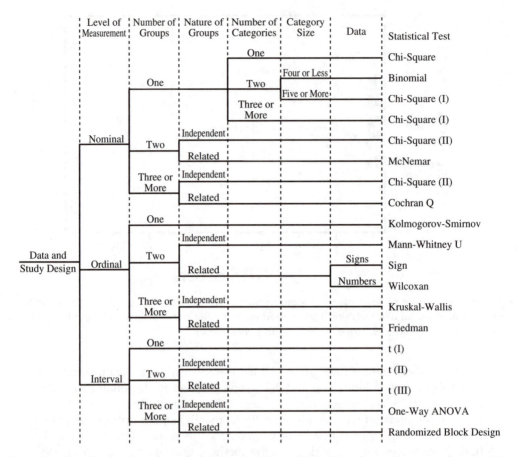

Figure 9.4 Tree diagram for selection of an appropriate statistical test depending upon characteristics of the study design and data to be analyzed. (Adapted from Sharp, V.F., *Statistics for the Social Sciences*, Little, Brown & Co., Boston, 1979. With permission.)

▼

The validity of a statistical test depends on certain assumptions about the data. If the data at hand do not satisfy these assumptions, the resulting P_a may be misleading.

▲

9.4.1 *Level of measurement*

What is the level of measurement: nominal, ordinal, or interval? **Nominal data** are used to categorize objects, individuals, conditions, etc., without ranking, as breed, sex, or blood line. **Ordinal data** are ranked but do not fall on a uniform scale. Terms such as *light*, *moderate*, and *heavy* are used to describe ordinal data. **Interval data** are ranked on a scale of equal units, such as temperature, erythrocyte counts, etc. Refer to the section on scales in Chapter 2 for a further discussion and examples of each data type.

9.4.2 *Number of groups*

How many groups are there in the study: one, two, or more? If you want to find out whether a single group is representative of a specified population, then you are looking at **one**

group. If you are interested in whether two samples come from the same population (the null hypothesis), then you are looking at **two groups**, whether they are two separate groups or the same group twice (as repeated measures over time). The same reasoning applies to **three or more groups**.

9.4.3   Nature of groups

What is the nature or character of your groups — independent or related? If the selection of an individual in one sample in no way influences the selection of an individual in another, then the groups are completely **independent**. In contrast, if groups have members that are matched or connected somehow to one another, then they are **related**.

Groups can be related when an individual serves as its own control, as **repeated measures** conducted before and after treatment. Another way that groups can be related is when individuals are paired by characteristics such as age, sex, or breed before being randomly assigned to each group. Because of the prior matching, you would now have groups that are alike in age, breed, or sex. Any difference that emerges among groups could not be attributed to these three variables. Pairing is an example of adjusting for **covariance**, where the initial values for animals in each experimental group will influence subsequent values. Covariance is also of concern in multivariate analysis (see Chapter 6), where variables other than the one under consideration may influence the outcome.

9.4.4   Number of categories

How many categories are there? This question refers only to nominal data. The number of categories refers to the number of subdivisions that a group or sample is broken down into. For instance, the canine population of a veterinary hospital may be separated into four categories based on sex: male, female, male neutered, and female neutered.

9.4.5   Category size

How many individuals or objects are in each of your categories? This question also refers only to nominal data.

9.4.6   Data

How do you plan to use your data? This question only applies to ordinal data divided into two related groups. The data can be expressed in one of two forms: numbers (such as grade of heart murmurs) or as plus and minus signs (such as strength of immunodiagnostic test reactions).

9.5   Parametric and nonparametric tests

Statistical tests are referred to as either **parametric** or **nonparametric**. When choosing a statistical test using the tree in Figure 9.4, we are also making a choice between a parametric or nonparametric test. Statistical tests appearing in the tree are organized as nonparametric or parametric in Table 9.2 (Sharp, 1979).

Parametric tests are more powerful than nonparametric tests; e.g., they have a higher probability of rejecting the null hypothesis when it should be rejected. Basic requirements for use of a parametric test are:

1. The groups in the samples are randomly drawn from the population.
2. The data are at the interval level of measurement.

Table 9.2 Nonparametric and Parametric Statistical Tests Listed in Figure 9.4

Nonparametric Tests
Binomial (test of proportion)
Chi-square (I) (goodness-of-fit test of observed vs. expected frequencies)
Chi-square (II) (contingency table analysis)
McNemar
Cochran Q
Kolmogorov–Smirnov
Mann-Whitney U
Sign
Wilcoxan
Kruskal-Wallis
Friedman
Spearman rho (p)[a]

Parametric Tests
t (I) (compares sample with population mean)
t (II) (unpaired t-test)
t (III) (paired t-test)
One-way analysis of variance
Randomized blocks design (two-way analysis of variance)
Pearson r[a]

[a] Spearman rho and Pearson r are measures of the degree of correlation between two variables. They do not appear in Figure 9.4.

Source: Sharp, V.F., *Statistics for the Social Sciences*, Little, Brown & Co., Boston, 1979. With permission.

3. The data are normally distributed.
4. The variances are equal.

Nonparametric tests have fewer and less stringent assumptions. Although they meet the first requirement of parametric tests, they do not meet the rest. They are distribution-free tests whose level of measurement is generally nominal or ordinal. Nonparametric tests must be used when sample sizes are very small, e.g., six or fewer (Sharp, 1979).

9.6   Sample size

It is intuitively obvious that the more subjects that are entered into a study, the greater confidence we can have that differences among groups are not due to random variation. The question is, how many subjects are enough? One or more of the following variables must be considered to optimize the power of a particular study. These variables are (1) the frequency of disease, (2) the amount of variability among individuals, (3) the difference in outcome between study groups, (4) P_a, and (5) P_b. Three common situations in which sample size must be considered follow.

▼

It is intuitively obvious that the more subjects that are entered into a study, the greater confidence we can have that differences among groups are not due to random variation. The question is, how many subjects are enough?

▲

9.6.1 Minimum sample size for demonstrating an extreme outcome

The best example of this situation in veterinary medicine is when we have to decide how many animals to sample to determine whether or not a particular disease is present in the herd. This is a common concern in disease eradication or control programs Here we only wish to detect the presence, rather than the prevalence, of disease in a herd. The type of error that we are trying to reduce is P_b, the likelihood of calling a herd negative when in fact it is positive (false negative result).

Example 9.3

Consider a herd of pigs in which 10% are infected with the pseudorabies virus and have detectable serum antibody. If a serum sample is drawn from one randomly selected animal in the herd, the probability that it will come from a pseudorabies-free animal is 0.90. Thus, P_b is 0.90 and we have a 90% chance of failing to detect infection in the herd. If two animals are sampled, then the chance that both samples were drawn from negative animals is 0.90×0.90, or 0.81.

Thus, the general formula for estimating P_b in the preceding example is

$$P_b = (1 - \text{prevalence of disease})^n$$

where P_b is the chance that none of the sampled animals is harboring the disease and n is the sample size. This equation can be turned around to estimate the required sample size for a given P_b:

$$n_{inf} = \frac{\log (P_b)}{\log (1 - \text{prevalence of disease})}$$

where n_{inf} is sample size for an **infinite population** (or very large relative to the sample size). If we set P_b at 0.05, then we would need to collect samples from approximately 29 animals to be 95% sure that at least one would be infected with pseudorabies virus.

The astute reader will have noticed that the previous formula is true only for very large herd sizes. For example, if the swine herd consisted of 29 animals or less, and all were tested, we would be more than 95% certain of the presence or absence of disease. The sample size requirements for state and federal disease control programs are based on formulas that adjust for herd size. The sample size estimate will also depend on test sensitivity and specificity. Perhaps the most important factor in estimating sample size to detect the presence or absence of disease is the accuracy of our estimate of existing prevalence. Since the required sample size increases as estimated prevalence decreases, it is best to assume a worst-case scenario, i.e., the lowest value for disease prevalence that we consider likely.

9.6.2 Minimum sample size for estimating a rate or proportion with a specified degree of precision

If we wish not only to detect disease, but also to estimate its prevalence, then a somewhat more complex calculation is used to estimate sample size. As you might expect, the sample size is larger than that needed to detect only the presence of disease. Sample size for an **infinite population** (n_{inf}) is estimated by the formula

$$n_{inf} = \frac{(P)\,(1-P)\,Z^2}{d^2}$$

where P is the estimated prevalence of infection (as a decimal), Z corresponds to the degree of confidence in our estimate (usually $Z = 1.96$ for 95% confidence in our estimate), and d is the maximum difference between observed and true prevalence that we are willing to accept (as a decimal) (Cochran, 1977, p. 75).

As before, sample size is inversely related to the amount of variability that we are willing to accept. Furthermore, test sensitivity and specificity, which are not included in this formula, will affect our estimate of the actual prevalence of the disease in the population.

To estimate the required sample size (n_{fin}) for estimating a rate or proportion when sampling from a **finite population** (N), the following conversion (Cochran, 1977, p. 76) can be made:

$$n_{fin} = \frac{n_{inf}}{1+(n_{inf}-1)/N}$$

9.6.3 Minimum sample size to detect differences among groups in studies of risk, prognosis, and treatment

As indicated previously, a variety of statistical tests are available for determining the significance of outcomes in clinical studies. Corresponding sample sizes vary with the test being used. If the investigator is sure of which test will be used, then it is often useful to do "what if" experiments by plugging in some hypothetical results and seeing whether statistically significant differences could be detected. By trial and error, and a reasonable estimate of the range of possible outcomes, one can estimate the sample size that will be needed. The best approach is to discuss the proposed experimental design with a biomedical statistician before the study is conducted. This individual may suggest alternative designs and would most certainly be of aid in estimating the required sample size.

9.7 Sampling strategies

Ideally an epidemiologic study should collect data from every individual in the **accessible population**, e.g., the population that is available for study. This may be possible when studying confined animal populations such as herds of cattle, stables of horses, etc. In other cases, the accessible population is too large or spread out over time, and a smaller sample of the population must be selected for study. Sampling should be conducted in such a way that the individuals selected for study are an unbiased representation of the population. Sampling strategies fall within two broad classes — **probability** and **non-probability** — each with several versions (Hulley and Cummings, 1988). Examples of each are described below.

Regardless of the sampling strategy employed, several factors associated with the data collection process may influence the validity of results. This is especially true of questionnaire surveys, where the investigator is dependent on the willingness of sampled individuals to respond to the survey. The overall response rate has a direct effect on the power of a study, whereas bias in responders vs. nonresponders may affect the validity of comparisons that are made. Finally, none of the sampling strategies described below ensure that the accessible population (for example, flea-infested dogs presented to a veterinary teaching hospital) is representative of the **target population** (all flea-infested dogs in the state, country, or world) to which the results will be generalized.

Given the variety of sampling options available, investigators should consult a biomedical statistician for advice on selecting the most appropriate sampling strategy.

9.7.1 Probability sampling

Probability sampling uses a random process to ensure that each member of a population has a specified chance of being selected. Probability sampling provides a scientific basis for saying that the intended sample represents the accessible population, and for computing confidence intervals and statistical significance. Several versions of probability sampling follow.

9.7.1.1 Simple random sampling

In **simple random sampling** every unit of the population to be sampled is enumerated in a list (**sampling frame**), and then a subset is randomly selected for study. A table of random numbers may be used to select individuals. The representativeness of the resulting sample is dependent on the accuracy of the sampling frame and success in finding and enrolling the selected individuals.

9.7.1.2 Systematic sampling

In **systematic sampling** subjects are selected for study through a periodic process, such as every 10th individual on a list. This approach might be used for sampling a large herd of cattle at the time of processing through a chute, or poultry on the processing line in a packing plant. Systematic sampling is technically a form of probability sampling, especially if the starting point is chosen at random. However, investigators should be alert for any natural periodicities in the population being sampled that might influence the representativeness of the sample population.

9.7.1.3 Stratified random sampling

In **stratified random sampling** the population is divided into subgroups according to characteristics such as age, breed, sex, or severity of clinical condition, and a random sample is taken from each of these **strata**. Stratified random sampling can be used to ensure consistency of precision across strata, or to ensure that geographically dispersed strata are proportionately represented. For example, in studying the incidence of adverse effects of early neutering, a feline population might be stratified by sex and age at gonadectomy (<5 and 5 months of age) and equal numbers of individuals then randomly selected from each stratum. This would yield incidence estimates for each sex/age at gonadectomy stratum with comparable precision. Alternatively, if we wish to estimate the regional prevalence of a disease among cattle, herd sampling could be proportional to the representation of dairy vs. beef cattle in the entire population.

9.7.1.4 Cluster sampling

Cluster sampling is the process of taking a random sample of natural groupings (**clusters**) of individuals from a population. Cluster sampling is useful for obtaining a representative sample from a widely dispersed population when it is impractical or costly to randomly sample the entire population. For example, a review of medical records of canine and feline cases of dental disease selected randomly from all cases seen in practices statewide would not be possible, as there is no statewide list of discharge diagnoses for private practices. The study could be conducted, however, by selecting a random sample of veterinary practices statewide and then reviewing all cases of canine and feline dental disease from each. **Two-stage cluster sampling** is used to draw a sample from populations that are organized into discrete subunits, such as city blocks in human communities, or pens of hogs in a finishing unit. The first stage consists of drawing a random sample of subunits (city blocks or pens) for sampling. The second stage consists of drawing a random sample of individuals from the subunits selected in the first stage.

Cluster sampling provides a way to reduce the difficulty and expense associated with population-based sampling, but there are some disadvantages. As naturally occurring groups tend to be relatively homogeneous, a relatively large number of clusters, heterogeneous for the variables of interest, should be sampled to ensure that the sample is representative of the population. Furthermore, because of the way the sample is selected, data analysis is more complex than for the previously described sampling strategies.

Example 9.4

Early-age (pediatric) neutering has been promoted as a way to reduce the population of dogs and cats in animal shelters. However, little is known about the perceived risks and benefits of early neutering among veterinary practitioners, and the actual long-term consequences. Spain et al. (2002) surveyed a simple random sample of 627 veterinary practitioners from a sampling frame of 1722 AVMA member veterinarians in canine and feline practices in the state of New York. Each received a pretested questionnaire, cover letter, and prepaid business reply envelope. Nonresponders were sent two reminders. The overall response rate to the survey was 66.9%. Respondents were asked to list what they believed were the general benefits and risks of neutering dogs and cats at 4 months of age. A total of 93 medical and behavioral benefits and 118 medical and behavioral risks were identified. The most common appear in Table 9.3 and Table 9.4.

The actual risks and benefits of early-age neutering of cats and dogs were assessed in follow-up studies (Spain et al., 2004a,b). Historical cohorts were selected through stratified random sampling of all cats and dogs gonadectomized and subsequently adopted at 6 weeks to 1 years of age from the Erie County, New York Society for the Prevention of Cruelty to Animals (SPCA) between July 1989 and November 1998. From 100 to 125 representatives of each species were randomly sampled from the sampling frame for each of four strata: male and female cats or dogs gonadectomized before 5.5 months of age and at or after 5.5 months of age. Follow-up data were sought from all adopters of sampled cats or dogs (who had not initially declined) through a questionnaire, with two follow-up mailings to nonresponders, as described above. A total of 1579 (84.2%) cat adopters and 1659 (79%) dog adopters completed the questionnaire. Medical records for all clinics (n = 71) for which five or more adopters gave authorization to review their cats' records were abstracted by study personnel for computer entry.

A total of 47 outcomes were evaluated for cats and 56 for dogs. Chi-square and Student's t-test were used for categorical and normally distributed continuous

Table 9.3 Perceived Medical and Behavioral Benefits of Early Neutering of Dogs and Cats among Veterinarians[a]

Perceived Benefits	% Listing
Medical (n = 93)	
Lowered risk of:	
Mammary cancer	63.1
Prostatic disease	31.6
Pyometra	23.7
Testicular cancer	14.5
Unplanned pregnancy	7.9
Anal gland cancer	4.0
Behavioral (n = 59)	
Lowered risk of:	
Aggression	52.8
Spraying, marking, or territorial behavior	51.9
Roaming behavior or getting hit by a car	16.5
Sexual behavior	8.9
Increased trainability	8.9

[a] Responses provided by at least 4% of veterinarians regarding specific benefits not listed on the survey form.

Source: Spain, C.V. et al., *J. Am. Anim. Hosp. Assoc.*, 38, 482–488, 2002. With permission.

Table 9.4 Perceived Medical and Behavioral Risks of Early Neutering of Dogs and Cats among Veterinarians[a]

Perceived Risks	% Listing
Medical (n = 118)	
Increased risk of:	
FLUTD[b] or a related complication	39.8
Urinary incontinence	16.7
Persistent juvenile vulva, vaginitis, or perivulvular dermatitis	13.0
Impairment of physical development or bone growth	13.0
Adrenal gland dysfunction	10.2
Obesity	6.5
Behavioral (n = 32)	
Increased risk of:	
Aggression in female dogs	25.0
Fearfulness or psychological trauma	25.0
Problems with socialization	16.7
Difficulty in training	16.7
Lower confidence level in male dogs	8.3
Submissive urination	4.2

[a] Responses provided by at least 4% of veterinarians regarding specific risks not listed on the survey form.

[b] FLUTD = feline lower urinary tract disease.

Source: Spain, C.V. et al., *J. Am. Anim. Hosp. Assoc.*, 38, 482–488, 2002. With permission.

Table 9.5 Medical Conditions Associated with Age at Gonadectomy in 1579 Cats

Condition	Age at Gonadectomy (mo)	Incidence Density[a]	Hazard Ratio[b]	95% CI	Overall p Value
Abscesses[c]	<3.5	0.88	0.53[d]	0.18–1.60	0.05
	3.5 to <5.5	0.26	0.08	0.01–0.71	
	5.5	1.26	1.0	NA	
Feline asthma	Continuous	0.14	0.77[e]	0.58–0.93	0.01
Gingivitis	<3.5	2.12	0.67	0.43–1.05	0.02
	3.5 to <5.5	1.61	0.45	0.24–0.87	
	5.5	3.24	1.0	NA	

Note: 95% CI = confidence interval for the hazard ratio; NA = not applicable (referent category).

[a] Incidence density/100 cat years at risk.

[b] Hazard ratio adjusted for cat's age at time of disease onset.

[c] For male cats only.

[d] Interaction between age at gonadectomy and follow-up time was significant; therefore, hazard ratios for abscesses were valid only near beginning of follow-up period.

[e] Hazard ratio/1-month decrease in age at gonadectomy.

Source: Spain, C.V. et al., *J. Am. Vet. Med. Assoc.*, 224, 372–379, 2004a. With permission.

data (respectively) where multivariable modeling was not required. Multivariable analyses were performed to determine whether age at gonadectomy was related to the occurrence of outcomes, while controlling for the effect of potentially confounding variables. Most behavioral outcomes were dichotomous, without time-to-event information, and were analyzed with unconditional logistic regression. Most medical outcomes were recorded as time-to-event data (i.e., time from adoption until diagnosis of the condition or end of follow-up) and were analyzed by use of multivariable survival analysis (Cox proportional hazards model).

A significant relationship with age at gonadectomy was found for three medical and five behavioral conditions in cats (Table 9.5 and Table 9.6), and four medical and eight behavioral conditions in dogs (Table 9.7 and Table 9.8). Overweight body condition (obesity) in dogs is not included in Table 9.2 but was significantly associated with age at gonadectomy (odds ratio per 1-month decrease in age at gonadectomy, 0.94; $p = 0.04$). The authors concluded that cats can be safely neutered at a young age without any serious medical or behavioral consequences. Likewise, male dogs can be safely neutered at an early age, but gonadectomy in female dogs should be postponed until at least 3 months of age because of the risk of urinary incontinence.

The authors discussed several potential biases in their studies, including (1) failure to detect extremely rare conditions because of low statistical power, (2) misclassification of medical or behavioral conditions, and (3) type I errors due to the large number of comparisons made. These data reveal a marked discrepancy between perceived and actual medical and behavioral risks associated with early neutering, and illustrate the potential risk of relying on expert opinion (authority) rather than objective evidence.

Table 9.6 Behavioral Conditions Associated with Age at Gonadectomy in 1579 Cats

Behavior	Age at Gonadectomy (mo)	Cats with Behavior (%)	Odds Ratio	95% CI	Overall p Value
Aggression toward veterinarians[a]	Continuous	2.5	0.77[b]	0.63–0.98	0.03
Hiding frequently[a,c]	Continuous	14.5	1.11[b]	1.02–1.20	0.01
Hyperactivity	<3.5	16.0	0.67	0.51–0.90	0.01
	3.5 to < 5.5	14.4	0.60	0.40–0.89	
	5.5	22.1	1.0	NA	
Sexual behaviors[a,c]	Continuous	12.2	0.93[b]	0.86–1.01	0.09
Shyness around strangers[c]	Continuous	56.3	1.04[b]	1.00–1.09	0.03
Urine spraying[a]	Continuous	2.1	0.79[b]	0.64–0.97	0.02

[a] Male cats only.

[b] Odds ratio/1-month decrease in age at gonadectomy.

[c] Not significant ($p > 0.05$) when considered a serious problem.

See Table 9.5 for remainder of key.

Source: Spain, C.V. et al., *J. Am. Vet. Med. Assoc.*, 224, 372–379, 2004a. With permission.

Table 9.7 Medical Conditions Other Than Obesity Associated with Age at Gonadectomy in 1659 Dogs

Condition	Age at Gonadectomy (mo)	Incidence Density[a]	Hazard Ratio[b]	95% CI	Overall p Value
Cystitis[c]	<5.5	1.38	2.76	1.08–7.14	0.02
	5.5	0.43	1.0	NA	
Hip dysplasia	<5.5	1.36	1.70	1.04–2.78	0.03
	5.5	0.98	1.0	NA	
Urinary incontinence[c]	Continuous	1.19	1.20[d]	1.06–1.35	< 0.01

Note: 95% CI = confidence interval for the hazard ratio; NA = not applicable (referent category).

[a] Incidence density/100 dog years at risk.

[b] Hazard ratio adjusted for dog's age at time of disease onset.

[c] For female dogs only.

[d] Hazard ratio/1-month decrease in age at gonadectomy.

Source: Spain, C.V. et al., *J. Am. Vet. Med. Assoc.*, 224, 380–387, 2004b. With permission.

9.7.2   Nonprobability sampling

In some cases, a nonprobability sampling design may be the only option available to the investigator. Reasons include cost, convenience, and the nature of the accessible population (those willing to submit data, for example). If a nonprobability sample is to be used, it is important that it approximate, as closely as possible, the kind of sample that would be obtained by probability sampling, as statistical tests are likely to be applied to the results. This is the same consideration when choosing an accessible population, e.g., that it be representative of the target population.

Table 9.8 Behavioral Conditions Associated with Age at Gonadectomy in 1659 Dogs

Condition	Age at Gonadectomy (mo)	Dogs with Behavior (%)	Odds Ratio	95% CI	Overall p Value
Aggression toward household members[a]	<5.5	29.0	1.32	1.05–2.10	0.02
	5.5	21.5	1.0	NA	
Barking that bothered household members[a,b]	Continuous	34.2	1.08[c]	1.02–1.12	<0.01
Barking or growling at visitors[a,b]	Continuous	65.4	1.08[c]	1.02–1.13	<0.01
Escaping from home (serious problem)	Continuous	9.6	0.93[c]	0.87–0.98	<0.01
Noise phobia[b]	Continuous	52.6	1.04[c]	1.01–1.08	<0.01
Separation anxiety	<5.5	14.2	0.72	0.55–0.94	0.02
	5.5	18.7	1.0	NA	
Sexual behaviors[b]	Continuous	27.3	1.05[c]	1.01–1.09	<0.01
Urination when frightened[c]	<5.5	9.4	0.74	0.54–1.01	0.06
	5.5	12.3	1.0	NA	

[a] Male dogs only.

[b] Not significant ($p > 0.05$) when considered a serious problem.

[c] Odds ratio/1-month decrease in age at gonadectomy.

See Table 9.7 for remainder of key.

Source: Spain, C.V. et al., *J. Am. Vet. Med. Assoc.*, 224, 380–387, 2004b. With permission.

9.7.2.1 Consecutive sampling

Consecutive sampling involves taking every patient from the accessible population who meets the selection criteria over a specified interval or number of patients. If the data to be gathered can be influenced by temporal disease patterns, then the sampling period should be of sufficient duration to accommodate this variation.

9.7.2.2 Convenience sampling

Convenience sampling is the process of selecting those members of the accessible population who are easily accessible. Patient selection is often based on willingness of owners to participate in the study. As such, there is always the risk that study subjects do not accurately represent the population at large. Investigators should address this concern in discussing study results.

9.7.2.3 Judgmental sampling

Judgmental sampling involves selecting from the accessible population those individuals judged most appropriate for the study. In this regard judgmental sampling is susceptible to the same biases as convenience sampling.

Example 9.5

Medical records data can be used by veterinary practitioners to better understand and anticipate health problems of importance in cats and dogs they examine and to better communicate with clients regarding the most prevalent disorders. Observational studies in companion animal research are often based on patients seen at veterinary teaching hospitals (VTHs). Since many of these animals are referred to the VTH with diseases that are difficult to diagnose and treat, they may not be representative of the general population seen at private veterinary practices. Lund et al. (1999) conducted a survey to estimate the prevalence of the most common disorders of dogs and cats examined at private veterinary practices in the U.S. A sample of 31,484 dogs and 15,226 cats was drawn from patients seen at 52 private veterinary practices that used the same computer-based practice management system. Referral and specialty practices were excluded from the survey. Practices that volunteered to participate in the study were randomly assigned, based on geographic region, to collect data on all cats and dogs examined by any veterinarian in the practice over four specific but not consecutive month-long periods during the year. Approximately 1300 codes for diagnoses, body condition score, and diet were used by participants to record findings of each canine or feline patient seen during the assigned interval and entered into each patient's computer-based medical record system by hospital staff. At the end of each of the four data collection periods computerized data were compiled into a single file and sent to the investigators, where it was uploaded into the research project database for further analysis. Prevalence estimates and frequencies for population description were generated using statistical software.

Fifty-two (82.5%) of 63 practices that were mailed study materials completed all four data collection periods. The most common disorders reported for dogs and cats are ranked in Table 9.9 and Table 9.10. Dental calculus and gingivitis were the most commonly reported disorders. About 7% of dogs and 10% of cats examined by practitioners during the study were considered healthy. Many conditions were common to both species (e.g., flea infestation, conjunctivitis, diarrhea, vomiting). Dogs were likely to be examined because of lameness, disk disease, lipoma, and allergic dermatitis. Cats were likely to be examined because of renal disease, cystitis, feline urologic syndrome, and inappetence.

This study actually used two sampling strategies to select patients for inclusion in the study. The practitioners who participated were a self-selected **convenience sample** of all practitioners using a particular practice management system. Those who agreed to participate in the study then collected data on a **consecutive sample** of all cats and dogs examined by any veterinarian in the practice during the prescribed data collection period. The authors caution that the generalizability of results is limited by a number of factors, including:

- The representativeness of participating practitioners, who constituted only about 3.5% of all companion animal practitioners who used the particular practice management system.
- The lack of case definitions and possibility of disease misclassification and underreporting of disorders requiring extensive or expensive diagnostic testing.
- Underreporting due to failure to code; 64% of total unique animal records lacked diagnostic codes, although some were probably client examinations not involving animal examination (pet food, fecals).
- Failure to distinguish between new (incident) and existing (prevalent) disorders, which limited use of data for monitoring disease trends.

Table 9.9 The 29 Most Common Disorders Reported for 31,484 Dogs Examined at Private Veterinary Practices in the U.S.

Disorder	Prevalence (%)	95% CI
Dental calculus	20.5	20.0–20.9
Gingivitis	19.5	19.1–20.0
Otitis externa	13.0	12.6–13.4
Healthy animal	6.8	6.5–7.1
Dermatitis	4.9	4.7–5.2
Flea infestation	4.4	4.2–4.6
Allergy	4.0	3.8–4.2
Lump	3.6	3.4–3.8
Pyoderma	3.4	3.2–3.6
Atopic/allergic dermatitis	3.1	2.9–3.3
Lameness	3.1	2.9–3.3
Conjunctivitis	3.0	2.8–3.2
Anal sac disease	2.5	2.3–2.6
Animal bite	2.5	2.3–2.7
Arthritis	2.4	2.3–2.6
Lipoma	2.3	2.1–2.5
Diarrhea	2.2	2.0–2.4
Heart murmur	2.2	2.1–2.4
Moist dermatitis	2.2	2.0–2.3
Periodontal disease	2.2	2.0–2.3
Vomiting	2.1	2.0–2.3
Obesity	2.0	1.8–2.2
Fungal otitis externa	2.0	1.8–2.1
Roundworm infection	1.9	1.8–2.1
Atopy	1.6	1.5–1.8
Cataract	1.6	1.4–1.7
Disk disease	1.6	1.5–1.7
Nuclear sclerosis	1.6	1.5–1.8
Pruritis	1.6	1.5–1.8

Note: CI = confidence interval.

Source: Lund, E.M. et al., *J. Am. Vet. Med. Assoc.*, 214, 1336–1341, 1999. With permission.

9.8   *Multiple comparisons*

Some studies, called **hypothesis testing**, are designed to evaluate the effect of one variable (as a risk factor, prognostic factor, or treatment) on an outcome. However, during the course of a study in which statistically significant results are found, it is often tempting to break groups down into smaller groups to search for additional associations. This process is referred to as **hypothesis generation** (or more disparagingly, *data dredging* or a *fishing expedition*).

One problem with such multiple comparisons is that the resulting subgroups contain fewer individuals than did the initial groupings. Consequently, the number of individuals in these groups may be too small to allow statistically significant differences to be detected. A second problem in making multiple comparisons is similar to the problem encountered in parallel testing — if enough comparisons are made, one is more likely to detect at least one that will be statistically significant, irrespective of the true state of affairs. Consequently, results derived from multiple comparisons should be considered as hypotheses to be tested in follow-up studies.

Table 9.10 The 25 Most Common Disorders Reported for 15,226 Cats Examined at Private Veterinary Practices in the U.S.

Disorder	Prevalence (%)	95% CI
Dental calculus	24.2	23.6–24.9
Gingivitis	13.1	12.5–13.6
Healthy animal	9.5	9.1–10.0
Flea infestation	9.2	8.7–9.6
Otodectes spp. infestation	7.4	7.0–7.9
Abscess	6.5	6.1–6.9
Respiratory tract infection	5.0	4.6–5.3
Cat bite	4.7	4.4–5.0
Tapeworm infection	3.3	3.1–3.6
Periodontal disease	3.0	2.7–3.2
Conjunctivitis	2.8	2.3–3.1
Feline military dermatitis	2.3	2.0–2.5
Otitis externa	2.3	2.1–2.6
Roundworm infection	2.3	2.1–2.6
Heart murmur	2.2	1.9–2.4
Vomiting	2.2	2.0–2.4
Renal disease	1.9	1.6–2.1
Diarrhea	1.8	1.6–2.0
Obesity	1.8	1.6–2.0
Animal bite	1.7	1.5–1.9
Dermatitis	1.7	1.5–1.9
Weight loss	1.6	1.4–1.8
Cystitis	1.5	1.3–1.7
Feline urologic syndrome	1.5	1.3–1.7
Loss of appetite	1.5	1.3–1.7

Note: CI = confidence interval.

Source: Lund, E.M. et al., *J. Am. Vet. Med. Assoc.*, 214, 1336–1341, 1999. With permission.

▼

If enough comparisons are made, one is more likely to detect at least one that will be statistically significant, irrespective of the true state of affairs.

▲

9.9 Summary

Statistical analyses, once a rarity in medical journals, are now routinely encountered in the medical literature, and veterinary journals are no exception. Such analyses often have immense practical importance, since research results are frequently the basis for decisions about patient care. Statistical analyses give us an idea of the level of confidence that we can have in our results.

Statistical tests reported in the medical literature are usually used to disprove the null hypothesis, e.g., the assumption that no difference exists between groups. By default, the alternative hypothesis would state that a difference exists. Research hypotheses are usually stated as either directional or nondirectional; e.g., either they specify in which direction a difference exists or they do not. If differences are detected, they are reported with the corresponding *p* value, which expresses the likelihood that the observed differences could have arisen by chance alone. The *p* values are expressed as one-tailed or two-tailed in accordance with whether the hypothesis being tested is directional or nondirectional, respectively.

The alternative hypothesis cannot be tested directly; it is accepted by default if the test of statistical significance rejects the null hypothesis. The null hypothesis is rejected in favor of the alternative hypothesis if the p value is less than the predetermined level of statistical significance. By convention, this is usually 5%; e.g., we are willing to erroneously conclude that an association between predictor and outcome variables exists less than 5% of the time. Since not everyone agrees with this criterion, it is preferable to specify the actual probability of this error, such as $p = 0.10$, $p = 0.005$, etc. The confidence interval provides a way of expressing the range over which a value is likely to occur.

Many of the rules that apply to the interpretation of statistical tests are similar to those discussed earlier in the context of diagnostic tests. In the usual situation, the outcome of a clinical study is expressed in dichotomous terms: either a difference exists or it does not. Since we are using samples to predict the true state of affairs in the population, there always exists a chance that we will come to the wrong conclusion. There are thus four possible outcomes of statistical tests: two are correct and two are incorrect. Alpha or type I error results when we conclude that outcomes were different when in fact they were not. Alpha error is analogous to the false positive result of diagnostic tests. Beta or type II error occurs when we conclude that outcomes were not different when in fact they were. Beta error is analogous to the false negative result of diagnostic tests. Power is the probability that a study will find a statistically significant difference when one exists. Power is analogous to diagnostic test sensitivity. P_b is the major determinant of sample size in disease eradication programs that rely on diagnostic tests to identify infected animals or herds, e.g., distinguish them from uninfected herds, even when the number of infected animals is low.

Statistics are also used to describe the degree of association between variables. The level of agreement between two or more test results (when expressed as categorical variables) is frequently expressed as the kappa (k) statistic, defined as the proportion of potential agreement beyond chance. The value of kappa ranges from –1.0 (perfect disagreement) through 0.0 (chance agreement only) to +1.0 (perfect agreement). The Pearson correlation coefficient, r, is a measure of the degree of linear association between two interval-level variables. The value of r may take any value between –1 and 1. If r is either –1 or 1, the variables have a perfect linear relationship. If r is near –1 or 1, there is a high degree of linear correlation. A positive correlation means that as one variable increases, the other increases. A negative correlation means that as one variable increases, the other decreases. If r is equal to 0, we say the variables are uncorrelated and that there is no linear association between them. In some cases, an association between variables may exist, but it is not strictly linear. Spearman's correlation coefficient, or Spearman rho, is the counterpart of the Pearson correlation coefficient for ordinal data.

The Pearson correlation coefficient is the square root of the coefficient of determination, r^2, which is a measure of closeness of fit of the data to the linear regression line. The value for r^2 expresses the amount of variation in the data that is accounted for by the linear relationship between two variables and may take any value between 0 and 1. The coefficient of determination is sensitive to the variability in data. As the amount of variability, or scatter, around the fitted regression line increases, the value of r^2 decreases. An r^2 value of 1 means that all values fall on the regression line.

All of the common statistical tests are used to estimate the probability of an alpha error, e.g., the likelihood of concluding that a difference exists when in fact it does not. The validity of each test depends on certain assumptions about the data. If the data at hand do not satisfy these assumptions, the resulting P_a may be misleading. Among the considerations in choosing a statistical test are (1) whether the data are nominal, ordinal, or interval, (2) the number of groups being compared, (3) whether the groups are independent or related, (4) the number and size of categories (for nominal data), and (5) how we intend to compare the data (for ordinal data).

It is intuitively obvious that the more subjects that are entered into a study, the greater confidence we can have that differences among groups are not due to random variation. The question is, how many subjects are necessary to ensure the power of anticipated or published studies? One or more of the following variables must be considered to optimize the power of a particular study: (1) the frequency of disease, (2) the amount of variability among individuals, (3) the difference in outcome between study groups, (4) P_a, and (5) P_b. Three common situations where sample size must be considered are (1) minimum sample size for demonstrating an extreme outcome, (2) minimum sample size for estimating a rate or proportion with a specified degree of precision, and (3) minimum sample size to detect differences among groups in studies of risk, prognosis, and treatment.

Sampling should be conducted in such a way that the individuals selected for study are an unbiased representation of the population. Sampling strategies fall within two broad classes — probability and nonprobability — each with several versions. Probability sampling includes simple random, systematic, stratified random, and cluster sampling. Nonprobability sampling includes consecutive, convenience, and judgmental sampling.

chapter 10

Medical ecology and outbreak investigation

10.1 Introduction

The previous chapters have focused on clinical epidemiology and the role of population characteristics in veterinary decision making. We have discussed the criteria by which clinically normal findings are distinguished from abnormal findings, factors affecting the interpretation and use of diagnostic tests, ways to measure the frequency of clinical events and their use to assess risk, prognosis, and treatment outcomes, and the role of chance in clinical research. In the following chapters we will discuss the dynamics of disease in populations, e.g., **medical ecology**. We will also learn how to conduct an outbreak investigation using all of the concepts, tools, and approaches discussed in previous chapters.

One of the things that distinguishes veterinary from human medicine is that veterinarians are frequently called on to diagnose and treat disease in populations as well as individuals. The health of an individual animal may be less important than that of the flock, kennel, or herd. However, the disease status of an individual animal frequently reflects that of the population from which it came. In other words, the animals that we see as clinicians may be regarded as **sentinels** for disease in the population.

▼

> The disease status of an individual animal frequently reflects that of the population from which it came. The animals that we see as clinicians may be regarded as sentinels for disease in the population.

▲

Practitioners are frequently called on to participate in local, state, and federal disease control programs. To perform in this capacity, veterinarians must understand and be able to communicate the scientific basis of these disease control programs to their clients. As veterinarians, we are expected to know how diseases are introduced, spread, and persist in animal populations. We must determine the cause of disease and also devise a plan to reduce disease frequency to an acceptable level. What is acceptable will depend on the cost of the disease and the cost of control.

10.2 Issues in the epidemiology of a disease

A number of issues emerge when considering the epidemiology of any disease. A distinction must be drawn between the **life cycle** of a disease agent, which describes the movement of a disease agent in the environment, and the **epidemiology of a disease** (or medical ecology), which describes the dynamics of a disease in the population. The life cycle of the disease agent is only part of the story. The major issues in the epidemiology of a disease are described below.

10.2.1 Occurrence

In Chapter 5 some of the measures of disease frequency were discussed. **Occurrence** refers to the frequency distribution of disease over **space** (spatial or geographic occurrence), time (temporal occurrence), or within a host population (demographics). This information is useful to gain a better appreciation of not only the significance of the disease, but also its probable cause, source, and mode of transmission.

10.2.2 Cause

Causes, or **determinants**, of disease include the etiologic agents directly responsible for disease and other factors that facilitate exposure, multiplication, and spread in the population. Disease determinants can be categorized as **agent, host,** and **environment** (or management) factors.

▼

> Disease determinants can be categorized as agent, host, and environment (or management) factors.

▲

10.2.3 Susceptibility

Host determinants of disease occurrence include both individual characteristics of hosts that render them susceptible or resistant to disease, and population characteristics, such as the level of **herd immunity**. Just as parasitic organisms have defined life cycle stages, a diseased population may be divided into **epidemiologic classes**. Typical epidemiologic classes are susceptible, incubating, sick, recovered, and immune. The proportion of the population in each of these classes will determine, in part, the dynamics of disease transmission within the population.

10.2.4 Source

Sources of disease agents include (1) recently infected individuals, (2) carrier animals (animals with inapparent infections that are also transmitters or potential transmitters of the infectious agent), (3) intermediate hosts and vectors, and (4) the environment. For every clinical case of a disease there may be numerous other inapparent infections. Some may be individuals in the incubation or prepatent phase of the disease. Others may be recovered individuals who continue to harbor the organism. If these individuals are also infectious, they may be a major source, or reservoir, of infection for susceptibles.

▼

> A diseased population may be divided into epidemiologic classes. Typical epidemiologic classes are susceptible, incubating, sick, recovered, and immune.

▲

10.2.5   Transmission

Diseases are broadly classified as **transmissible** or **nontransmissible** (Toma et al., 1999). Within these two broad categories there are a number of specific modes of transmission. A distinction must be made between the **mode of transmission** and the **route of infection**. It would be incorrect to say that the mode of transmission is via the respiratory tract since we have not indicated whether the organisms gained access via droplet transmission (direct transmission) or droplet nuclei or dust (airborne transmission). The respiratory tract is really a route of infection rather than a mode of transmission.

10.2.6   Cost

In food-producing and other animals raised and managed for profit, the impact of disease is frequently described in terms of performance or economics, rather than morbidity and mortality. Likewise, decisions as to whether to treat or cull the animal may be determined in large part by economics. Any assessment of cost should include the cost of disease control.

10.2.7   Control

Ultimately the practitioner must devise a plan for the reduction of disease risk or frequency in the population. This may be accomplished through disease prevention, control (treatment), or eradication.

10.3   Outbreak investigation

Outbreak investigation, sometimes referred to as field epidemiology, is similar, in principle, to examination of a patient in a hospital setting. In both instances history, physical, and laboratory examinations are used to try to identify the cause(s) of disease at the individual or herd level. Working hypotheses at the herd level are (1) diseases usually have multiple causes, and (2) disease events are not randomly distributed in a population. Typically, disease frequency and distribution data are collected and analyzed to identify disease patterns (occurrence), which are then analyzed to suggest determinants of disease.

By tracing the steps involved in an outbreak investigation we can better appreciate the importance of the issues in the epidemiology of a disease. The steps are analogous to the systematic approach (**SOAP**) used with individual patients. Components of an epidemiologic workup are described in the following subsections.

10.3.1   Descriptive phase (subjective, objective data)

The distribution of cases during an outbreak follows certain patterns in time (chronology), space (geography), and hosts (demography). The chronological distribution of disease events can be recognized by plotting the frequency of new cases over time, resulting in an epidemic curve. The geographic distribution can be recognized using various types of maps, most commonly spot maps. The demographic patterns of disease distribution can be identified by comparing frequency rates in different strata based on age, sex, breed, etc., and depicted as attack rate tables or graphs. Among the questions asked during this phase of outbreak investigation are the following:

1.   What are the characteristics of the clinical syndrome, e.g., the case definition?
    a.   What signs were/are observed in live and dead animals?
    b.   What was the incubation period?

  c. How long did signs last?

  d. What is the prognosis for diseased animals?

2. What are the temporal, spatial, and demographic patterns of disease?

  a. When did the cases occur?

  b. Where did the cases occur?

  c. What was the incidence of disease? For example, how many animals were at risk and how many were affected?

  d. What are the characteristics of the affected and unaffected animals?

  e. How rapidly did the disease spread and what is the likely mode of transmission?

  f. Are any other domestic animals or wildlife affected? Is there any concurrent human illness?

3. What is the herd history?

  a. Describe the management and husbandry practices, including housing, feed, water.

  b. Describe disease control/hygiene practices, including vaccination, parasiticides/dewormers, other treatments, vermin and pest control, and waste disposal.

  c. Describe the herd's production/disease history.

  d. Has there been contact with other domestic animals or wildlife?

  e. Has there been any animal movement or introductions recently?

  f. Have there been any health problems in adjacent herds?

4. What is the environmental history?

  a. What has the weather been like?

  b. Describe the geographic location, e.g., topography, soil type, vegetation.

  c. Have fertilizers, herbicides, pesticides been used recently?

The answers to the above questions should help guide sample collection and the selection of appropriate diagnostic test procedures.

10.3.2 Analytic phase (assessment)

During this phase the descriptive data are compared and analyzed in light of what is known about diseases on the differential list and whatever laboratory test results had been requested.

1. What associations exist? For example, what risk factors appear to be associated with the disease?

2. What is the probable source of the etiologic agent and how is it being spread?

3. What is the probable cause of the disease?

4. How much does the disease cost?

10.3.3 Intervention (plan)

What are you going to do? This is why you became involved in the first place.

1. Are current measures adequate to control the outbreak? What else should be done?

2. What immediate and long-term preventive options are available?

3. What are the economic benefits/consequences of these options?

In the following chapters each of the issues in the epidemiology of a disease is discussed. Case studies are included to illustrate how outbreak investigations are conducted.

10.4 Summary

A number of issues surface when considering the epidemiology of any disease. These include its cause, occurrence, source and transmission, determinants of the susceptibility of individuals and populations, the cost of the disease, and measures that can be used to achieve control.

Outbreak investigation is similar, in principle, to examination of a patient in a hospital setting. In both instances history, physical, and laboratory examinations are used to try to identify the cause(s) of disease at the herd or individual level. Working hypotheses at the herd level are (1) diseases usually have multiple causes, and (2) disease events are not randomly distributed in a population. Typically, disease frequency and distribution data are collected and analyzed to identify disease patterns (occurrence), which are then analyzed to suggest possible causes. Disease determinants are generally divided into three categories: agent, host, and environment.

An epidemiologic workup is similar to the clinical assessment of individual patients and includes descriptive, analytical, and intervention phases. During the descriptive phase data are collected from the herd and the patterns of disease occurrence over time, space, and among hosts are described. During the analytic phase the descriptive data are compared and analyzed in light of what is known about diseases on the differential list. During the intervention phase an optimal disease control plan is selected based on the best combination of immediate and long-term objectives.

chapter 11

Measuring and expressing occurrence

11.1 Introduction

Earlier in the text we discussed frequency of clinical findings and disease and made a distinction between incidence and prevalence. Occurrence refers to the frequency distribution of disease over space (spatial or geographic occurrence), time (temporal occurrence), or within a host population. Not only is this information useful for gaining a better appreciation of the significance of the disease, but it may suggest the probable cause, source, and mode of transmission of the condition.

11.2 Case definition

The first step in any disease investigation is identification of the cases and noncases. This is not as easy as it might first appear. In studies of the characteristics of experimentally induced disease, animals are easily separated into cases and noncases on the basis of their exposure history. When faced with a disease outbreak, however, we usually do not know the nature of the exposure, or which animals were exposed. We only have our perceptions of which animals are sick and which are not.

11.2.1 Based on disease signs, symptoms, and epidemiology

Cases may be defined on the basis of a discrete set of signs and symptoms. However, few animals show the complete range of disease signs, and minimal criteria for a diagnosis often have to be established. Biological variation among true cases and noncases has the effect of including cases among the noncases and vice versa. Furthermore, in any population there will always be animals with inapparent infections. Some cases will be incorrectly assigned to the noncase group. Clinical signs alone are seldom restrictive enough to exclude animals who are not suffering from the disease in question, but who may exhibit signs consistent with it. In these cases, epidemiologic criteria, such as the occurrence of the disease, may be added to the case definition.

11.2.2 Based on performance

Cases do not have to be defined on the basis of a clinically defined syndrome. Frequently we are interested in identifying risk factors associated with substandard performance. Producers usually become aware of a disease condition by its adverse effect on animal performance.

11.3   Reporting disease occurrence

The occurrence of disease in a population may be reported in three different ways:

1. **Host characteristics**, such as age, sex, and breed
2. **Time**, which includes date of onset
3. **Place**, from within a housing unit to geographic distribution

Scrutiny of the results of such classification enables one to recognize characteristics common among affected individuals and rare among the healthy (Morton et al., 1990).

11.3.1   Host distribution

11.3.1.1   Attack rate

Earlier in this book we discussed incidence and prevalence, incidence being the number of new cases occurring in a susceptible population over a defined time interval, and prevalence being the number of sick individuals at any given point in time. A third rate that is frequently used, particularly during outbreak investigations, is the **attack rate**. An attack rate measures the proportion of the population that develops disease among the total exposed at the beginning of the outbreak (Morton et al., 1990). The attack rate equals

$$\frac{\text{Number who become sick}}{\text{Number at risk at beginning of outbreak}}$$

The attack rate is essentially an incidence rate where the time period of interest is the duration of the epidemic.

11.3.1.2   Crude vs. adjusted rates

Comparison of disease rates among different groups is fundamental to determining the cause, source, and probable mode of transmission of a disease. Since comparison of crude rates (see Chapter 5) can lead to erroneous conclusions, it is necessary to adjust for any host factors that might interfere with an accurate comparison. Rates are commonly adjusted for age, breed, and sex (see Chapter 5).

11.3.2   Temporal distribution

Most diseases have characteristic patterns of temporal occurrence. When disease is first recognized in a population, frequency data should be used to construct an **epidemic curve**. An epidemic curve gives a convenient pictorial depiction of the epidemic, and certain limited deductions may be drawn. Specifically, we want to know whether the disease is sporadic, endemic, or epidemic. The answer to this question often gives important clues as to the mode of transmission of a disease agent and its identity and suggests what subsequent steps should be taken.

11.3.2.1   Sporadic disease

A disease is **sporadic** when it occurs rarely and without regularity in a population unit. A sporadic pattern of occurrence elicits the question: Where is the disease when it apparently is not around? One explanation might be that infection exists in the population inapparently and only in occasional animals do signs of disease evidence themselves. An example might be fleabite dermatitis in cats and dogs. Most have fleas, but few develop severe reactions to infestation. A second explanation might be that the infection is generally absent and the disease is noted only when it is introduced into the population with an infected animal (as bovine tuberculosis), a suitable vector (as West Nile virus), or occasional contact with an environmental source, either animal (as plague) or inanimate (as tetanus).

11.3.2.2 Endemic disease

A disease is **endemic** when it occurs with predictable regularity in a population with only minor fluctuations in frequency pattern over time. A disease may be endemic at any level of occurrence, as reflected in terms used to describe the levels of occurrence of endemic disease: (1) **holoendemic**, when most animals are affected; (2) **hyperendemic**, when a high proportion of animals are affected; (3) **mesoendemic**, when a moderate proportion of animals are affected; or (4) **hypoendemic**, when a relatively small proportion of animals are affected. Herd infestations with internal parasites tend to occur as endemic diseases.

11.3.2.3 Epidemic disease (outbreak)

A disease is **epidemic** when its frequency within the population during a given time interval is clearly in excess of its expected frequency. The epidemic occurrence of disease is not based on absolute numbers or rates; it is a purely relative term. Thus, whether an observed frequency of any particular disease constitutes an epidemic would vary from one place and population to another. An epidemic implies a clustering of disease in space as well as time. **Outbreak** is a somewhat less precise term, roughly synonymous with epidemic. The shape of the epidemic curve may provide clues as to the nature of exposure of susceptible individuals and the etiologic agent. A **point source epidemic** will typically have an epidemic curve that is skewed to the right; exposure occurs over a relative short period, and the tail reflects variable incubation periods. **Propagating epidemics** often have a curve skewed to the left, reflecting long-term exposure to the disease agent. A **pandemic** is a large-scale epidemic over a wide geographic region. Conditions leading to an epidemic are essentially the same as those outlined for sporadic disease. Whether a disease presents as sporadic or epidemic is also a function of the efficiency of transmission of infection from infected to susceptible animals.

Stylized temporal patterns of disease occurrence are depicted in Figure 11.1, and specific examples in Figure 11.2 and Figure 11.3. Figure 11.2 depicts sporadic occurrence (incidence during December 1983) of new cases of clinical mastitis in dairy cows, followed by several outbreaks. The initial sporadic cases were attributed to opportunistic infections with *Serratia liquefaciens* in teats damaged by severe cold. Subsequent epidemics were attributed to mechanical spread to other cows with damaged teats during the milking procedure (Bowman et al., 1986).

Figure 11.3 depicts an epidemic of infertility in a 940-cow dairy herd attributed to trichomoniasis (Goodger and Skirrow, 1986). Overall prevalence of infection (crude rate) during January 1985 was 10.67%, based on culture results. During the latter half of 1984 the temporal occurrence was consistent with the definition of a propagating epidemic, suggesting unabated spread of the agent to susceptible animals.

11.3.3 Time series analysis

Time series analysis is concerned with the detection, description, and measurement of patterns or periodicities from temporal disease occurrence data (Schwabe et al., 1977). The purpose of time series analysis is to identify periods of high or low risk so that causal associations can be explored. Patterns of disease occurrence (incidence) are influenced by

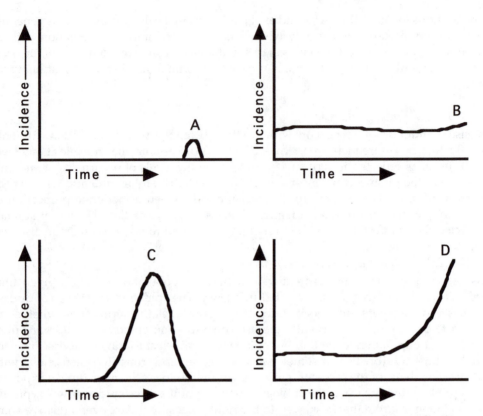

Figure 11.1 Examples of patterns of disease occurrence: (A) sporadic, (B) endemic, (C) point source epidemic, and (D) propagating epidemic. (From Schwabe, C.W. et al., *Epidemiology in Veterinary Practice*, Lea & Febiger, Philadelphia, 1977. With permission.)

one or more of the following: (1) secular trend, (2) seasonal fluctuation, (3) cyclic variation, and (4) irregular variation (Carter et al., 1986).

Patterns of disease occurrence are influenced by one or more of the following: (1) secular trend, (2) seasonal fluctuation, (3) cyclic variation, and (4) irregular variation.

Secular trends are overall long-term rises or declines in incidence rate that occur gradually over long periods. A secular trend can be identified from time series data by (1) visual observation of plotted raw data, (2) least squares regression, or (3) the moving average method (Figure 11.4 and Figure 11.5). **Least squares regression** is a statistical technique that derives a line with the least mean squared deviation from all data points. Details and assumptions of the procedure are beyond the scope of this book, but can be found in standard statistical texts. It is a standard option on statistical calculators and statistical packages for computers. A **moving average** is a series of data averages centered at each successive measurement point on the timescale (Schwabe et al., 1977). Twelve-month moving averages can be used to smooth out or eliminate irregular variations and those with periodicities of 12 months or less. The result is an approximate secular trend line.

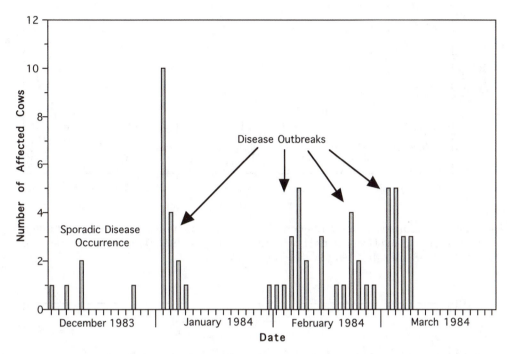

Figure 11.2 Temporal distribution of clinical mastitis treated in a herd. Sporadic incidence during December 1983 is followed by a series of epidemics from January through March 1984. (From Bowman, G.L. et al., *J. Am. Vet. Med. Assoc.*, 189, 913–915, 1986. With permission.)

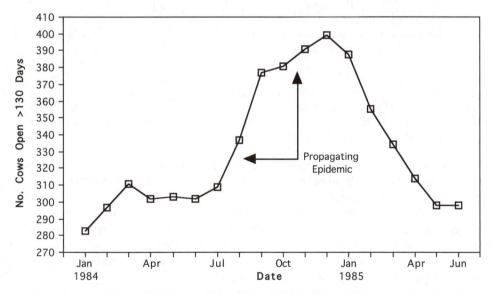

Figure 11.3 A propagating epidemic of infertility in a 940-cow dairy herd. (From Goodger, W.J. and Skirrow, S.Z., *J. Am. Vet. Med. Assoc.*, 189, 772–776, 1986. With permission.)

Seasonal fluctuations are regular changes in incidence rates with periods shorter than a year. Three-month moving averages help smooth out short-term data fluctuations and approximate seasonal fluctuations in disease incidence. The twelve-month moving average can also be used to calculate another index of seasonal disease incidence known as

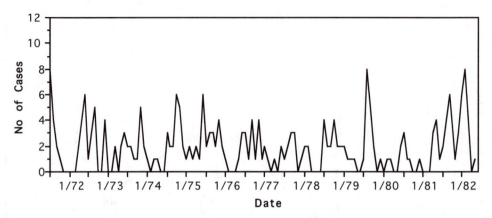

Figure 11.4 The occurrence and distribution of *Salmonella* cases among horses admitted to the Veterinary Medical Teaching Hospital, UC Davis, July 1971 to June 1982. (From Carter, J.D. et al., *J. Am. Vet. Med. Assoc.*, 188, 163–167, 1986. With permission.)

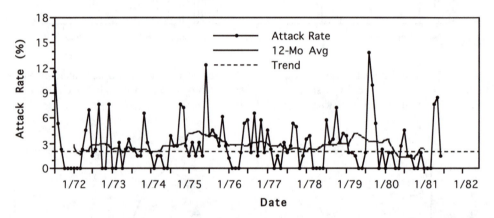

Figure 11.5 Monthly attack rate (incidence), 12-month centered moving average, and trend of salmonellosis in horses at the Veterinary Medical Teaching Hospital, UC Davis, July 1971 to June 1981. Monthly attack rate = (new cases) ÷ (daily average inpatients for the month). (From Carter, J.D. et al., *J. Am. Vet. Med. Assoc.*, 188, 163–167, 1986. With permission.)

the specific seasonal, or seasonal index. **Specific seasonals** are a ratio in which the observed monthly incidence rate is divided by the 12-month moving average incidence rate centered on the middle of that month (Schwabe et al., 1977). If specific seasonals are available for a number of years, then they can be averaged (by mean or median) for each month to derive **typical seasonals**, which are indices of the amount of variation attributable to seasonal influences (Figure 11.6). Seasonal indices are expressed as percentage deviation from 1. Thus, if the seasonal index were half the average for that month, then it would be 50%; if it were twice the average, it would be 200%.

Subtraction of typical seasonals from specific seasonals leaves the combined cyclical and irregular variation in disease occurrence. **Cyclical changes** refer to the rise and fall of disease incidence developing at intervals longer than 1 year. **Irregular variation** reflects random or unpredictable variation in disease occurrence among individuals in a population. Both cyclical and irregular variation are associated with disease outbreaks.

Examples of the application of time series analysis can be found in the following example.

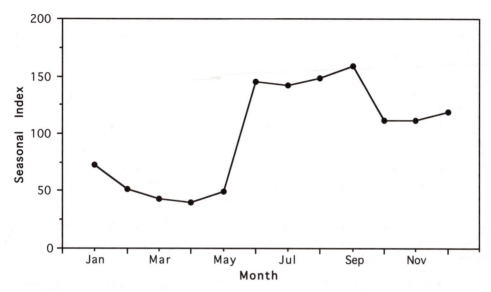

Figure 11.6 Seasonal index of *Salmonella* serotypes causing clinical disease in horses at the Veterinary Medical Teaching Hospital, UC Davis, July 1971 to June 1981. (From Carter, J.D. et al., *J. Am. Vet. Med. Assoc.*, 188, 163–167, 1986. With permission.)

Example 11.1

In 1982 the entire Large Animal Clinic of the Veterinary Medical Teaching Hospital (VMTH) at the School of Veterinary Medicine, University of California at Davis, was forced to close temporarily because of a serious outbreak of *Salmonella saint-paul* infection in horses (Carter et al., 1986). An epidemiologic study of clinical salmonellosis during the 11-year period up to and including the outbreak (July 1971 through June 1982) revealed 245 cases of equine salmonellosis caused by 18 serotypes (Figure 11.4). The distribution of serotypes over time revealed disappearance of some serotypes and the introduction of others.

A time series analysis of monthly attack rates (number of new cases divided by daily average equine inpatient population for the month) revealed no significant overall increase or decrease in the rates (secular trend) over the 11-year period (Figure 11.5).

Seasonal fluctuations occurred, with highest incidence of salmonellosis from June through September, and lowest incidence from January through May (Figure 11.6). Cyclical changes appeared as three major outbreaks and several smaller outbreaks over the 11-year period (Figure 11.7). There was no regular pattern in the cycles that would be useful for forecasting salmonellosis outbreaks at the VMTH.

The results of the time series analysis of this outbreak may be summarized as follows: The incidence of salmonellosis in the VMTH has been stable over the past decade, neither increasing nor decreasing. There has been a definite seasonal trend, with highest incidence from June through September and lowest incidence from January through May. Over the 10-year period from 1971 to 1981 there have been three major outbreaks and several smaller outbreaks. The

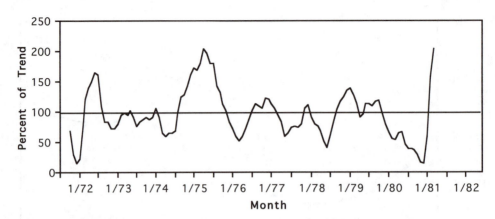

Figure 11.7 Cycles of salmonellosis in horses at the Veterinary Medical Teaching Hospital, UC Davis, July 1971 to June 1981. (From Carter, J.D. et al., *J. Am. Vet. Med. Assoc.*, 188, 163–167, 1986. With permission.)

contribution of any factors found to be associated with increased risk of salmonellosis should be interpreted in light of the temporal patterns of disease.

11.3.4   Spatial distribution

There are a number of ways of depicting the spatial distribution of disease frequency. **Areal maps** depict the distribution and frequency of disease within defined areas or boundaries, as counties, states, or ecological zones. Another approach is the simple **spot (or dot) map**, where each dot either represents a case or is scaled to represent the frequency of disease. There are many variations of spot maps, however, and one should always examine them carefully so as not to misinterpret the information provided. **Overlay mapping,** where two or more spatial distribution maps are superimposed on one another, provides a simple technique for exploring the association among spatially distributed variables.

11.4   Case study

11.4.1   The epidemic of West Nile virus in the U.S., 2002

Presented is a description of host, spatial, and temporal distribution of an emerging infectious zoonotic disease (O'Leary et al., 2004).

11.4.1.1   Introduction

West Nile virus (WNV), which is indigenous to the eastern hemisphere, was first recognized in the U.S. in 1999 during an outbreak in New York City. Through 2001, 10 states reported a total of 149 human WNV illnesses and 18 deaths, while thousands of animal infections were reported from 27 states and the District of Columbia. In 2002, a multistate WNV epidemic resulted in an unprecedented number of neuroinvasive human illnesses and avian and equine infections that often preceded the identification of human illnesses.

11.4.1.2   Purpose of the study

This study was conducted to define the host (demographic), spatial, and temporal patterns of neuroinvasive WNV during the 2002 WNV outbreak, and the value of WNV surveillance data for predicting human illness.

11.4.1.3   Epidemiologic methodology

11.4.1.3.1   Surveillance methods.   Data submitted to the U.S. Centers for Disease Control and Prevention's (CDC) **ArboNET surveillance system** by 54 state and local health agencies were used for this study. ArboNET includes surveillance data on human cases of WNV illness and WNV-infected birds, nonhuman mammals, and mosquitoes collected and interpreted according to guidelines published by CDC. Case definitions were based on standardized clinical and laboratory-based criteria. Active case surveillance was encouraged by CDC after the first case of WNV occurred within a jurisdiction.

11.4.1.3.2   Laboratory methods.   Acute-phase serum and cerebrospinal fluid samples and appropriately timed convalescent-phase serum samples were collected from suspected case patients. **Laboratory-confirmed evidence** of a recent WNV infection included presence of WNV-specific IgM antibody in cerebrospinal fluid; a fourfold or greater change in neutralizing antibody titer in paired sera; presence of WNV-specific IgM and neutralizing antibodies in a single serum sample; isolation of WNV in culture; or demonstration of WNV genomic sequences in serum, cerebrospinal fluid, or other bodily fluids or tissues. **Laboratory-probable evidence** of WNV infection included the presence of either IgM or neutralizing antibodies against WNV in a single serum sample.

11.4.1.3.3   Data collection and analysis.   Included in the analysis were human cases with illness onset during 2002 and reported to ArboNET between January 1, 2002 and April 15, 2003. West Nile virus cases of encephalitis, meningitis, and meningoencephalitis were combined as **neuroinvasive WNV illness**. Incidence was calculated as cases per million population using 2000 U.S. Census data and mapped using commercial geographic information system (GIS) software. Crude relative risks and their 95% confidence intervals (CIs), chi-squared tests, Spearman's rank correlation, and Mantel–Haenzel chi-squared statistics were calculated. **Two-sided p-values** were reported. Animal infections with WNV were reported to ArboNET by health departments via an Internet secure data network.

11.4.1.4   Assumptions inherent in the methodology

It was assumed that contributors to ArboNET adhered to recommended guidelines.

11.4.1.5   Basic epidemiologic findings

In 2002, 4156 human WNV illnesses from 739 counties in 39 states and the District of Columbia were reported. In addition, 16,741 WNV-infected dead birds were reported from 42 states and the District of Columbia; 14,571 infected nonhuman mammals (including 14,539 equids) were reported from 41 states; and 6604 infected pools of mosquitoes from 29 species were reported from 37 (81%) of 45 jurisdictions performing mosquito surveillance.

11.4.1.5.1   Patient demographic and clinical information.   Of 4156 reported WNV human illness cases, 2259 (54%) were classified as confirmed and 1897 (46%) as probable. Complete demographic and clinical data were available for 4146 (99%) of these cases and are summarized in Table 11.1. Of note is that 71% of cases were neuroinvasive, while 28% experienced uncomplicated WNV fever only. The case fatality rate was highest (12%) for WNV cases manifesting as encephalitis or menigoencephalitis, compared with 2% for cases with meningitis and 1% with fever only. The median age for fatal cases overall was 77.5 years (range, 19 to 99 years).

Of the 2942 reported cases of neuroinvasive illness, 84% were from only 11 north-central and southern states. Mississippi had the highest incidence of neuroinvasive illiness (57 cases per million persons). Los Angeles County, California, was the only county west of the Rocky Mountains to report a human case (Figure 11.8).

Table 11.1 Demographic and Clinical Information for 4146 Human West Nile Virus Illness Cases Reported to Centers for Disease Control and Prevention, U.S., 2002

| | Clinical Syndrome | | | |
	Encephalitis or Meningoencephalitis	Meningitis	Fever	Unspecified
No. cases (%)	2220 (54)	722 (17)	1157 (28)	47 (1)
No. males (%)	1239 (56)	361 (50)	582 (50)	26 (55)
Age				
Median	64 years	46 years	49 years	43 years
Range	1 month–99 years	3 months–91 years	1–97 years	0–89 years
Group (%)				
0–39	359 (16)	253 (35)	306 (26)	21 (45)
40–69	974 (44)	367 (51)	678 (59)	21 (45)
70 and older	887 (40)	102 (14)	173 (15)	5 (10)
No. deaths (%)	261 (12)	15 (2)	7 (1)	1 (2)
No. males (%)	164 (63)	11 (73)	7 (100)	0 (0)
Age				
Median	78 years	74 years	72 years	89 years
Range	19–99 years	40–91 years	59–89 years	89 years

Source: O'Leary, D.R. et al., *Vector Borne Zoonotic Dis.*, 4, 61–70, 2004. With permission.

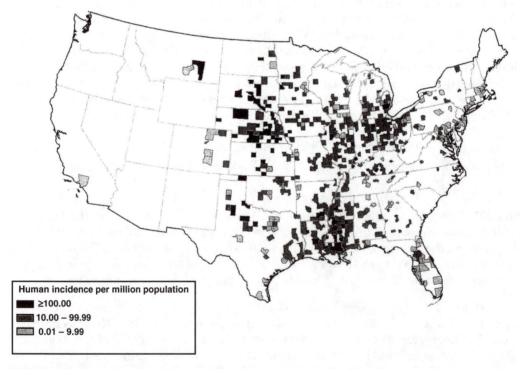

Human incidence per million population
- ≥100.00
- 10.00 – 99.99
- 0.01 – 9.99

Figure 11.8 Reported incidence of neuroinvasive human West Nile virus illness, by county and state, United States, 2002 (n = 589 counties). (From O'Leary, D.R. et al., *Vector Borne Zoonotic Dis.*, 4, 61–70, 2004. With permission.)

Reported date of onset of neuroinvasive illness ranged over a 30-week period from May 19 (District of Columbia) to December 14 (Mississippi) (Figure 11.9), with 74% occurring during the 6-week period from August 11 through September 21. The **epidemic peak** occurred during the week ending August 24, when 451 cases of neuroinvasive illness

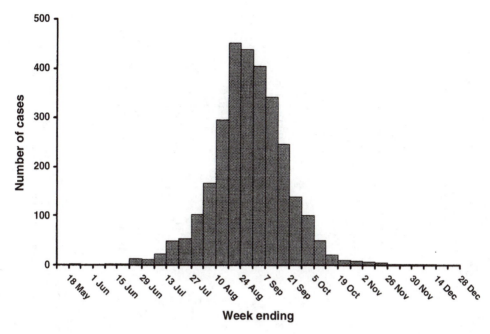

Figure 11.9 Reported number of neuroinvasive human West Nile virus illness cases by week of illness onset, United States, 2002 (n = 2,942 cases). (From O'Leary, D.R. et al., *Vector Borne Zoonotic Dis.*, 4, 61–70, 2004. With permission.)

occurred. The duration of the epidemic was longer in the southern U.S., where neuroinvasive illnesses were reported weekly from mid-June through mid-December.

11.4.1.5.2 Age-specific neuroinvasive illness incidence and mortality. The incidence of neuroinvasive illness and fatality-to-case ratios increased significantly with age (Table 11.2). Older individuals were as much as 12 times more likely to suffer neuroinvasive illness and 48 times more likely to die as a result of illness than their younger counterparts. Incidences of neuroinvasive illness and associated fatalities were significantly higher for middle-aged and older males than for females.

11.4.1.5.3 Surveillance events preceding neuroinvasive human illnesses. Of 589 counties reporting human neuroinvasive illnesses, 527 (89%) first detected WNV transmission in nonhuman species. **West Nile virus-infected dead birds** were the first positive surveillance event in 72% of counties, followed by infected nonhuman mammals in 18%, infected mosquitoes in 6%, and seroconversion among **sentinel birds** in 2%. In 2% of counties multiple types of nonhuman surveillance events occurred on the same day. The median **lead time** between detection of infected birds in a county and the first human illness was 38.5 days (range, 2 to 252 days). In 85% of these counties the lead time exceeded 14 days, the approximate upper limit of WNV incubation in humans. The majority (77%) of counties reporting infected nonhuman species did not report any neuroinvasive human illnesses.

11.4.1.6 Conclusions and measures taken
The 2002 West Nile virus outbreak was the largest recognized epidemic of a neuroinvasive arboviral illness in the western hemisphere, and the largest epidemic of neuroinvasive WNV illness ever recorded. The strong association of neuroinvasive illness and mortality with advancing age was consistent with previous reports. However, the slightly higher incidence and mortality for males observed in this study have not been consistently

Table 11.2 Relative Risk Estimates for Neuroinvasive West Nile Virus Illness[a] and Fatality by Age Group and Sex, U.S., 2002

	Neuroinvasive West Nile Virus Illness				Fatal Neuroinvasive West Nile Virus Illness	
	Population at Risk[b]	Number (%)	Incidence per Million Population[c]	Relative Risk (95% CI)[d]	Number (Fatality-to-Case Ratio (%))[c]	Relative Risk (95% CI)[d]
All cases						
Age category (yr)						
0–9[e]	35,677,630	42 (1)	1	Reference	0 (0)	Reference
10–19[e]	36,554,351	74 (3)	2	Reference	1 (1)	Reference
20–29[e]	34,481,647	177 (6)	5	Reference	2 (1)	Reference
30–39[e]	39,028,636	319 (11)	8	Reference	4 (1)	Reference
40–49	38,277,913	451 (15)	12	2.8 (2.5–3.2)	7 (2)	1.4 (0.5–3.7)
50–59	27,933,078	431 (15)	15	3.7 (3.2–4.2)	16 (4)	3.3 (1.4–7.8)
60–69	18,363,781	459 (16)	25	6.0 (5.3–6.7)	41 (9)	8.5 (3.9–18.4)
70–79	14,735,227	594 (20)	40	9.6 (8.6–10.7)	100 (17)	17.5 (8.4–36.8)
80–89	7,020,171	353 (12)	50	12.0 (10.5–13.6)	90 (25)	29.6 (14.2–62.0)
90 and older	1,323,508	42 (1)	33	7.6 (5.5–10.3)	15 (36)	48.0 (21.5–105.2)
Total	253,395,942	2942 (100)	12		276 (9)	
Male						
Age category (yr)						
0–39	74,030,546	323 (20)	4	1.1 (0.9–1.3)	5 (2)	2.2 (0.5–10.0)
40–69	41,047,519	741 (46)	18	1.3 (1.2–1.5)	45 (6)	1.8 (1.1–3.2)
70 and older	9,015,501	536 (34)	59	1.8 (1.6–2.1)	125 (23)	1.3 (1.0–1.7)
Total	124,093,566	1600 (100)	13	1.2 (1.1–1.3)	175 (11)	1.5 (1.2–1.9)
Female						
Age category (yr)						
0–39[f]	71,711,718	289 (21)	4	Reference	2 (1)	Reference
40–69[f]	43,527,253	600 (45)	14	Reference	19 (3)	Reference
70 and older[f]	14,063,405	453 (34)	32	Reference	80 (18)	Reference
Total[f]	129,302,376	1342 (100)	10	Reference	101 (8)	Reference

[a] Includes encephalitis, with or without meningeal signs, and meningitis.
[b] Population figures are from the 2000 U.S. Census and exclude the 14 states that did not report neuroinvasive human West Nile virus illnesses in 2002: AK, AZ, DE, HI, ID, ME, NV, NH, NM, OR, UT, VT, WA, WY.
[c] Neuroinvasive illness incidence and fatality rates, respectively, increased significantly with age (Spearman's rank correlation, one-sided, $p = 0.02; 0.01$).
[d] CI = confidence interval.
[e] Persons in these four age groups were combined to serve as the reference population.
[f] Females in all age groups were combined to serve as the reference population.
Source: O'Leary, D.R. et al., *Vector Borne Zoonotic Dis.*, 4, 61–70, 2004. With permission.

observed in other outbreaks. Either or both of these apparent associations could be the result of surveillance artifacts, e.g., misclassification and reporting biases inherent to the reporting system, and should be interpreted cautiously.

The 2002 WNV outbreak exhibited a marked westward geographic expansion of WNV across the U.S. when compared to the geographic distribution of previous years. The **emerging long-term epidemiologic pattern** of WNV may be similar to either St. Louis encephalitis (SLE) or Japanese encephalitis virus, two related but epidemiologically distinct flaviviruses. Like WNV, SLE is maintained and amplified in transmission cycles that involve passerine birds as **amplifying hosts** (see Chapter 13) and culicine mosquitoes as vectors. Since 1933, when it was first recognized in the U.S., SLE has presented as sporadic cases, case clusters, or regional outbreaks resulting in dozens to hundreds of neuroinvasive illnesses. In contrast, Japanese encephalitis occurs only in Asia, where intense seasonal transmission can occur in rural transmission cycles involving culicine mosquitoes, aquatic birds, and pigs, and where annual epidemics may involve thousands of cases.

West Nile fever (vs. neuroinvasive WNV infections) is probably significantly underdiagnosed in the U.S. It is estimated that approximately 20 West Nile fever illnesses occur for every neuroinvasive illness. However, the value of increased testing and surveillance for West Nile fever is unknown. Similarly, the value of animal surveillance data as an alert system for reducing human risk of WNV neuroinvasive illnesses is compromised by the short lead time afforded and low specificity (high proportion of false positives). The authors suggest that for the foreseeable future, WNV prevention and control strategies should be based on high-quality nonhuman and human surveillance combined with more traditional approaches, such as vector mosquito control and ongoing public education on personal mosquito protection and elimination of periresidential mosquito habitat.

11.5 Summary

Occurrence refers to the frequency distribution of disease over space (spatial or geographic occurrence), time (temporal occurrence), or within a host population. Not only is this information useful to gain a better appreciation of the significance of the disease, but it may suggest the probable cause, source, and mode of transmission. The first step in any disease investigation is identification of the cases and noncases. Cases may be defined on the basis of a discrete set of signs and symptoms, performance indicators, or epidemiologic criteria. Epidemiologic criteria, such as the occurrence of the disease, may be added to the case definition.

The occurrence of disease in a population may be reported in three different ways: (1) host characteristics, such as age, sex, and breed; (2) time, which includes date of onset; or (3) place, from within a housing unit to geographic distribution. An attack rate measures the proportion of the population that develops disease among the total exposed at the beginning of the outbreak. Attack rates are often used to report disease frequency during outbreak investigations. The attack rate is essentially an incidence rate where the time period of interest is the duration of the epidemic. Since comparison of crude rates can lead to erroneous conclusions, it is necessary to adjust for any host factors that might interfere with an accurate comparison. Rates are commonly adjusted for age, breed, and sex.

Most diseases have characteristic patterns of temporal occurrence. A disease is sporadic when it occurs rarely and without regularity in a population unit. A disease is endemic when it occurs with predictable regularity in a population, with only minor fluctuations in frequency pattern over time. A disease may be endemic at any level of occurrence. A disease is epidemic when its frequency within the population during a given time interval is clearly in excess of its expected frequency.

Time series analysis is concerned with the detection, description, and measurement of disease patterns or periodicities from temporal occurrence data. The purpose of time series analysis is to identify periods of high or low risk so that causal associations can be explored. Patterns of disease occurrence (incidence) are influenced by one or more of the following: (1) secular trend, (2) seasonal fluctuation, (3) cyclic variation, and (4) irregular variation. Secular trends are overall long-term rises or declines in incidence rate that occur gradually over long periods. Seasonal fluctuations are regular changes in incidence rates with periods shorter than a year. Cyclical changes refer to the rise and fall of disease incidence developing at intervals longer than 1 year. Irregular variation reflects random or unpredictable variation in disease occurrence among individuals in a population. Both cyclical and irregular variation are associated with disease outbreaks.

There are a number of ways to depict the spatial distribution of disease frequency. Areal maps depict the distribution and frequency of disease within defined boundaries, as counties, states, or ecological zones. Another approach is the simple spot (or dot) map, where each dot either represents a case or is scaled to represent the frequency of disease. Overlay mapping can be used to explore the association among spatially distributed variables.

chapter 12

Establishing cause

12.1 Introduction

Epidemiologic investigation of a disease outbreak of unknown etiology will usually incriminate a number of factors, or **determinants**, of the disease. Usually only one factor (the etiologic agent) is causal, and its relationship to the disease syndrome may be confirmed by some variation of **Koch's postulates**. Other factors, termed host and environmental determinants, may facilitate the introduction and spread of the etiologic agent within animal populations. In this chapter we examine how these determinants are identified and how their relationship to disease is established.

12.2 Multiple causation of disease

Determinants of disease include both the etiologic agent(s) directly responsible for disease and other factors that facilitate exposure, multiplication, and spread in the population. These determinants can be categorized as **agent, host**, and **environment** (or management) factors. The way in which these factors interact to cause disease has been referred to as the **web of causation**, which is another expression of the concept of multiple causality.

▼

Determinants of disease include the agent, host, and environment.

▲

12.2.1 Agent factors

The biological properties of agents, such as pathogenicity and virulence, strains and genetic variability, are primary determinants of the ability of an agent to cause disease. Contributors to the pathogenicity and virulence of disease agents are generally covered in microbiology texts and are not discussed further here.

12.2.2 Host factors: susceptibility

The susceptibility of individual animals to disease is a second determinant of disease occurrence. Natural variation affects the response of individual animals to exposure to a disease agent. Most of the statistical examples that were discussed earlier have focused on this type of variation. Some animals have **innate resistance** to infection or disease due to age, sex, or breed. **Acquired resistance** in the individual may be the result of prior natural or artificial (vaccination) exposure to the agent. In some cases, animals are latently infected with an agent that has the potential to cause clinical disease. The triggering mechanism may be an altered immune response brought on by stress. An example is the predictable outbreak of shipping fever complex seen in cattle shortly after being transported to a new location.

Populations also differ in susceptibility. Resistance in populations is called **herd immunity** (or **population immunity**) and is related to the proportion of resistant animals in the population. **Innate herd immunity** reflects a population that is resistant to an infection for some reason other than prior natural exposure or immunization. **Acquired herd immunity** results from the development of protective immunity in a population after natural exposure or immunization.

▼

Populations differ in susceptibility. Resistance in populations is called herd immunity and is related to the proportion of resistant animals in the population.

▲

Increased herd immunity has the effect of limiting the spread of directly transmitted diseases by reducing the proportion of **effective contacts**, e.g., contacts between infected and susceptible animals that result in transmission of a disease agent. Increased herd immunity may also limit the spread of indirectly transmitted and airborne disease agents by reducing environmental contamination. In either case, the **effective reproductive number** (see Chapter 13) for a disease agent may fall below that required for its maintenance in the population, leading to its eventual eradication.

It follows that the higher the **intrinsic reproductive number** (R_0; see Chapter 13) of a disease organism, the higher the level of herd immunity that must be achieved for its eradication. Very high levels of artificially induced herd immunity are required to eradicate diseases whose intrinsic reproduction rates are high (Table 12.1). The relatively small value of R_0 for smallpox, and corresponding low level of herd immunity that must be artificially induced, may partially explain the success of the global eradication campaign. Other factors are the obviousness of the disease and availability of an effective vaccine. In contrast, the high values of R_0 for malaria suggest that eradication through vaccination will be much more difficult to achieve. Furthermore, carriers may easily escape detection, and prototype vaccines do not prevent infection, only disease. The cyclical nature of wildlife disease epidemics may be related to the destabilizing effect of population fluctuations upon herd immunity.

Example 12.1

In Kazakhstan and elsewhere in central Asia, the bacterium *Yersinia pestis* circulates in natural populations of gerbils, which are the source of human cases of **bubonic plague**. In an effort to improve plague surveillance strategies in the region, Davis et al. (2004) conducted time series analysis of field data on plague prevalence among great gerbils and gerbil population abundance collected over a 40-year period. Their analysis revealed that plague invades, fades out, and reinvades in response to fluctuations in the abundance of its main reservoir host, the great gerbil (*Rhombomys opimus*) (Figure 12.1A and B). Two types of host abundance thresholds for plague invasion and persistence in this wildlife species were identified: (1) an **invasion threshold** dependent on the abundance of susceptibles and (2) a **persistence threshold**, or critical community size, that

Table 12.1 Relationship between a Pathogen's Intrinsic Reproductive Number (R_o) and the Proportion of the Host Population That Must Be Vaccinated (Herd Immunity) to Achieve Eradication of Some Directly and Indirectly Transmitted Human Diseases

Disease	Location and Time of Data Collection	R_o	P (%)
Smallpox	Developing countries before global eradication campaign	3.5	72
Measles	England and Wales (1950–1968)	16–18	95
	Ghana (1960–1968)	14–15	94
Pertussis	England and Wales (1944–1978)	16–18	95
	Maryland (1908–1917)	13	93
German measles	England and Wales (1979)	6	84
	West Germany (1972)		
Chicken pox	Parts of U.S. (1913–1921, 1943)	7–11	91
	England and Wales (1944–1968)	10–12	92
Diphtheria	Parts of U.S. (1910–1919)	4–5	80
Scarlet fever	Parts of U.S. (1908–1919)	6–7	86
Mumps	England and Wales (1960–1980)	11–14	93
	Netherlands (1970–1980)		
Poliomyelitis	U.S. (1955)	5–6	84
	Netherlands (1960)	6–7	86
Malaria (*Plasmodium falciparum*)	Northern Nigeria (1970s)	80	99
Malaria (*Plasmodium malariae*)	Northern Nigeria (1970s)	16	94
HIV (Type I)	England and Wales (male homosexuals; 1981–1985)	2–5	80
	Kampala, Uganda (heterosexuals; 1985–1987)	10–11	91

Note: R_o = the number of secondary infections produced by one case in a totally susceptible population; P (%) = the proportion of the population that must be protected by immunization to achieve eradication, i.e., $R_o (1 - P) < 1$.

Source of data: May, R.M., *Am. Sci.*, 71, 36–45, 1983; Anderson, R.M. and May, R.M., *Infectious Diseases of Humans: Dynamics and Control*, Oxford University Press, Oxford, 1991. With permission.

permits new susceptibles to be recruited at a high enough rate for infection to persist. Based on these findings, the authors proposed a two-stage approach to plague surveillance: use host abundance data (based on burrow occupancy) to identify periods when plague might emerge (with a 2-year delay) and (2) limit bacteriologic testing to predicted high-risk periods.

12.2.3 Environmental (management) factors

According to most general practitioners, environmental or management factors are the most important determinants of disease occurrence. Management factors also comprise a category of factors that are difficult to quantify and manipulate. Examples are the influence of milking hygiene on the occurrence of bovine mastitis or management practices on neonatal calf mortality.

12.3 Sources of bias in evaluating cause–effect relationships

Conducting an epidemiologic investigation is much like playing the role of Inspector Hercule Poirot in an Agatha Christie mystery. Observational data (evidence at the crime scene) are used retrospectively (after the fact) to identify a causal association (the guilty)

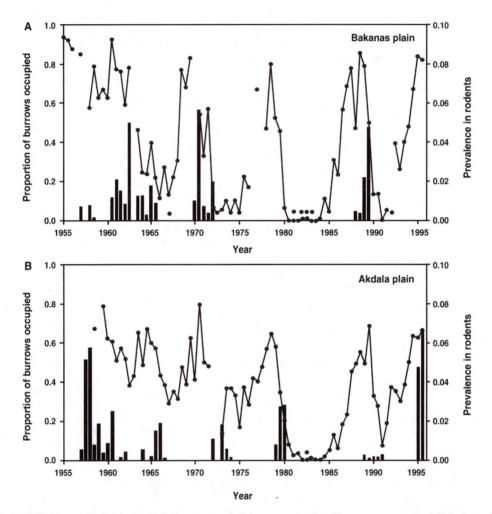

Figure 12.1 A and B: Spring and fall estimates of the proportion of burrows occupied (filled circles connected by solid lines) and prevalence of plague (vertical bars) in great gerbil populations from two sites in the Prebalkhash plague focus of Kazakhstan. In some seasons (marked by an asterisk), no great gerbils were tested for plague. (From Davis, S. et al., *Science*, 304, 736–738, 2004.)

and infer the nature of that association (the motive). The problem for both the detective and the epidemiologist is that the investigation may implicate several causal variables that are directly or indirectly associated with the outcome. Ignoring the potential relationships among variables can lead to biased estimates of the effect of exposure on outcome. Investigators have several tools at their disposal for sorting out these effects, which are discussed below.

▼

Conducting an epidemiologic investigation is much like a criminal investigation. Several causal variables that are directly or indirectly associated with the outcome may be implicated. Ignoring the potential relationships among these variables can lead to biased estimates of the effect of exposure on outcome.

▲

12.3.1 Confounding

Confounding occurs when two or more variables found to be associated with an outcome (as disease) are also associated with each other. As a result, it is impossible, from a cursory examination, to determine which variable is responsible for the observed outcome. The confounder's association with the outcome may be causal, or it may simply be associated with the true cause. For example, prior to the discovery of the role of freshwater stream snails and their associated trematode parasites as intermediate hosts and vectors for *Neorickettsia (Ehrlichia) risticii*, causative agent of equine monocytic ehrlichiosis, or Potomac horse fever (Reubel et al., 1998; Pusterla et al., 2000), a number of other factors were believed to contribute in some way to the risk of contracting the disease. These included ticks, biting flies, mosquitoes, white-footed mice, and duration of access to pasture (Gordon et al., 1988). It is now apparent that the relationship of these previously suspected factors was only through a passive association with the true cause.

12.3.2 Interaction or effect modification

Interaction occurs when one variable modifies the effect of another. For example, if the severity of disease from exposure to an agent is greater in the very young or the very old, we say that there is an interaction between the two variables, or **effect modification** of age upon disease. Other common variables that can modify the magnitude of cause–effect relationships are breed and sex. Interaction can be detected by performing stratified (**Mantel–Haenszel**) two-by-two analyses, stratifying on the suspected effect modifier. For example, if we wish to evaluate the effect of a particular agent on calf survival from birth to weaning, we might construct a series of two-by-two tables stratified by age groups. If there is a notable difference in risk (relative risk or odds ratio) between one or more age groups (**strata**), then interaction between age and pathogenicity should be considered.

If interaction among predictor variables exists, then the Mantel–Haenszel summary odds ratio, which assumes uniform risk among subgroups or strata, may be biased. If more than one major predictor variable (risk factor, exposure) exists, or if interaction is present, then multivariable logistic regression should be used to estimate the contribution of each risk factor to the outcome.

12.3.3 Multicollinearity

Multicollinearity occurs when two or more predictor variables (**covariates**) are also highly correlated with each other, independent of the outcome variable. Examples might be the use of erythrocyte counts and hemoglobin levels to assess anemia, or two related serologic tests as predictors of the same disease. In each case, the two predictor variables are really measuring the same thing, such that we would expect values for both to increase or decrease together. Many medical measurements are highly correlated, and it is standard practice to perform several corroborating tests in diagnosing an illness.

Multivariable logistic regression, which is often used to estimate the contribution of multiple risk factors to disease outcomes, cannot distinguish between two predictor variables that are highly correlated. For this reason, univariate (two-by-two) analysis should always be performed first to identify those predictor variables associated with the outcome. The relationship between individual predictor variables can then be assessed with two-by-two tables or by examining a correlation matrix of predictor variables. The presence and degree of multicollinearity can be assessed by asking how well each independent (X) variable can be predicted from the other X variables (ignoring the Y variable).

12.3.4   Procedure for evaluating interaction and confounding

For the following discussion, it is assumed that the odds ratio (OR) is the parameter of interest. This is usually the case when evaluating the contributions of a number of potential risk factors to disease occurrence. The simplest analytic tool for evaluating interaction and confounding is the Mantel–Haenszel stratified analysis. It divides the analysis into separate tables for each value of the stratifying variable (such as age group), and then combines the results in a way (the **adjusted odds ratio**) that removes the effect of confounding. By stratifying on a variable, we eliminate the effect of confounding by that variable. The adjusted OR is only valid, however, if the ORs in individual strata are similar in value. If they are not, then interaction is present. If interaction is present, then two options are available:

1. Set up the stratification in a different way by combining groups, etc., to reduce the number of differing strata to a minimum.
2. If strata still differ, report the result for each of the differing strata (age groups) separately, rather than in a combined result.

If there is no statistically significant interaction among predictor variables, then the next question is whether or not the stratifying variable confounds the exposure–disease relationship. To assess confounding, the crude OR is compared with the Mantel–Haenszel adjusted OR. The adjusted OR is always a more valid estimate of the true OR than the crude OR; the adjusted OR, however, tends to be less precise (i.e., the confidence intervals tend to be a little wider than the crude OR). There is no statistical test for confounding; the analyst must choose between the more valid but less precise estimate (the adjusted OR) and the less valid but more precise estimate (the crude OR). Some investigators may choose an arbitrary rule for deciding whether the level of confounding is important by comparing the crude and adjusted parameters. For example, the decision may be: if the crude and adjusted parameters differ by more than 5 or 10%, the stratifying variable will be considered a confounder. If the stratifying variable does not modify or confound an exposure–disease relationship, then it could be ignored in any further analyses.

In summary, the steps for evaluating the role of the stratifying variable are (Dean et al., 2000):

1. Is there interaction? If there is interaction, do not use the adjusted or the crude OR. Instead, present the ORs from each stratum. If there is no interaction:
2. Is there confounding? If the crude OR and adjusted OR are similar, then there is no need to stratify on the variable. If the crude OR and adjusted OR are different, use the adjusted OR because it is more valid than the crude OR.

If the parameter of interest is the relative risk (RR) or attributable risk (AR), the same approach for evaluating interaction and confounding is used.

12.3.5   The choice of multivariable vs. stratified analysis

When should multivariable logistic regression be used? Answer: If the outcome variable is dichotomous (e.g., ill or not ill) and there is more than one major predictor variable (risk factor, exposure) of interest, or if interaction is present. With only one predictor variable and no interaction, Mantel–Haenszel stratified analysis can compensate for the confounding if the number of confounders is small. If there are many confounders, the number of strata becomes large and each one contains small numbers, so that Mantel–Haenszel analysis becomes impractical.

As a general rule, simple and stratified univariate analyses should be done before embarking on logistic regression. It gives a feeling for the data set in a simple setting. If the results of logistic regression differ radically from the univariate analysis, it is an indication to check the logistic regression methods to be sure that there is not some underlying misconception or mistake (Dean et al., 1995).

12.4   Establishing cause

In 1882 Koch set forth the following postulates for determining that an infectious agent is the cause of a disease (Fletcher et al., 1996):

1.   The organism must be present in every case of the disease.
2.   The organism must be isolated and grown in pure culture.
3.   The organism must, when inoculated into a susceptible animal, cause the specific disease.
4.   The organism must then be recovered from the animal and identified.

Koch's postulates were an important step in removing disease causation from the anecdotal evidence and superstitions of the time. However, the causes of many diseases cannot be established by means of Koch's postulates.

▼

The causes of many diseases cannot be established by means of Koch's postulates.

▲

Example 12.2

Enzootic pneumonia of calves is an infectious respiratory disease of calves maintained in confinement, either indoors or outdoors. Morbidity rates may approach 100% and mortality rates frequently exceed 20%. The cause is not a single etiologic agent but rather a triad of (1) management-related stress factors plus (2) a primary infection by any of several viruses followed by (3) a super-infection with any of a variety of bacteria. For most disease syndromes there are many potential causes, and a single etiologic agent may cause a disease syndrome common to several other diseases. Koch's postulates are useful only in those special circumstances in which one particular cause dominates, and when that cause is physically transmissible (Fletcher et al., 1982). Fortunately, other criteria may be applied to test the strength of a presumed cause–effect relationship. A description of these criteria follows.

12.4.1   Strength of study designs

In Chapter 1 a variety of epidemiologic study designs were described. Generally, as one goes down the list in Table 1.4 the relative strength of study designs increases. Generally speaking, we can be more confident that a causal association exists as the strength of the study design increases.

12.4.2   Temporal relationship between cause and effect

Demonstration of a **temporal relationship** between a hypothesized cause and effect is fundamental for concluding that a causal association exists. It is difficult to establish a temporal relationship in cross-sectional studies, in which both the outcome and suspected cause are measured at the same time. Longitudinal studies are particularly well suited for demonstrating causal associations, even if only two sampling periods occur. **Paired sampling** is a technique that has proved useful in establishing cause in clinical practice and outbreak investigation.

12.4.3   Strength of the association

The stronger the association between a presumed causal factor and outcome, the more likely that a cause-and-effect relationship exists. As discussed in previous chapters, the **strength of association** between variables can be assessed by estimating relative risk, odds ratios, and correlation coefficients, and through a number of statistical tests. However, we should not forget that association is a statistical concept that does not necessarily imply a cause–effect relationship (Toma et al., 1999). The case for causation can be strengthened if statistical associations also make biological sense (see "Biological Plausibility" below).

12.4.4   Dose–response relationship

A cause–effect relationship is more likely to exist if it can be shown that varying amounts of the suspected cause are related to varying amounts of the effect. This is termed a **dose–response relationship**, or **biological gradient**. Dose can be measured in terms of absolute quantities, such as exposure to variable amounts of a substance, or length of time over which exposure has occurred.

12.4.5   Biological plausibility

Epidemiologic study designs are especially appropriate for the study of risk and prognostic factors (including treatment responses) for naturally occurring disease. Epidemiologic studies cannot, however, prove that a cause–effect relationship exists, but only that an association exists that is unlikely to have arisen by chance alone. Statistical correlation does not prove causality. Research on mechanisms of disease provides the biological basis for believing that associations are in fact causal. On the other hand, information derived from research on mechanisms of disease cannot assume that a particular phenomenon will behave in nature as it does in the laboratory. For this, epidemiologic studies must be conducted. Absence of a biological explanation does not necessarily mean that a causal association is absent. It may simply mean that current medical knowledge is incomplete.

12.4.6   Consistency

Evidence for a causal relationship is strengthened when several studies conducted under different conditions all come to the same conclusion. On the other hand, inconsistency in clinical findings may sometimes be attributed to differences in study design.

12.4.7   Elimination of other possibilities (rule out)

A differential list ranks the possible causes for an observed disease or other outcome. Sometimes the cause of disease, or a disease outbreak, is suggested by our inability to rule it out from a differential list of possible causes.

12.4.8   Reversible associations

If removal of a factor results in decreased risk or frequency of disease, then it is more likely to be causal. This concept is the basis for current approaches to therapy and clinical trials.

Example 12.3

In Chapter 9 a study that examined the long-term risks and benefits of early-age gonadectomy of cats and dogs (Spain et al., 2004a,b) was described. The authors applied six of the eight criteria described above to assess whether associations between age at gonadectomy and the outcomes were likely to represent a cause-and-effect relationship. They specifically mentioned four of the criteria:

1. **Temporal relationship between cause and effect**: The likelihood that the outcomes occurred after gonadectomy rather than being already present at the time of adoption and surgery
2. **Strength of the association**: Magnitude of the hazard or odds ratio and their statistical significance
3. **Biologic plausibility**: Presence (or absence) of a plausible biological mechanism
4. **Consistency**: Consistency of the results with other studies (if any)

Although the authors identified several potential sources of bias that might have influenced the results, the study was well designed and executed. Thus, **strength of study design** might be added to the criteria that could be applied to establish the presence or absence of causal associations. Further, for those outcomes where age at gonadectomy was treated as a continous variable, this relationship might be considered evidence of a **dose–response relationship**, with decreasing age at gonadectomy being the dose variable, or biological gradient. As this was a cohort study, there was only one variable: age at gonadectomy. Thus, consideration of other rule outs (causal factors) was not an option. Similarly, gonadectomy as performed was irreversible, so evidence of a reversible association between gonadectomy and outcomes could not be obtained.

12.5 Case study

12.5.1 Case control study of factors associated with excessive proportions of early fetal losses associated with mare reproductive loss syndrome in central Kentucky during 2001

Direct and indirect epidemiologic evidence are used to identify the likely cause of an outbreak and suggest ways to prevent future occurrences (Dwyer et al., 2003).

12.5.1.1 Introduction

Central Kentucky is one of the largest thoroughbred breeding epicenters in the world, with more than 20,700 mares bred in 2001. The equine industry contributes $3.4 billion to the Kentucky economy and is one of the largest industries in the state. Thus, farm veterinarians and managers, diagnostic laboratory personnel, and extension veterinarians take care in monitoring for outbreaks of any type of disease, including outbreaks of abortion.

In the spring of 2001, private and public veterinarians became aware of a marked increase in the number of early fetal losses (EFLs) and late-term abortions (LTAs) on thoroughbred farms in central Kentucky. The syndrome was named **mare reproductive loss syndrome** (MRLS). No infectious or contagious agents could be incriminated, and extensive pasture sampling and testing revealed no endophyte-infected pastures or known mycotoxins. The timing of reproductive losses coincided with several unusual environmental phenomena during April and May: an unprecedented dry period with warm weather alternating with periods of frost, and the emergence of multitudes of **Eastern tent caterpillars** (*Malacosoma americanum*) living primarily in black cherry trees, which are abundant in Kentucky, and other fruit trees (e.g., apple, crabapple, and pear). In areas of high concentrations, these caterpillars covered fence lines, filled feed buckets, blanketed driveways, and were found on the walls of barns, stalls, and homes.

12.5.1.2 Purpose of the study

This investigation was conducted to identify factors associated with MRLS in central Kentucky during 2001 and areas for further research and investigation.

12.5.1.3 Epidemiologic methodology

12.5.1.3.1 Study design.   A case control study was conducted to identify factors related to MRLS during 2001. It became apparent early in the course of the study that the principal manifestation of MRLS on farms recruited for the study was EFLs. Therefore, although the occurrence of LTAs was recorded, the focus of analyses of data obtained through the case control study was EFLs. **Case farms** included those on which owners and managers perceived EFLs to be in excess of what they considered normal for their farms, in comparison with the previous few years. **Control farms** were those for which owners and managers reported losses typical for their farms.

A general questionnaire was designed to collect farm- and pasture-level data on case and control farms. An additional questionnaire was administered on six case farms and was designed to collect data (including age, parity, breeding status, and any medications that had been administered and may have been associated with EFL) on individual animals. Case horses were horses confirmed by means of ultrasonographic examination at 60 days of gestation or later to no longer be pregnant. Control horses were horses confirmed to still be pregnant after 60 days of gestation.

12.5.1.3.2 Study implementation.   A training session was held for all study personnel during which questionnaires were reviewed and terminology defined. To ensure confidentiality, farms were identified by farm number only. Only the project coordinator had the key to all farm names and identification codes. Data definitions included high caterpillar concentration (blankets of caterpillars on fences, waterers, or other surfaces), moderate caterpillar concentration (many caterpillars in trees, with some in pastures or barns), and low caterpillar concentration (few caterpillars observed). Other terms that were defined included feeding hay outside (horses fed on the ground or in feeders) and frequent presence of waterfowl (waterfowl often seen or evidence thereof seen on the horse premises or in the immediate vicinity). A typical farm interview lasted 2 to 3 hours in addition to travel time.

12.5.1.3.3 Statistical analyses.   A single investigator reviewed completed questionnaires and validated questionable responses as needed. Proportions of case and control farms exposed to each factor of interest were calculated and compared. Potential associations between farm EFL status (case or control) and individual farm-level variables were further evaluated with logistic regression. On the basis of *a priori* hypotheses suggested by the unusual environmental conditions, the presence of cherry trees, caterpillar concentration, and farm size were included as **covariates** in each model to simultaneously adjust for the potential effects of these variables while evaluating the other variables of interest.

When proportions of pastures exposed to factors of interest differed by >10% between affected and control pastures, these variables were considered eligible for multivariable logistic regression modeling. A p value of 0.05 was required for a variable to remain in the final model.

Odds ratios for horse-level factors of interest and their statistical significance were calculated. Variables with an odds ratio of 2 or 0.5 and a p value of 0.20 were considered eligible for multivariable logistic regression modeling, with EFL status as the response variable. A p value of 0.05 was required for a variable to remain in the final model.

12.5.1.4 Assumptions inherent in the methodology

It was assumed that the case definition, sampling strategy, questionnaire design, and data definitions would ensure representativeness and accuracy of data, and comparability across data collectors. The most likely direct and indirect causal factor(s) were inferred based on (1) temporal relationship, (2) strength of association, (3) biologic plausibility, (4) consistency of findings with other studies, and (5) apparent reversible association.

12.5.1.5 Basic epidemiologic findings

A total of 133 (88%) of 150 farms eligible for inclusion in the study participated, representing 10 counties. Reasons cited for nonparticipation were lack of time because of being too busy with breeding stallions, illness of the farm manager or family members, or the farm manager being absent from the farm. Of the 133 farms that participated in the survey, 97 were classified as case farms and 36 as controls.

Table 12.2 and Table 12.3 list statistically significant farm- and pasture-level factors associated with excessive proportions of EFLs. **Farm-level factors** associated with excessive proportions of EFLs included having 50 mares on the farm ($p = 0.01$), the presence of a high concentration of caterpillars ($p < 0.001$), and the frequent presence of waterfowl ($p < 0.001$). The only factor associated with a lower risk of EFLs was feeding hay outside, whether on the ground or in a manger or other device ($p = 0.006$). Two **pasture-level factors** were significantly associated with excessive EFLs: the presence of moderate or high caterpillar concentrations ($p < 0.001$) and pastures containing barren or maiden mares bred in 2001 ($p = 0.004$). Mare-level data were collected from 340 mares on six farms, and statistically significant factors are listed in Table 12.3. **Mare-level factors** associated with excessive proportions of EFLs included being bred in February ($p = 0.003$; Table 12.4) and having been exposed to cherry trees ($p = 0.04$). An extensive list of farm-, pasture-, and mare-level variables was found to have no statistically significant association with the risk of excessive EFLs.

12.5.1.6 Conclusions and measures taken

Of the five factors associated with an increased risk of EFLs, exposure to moderate or high caterpillar concentrations stood out, as it was identified at both the farm and pasture levels and had the highest odds ratio. Black cherry trees were probably passively associated with excessive EFLs as a **confounder**, as they are the preferred food choice for the caterpillars. The association of excessive EFLs with farm size was probably due to breeding a larger percentage of barren and maiden mares on these farms during the high-risk period in February. The increased risk associated with waterfowl could not be explained biologically. The authors hypothesized that the association may be an artifact due to the way the

Table 12.2 Farm-Level Factors Associated with Excessive Proportions
of Early Fetal Losses on Horse Farms in Central Kentucky during 2001

Factor	Case Farms (%)	Control Farms (%)	Adjusted OR[a]	95% CI
Farm size, 50 mares	66.0	38.9	3.2	1.3–7.7
High caterpillar concentration	67.0	22.2	6.4	2.5–16.9
Frequent presence of waterfowl	60.8	25.0	5.6	2.2–14.3
Feeding hay outside	82.1	91.4	0.19	0.06–0.61

Note: OR = odds ratio; CI = confidence interval for OR.

[a] Each factor was examined individually using logistic regression with farm size, presence of cherry trees, and caterpillar concentrations included as covariates when these factors were not the factor of interest.

Source: Dwyer, R.M. et al., *J. Am.Vet. Med. Assoc.*, 222, 613–619, 2003.

Table 12.3 Pasture-Level Factors Associated with Excessive Proportions
of Early Fetal Losses on Horse Farms in Central Kentucky during 2001

Factor	Case Pastures (%)	Control Pastures (%)	Adjusted OR	95% CI
Moderate or high caterpillar concentration	87.4	40.5	7.1	2.6–19.8
Pasture primarily contains maiden or barren mares	67.4	27.7	6.5	1.8–23.4

Note: Factors were analyzed by means of multivariable logistic regression with backward elimination. See Table 12.2 for key.

Source: Dwyer, R.M. et al., *J. Am.Vet. Med. Assoc.*, 222, 613–619, 2003.

Table 12.4 Individual Horse-Level Factors Associated with Excessive Proportions
of Early Fetal Losses on Horse Farms in Central Kentucky during 2001

Factor	Case Mares (%)	Control Mares (%)	Adjusted OR	95% CI
Bred in February	50.0	10.5	5.4	2.5–12.0
Exposed to cherry trees in or around pasture	96.1	74.2	7.6	1.1–51.4

Note: Factors were analyzed by means of multivariable logistic regression with backward elimination. See Table 12.2 for key.

Source: Dwyer, R.M. et al., *J. Am.Vet. Med. Assoc.*, 222, 613–619, 2003.

question was framed or answered, but that follow-up is warranted to determine whether waterfowl are an environmental marker for another cause of EFLs. Feeding hay outside was protective in the farm-level analysis, but insignificant in the pasture-level analysis. This discrepancy may be due in part to the way the pasture-level survey question was framed, as it only asked whether supplemental hay was fed, without regard to the location. The authors suggest that feeding hay outside may reduce pasture forage consumption, thereby reducing exposure to caterpillars. Results suggest that limiting exposure to Eastern tent caterpillars and cherry trees and feeding hay to mares outside may help decrease the risk of excessive proportions of early fetal losses associated with mare reproductive loss syndrome. The list of management factors not associated with excessive EFLs was also helpful, as it allowed farm managers to focus on those factors most likely to reduce the incidence of EFLs.

12.6 Summary

Epidemiologic investigation of a disease outbreak of unknown etiology will usually incriminate a number of factors, or determinants, in the disease. Determinants of disease include both the etiologic agent(s) directly responsible for disease and other factors that facilitate exposure, multiplication, and spread in the population. These determinants can be categorized as agent, host, and environment (or management) factors. The way in which these factors interact to cause disease has been referred to as the web of causation, which is another expression of the concept of multiple causality.

The biological properties of agents, such as pathogenicity and virulence, strains and genetic drift, are primary determinants of the ability of an agent to cause disease. The susceptibility of individual animals to disease is a second determinant of disease occurrence. Natural variation affects the response of individual animals to exposure to a disease agent. Some animals have innate resistance to infection or disease due to age, sex, or breed. Acquired resistance in the individual may be the result of prior natural or artificial (through immunization) exposure to the agent.

Populations also differ in susceptibility. Resistance in populations is called herd immunity and is related to the proportion of resistant animals in the population. Resistance may be innate or acquired. Increased herd immunity has the effect of limiting the spread of diseases by reducing the proportion of effective contacts, e.g., contacts between infected and susceptible animals that result in transmission of a disease agent. As a result, the reproductive number for a disease agent may fall below that required for its maintenance in the population, leading to its eventual eradication. It follows that the higher the intrinsic reproductive number (R_o) of a disease organism, the higher the level of herd immunity that must be achieved for its eradication.

According to most general practitioners, environmental or management factors are the most important determinants of disease occurrence. Management factors also comprise a category of factors that are difficult to quantify and manipulate.

Conducting an epidemiologic investigation is much like a criminal investigation. Several causal variables that are directly or indirectly associated with the outcome may be implicated. Ignoring the potential relationships among these variables can lead to biased estimates of the effect of exposure on outcome. Confounding occurs when two or more variables found to be associated with an outcome (as disease) are also associated with each other. As a result, it is impossible, from a cursory examination, to determine which variable is responsible for the observed outcome. Interaction, or effect modification, occurs when one variable modifies the effect of another. Multicollinearity occurs when two or more predictor variables (covariates) are also highly correlated with each other, independent of the outcome variable. The effects of these associations can be sorted out through the application of Mantel–Haenszel stratified analysis and multivariable logistic regression.

A number of criteria may be applied to evaluate the strength of a presumed cause–effect relationship. These include (1) the strength of the study design, (2) demonstration of a temporal relationship, (3) the strength of the association, (4) demonstration of a dose–response relationship, (5) biological plausibility, (6) consistency of findings with studies conducted in different settings and with different patients, (7) elimination of other possibilities on the rule-out list, and (8) demonstration of a reversible association between presumed cause and effect.

chapter 13

Source and transmission of disease agents

13.1 Sources of infection

13.1.1 Iatrogenic infections

Some of the cases of salmonella infection among horses at the UC Davis Veterinary Medical Teaching Hospital discussed in Chapter 11 were **nosocomial**, e.g., hospital acquired. **Iatrogenic illnesses**, e.g., those illnesses induced in a patient by a clinician's actions, extend the concept of nosocomial infections one step further by including any clinician-induced illness, infectious or otherwise, regardless of where it was acquired. Drug overdoses, the inappropriate use of particular therapeutic regimens, and adverse drug reactions are examples of iatrogenic illnesses.

In some cases, as when attenuated vaccines are used, reactions are unavoidable. In these cases, the owner is advised that the patient may exhibit a brief period of mild illness following vaccination. Occasionally, however, a vaccine strain is suspected as the cause of an outbreak. Given the ubiquity of disease agents in the environment, it is often difficult to directly implicate the vaccine as the source of the disease agent. The recent availability of tools for the molecular characterization of microorganisms has given birth to a new branch of epidemiology — **molecular epidemiology** — which may be employed to trace the origin of a particular isolate.

▼

> Iatrogenic illnesses extend the concept of nosocomial infections one step further by including any clinician-induced illness, infectious or otherwise, regardless of where it was acquired.

▲

Example 13.1

The transmissible spongiform encephalopathies (TSE) are a group of fatal neurodegenerative diseases, which include scrapie in sheep and goats, bovine spongiform encephalopathy (BSE) in cattle, and Creutzfeldt–Jakob disease (CJD) in humans. These disorders are characterized by a posttranslational conversion and brain accumulation of an insoluble, protease-resistant isoform (PrP^{Sc}) of the host-encoded prion protein (PrP^{C}). Several TSE strains have been isolated in both animal and human disorders. In Italy, a sudden increase in outbreaks of confirmed cases of scrapie was observed between August 1996 and October 1997 in sheep and goats vaccinated previously against *Mycoplasma agalactiae*. In January 1999, a new outbreak was reported in a mixed flock of Comisana sheep and half-bred goats exposed to the same vaccine, with all available evidence that the epidemic represented a further iatrogenic form of scrapie. Zanusso et al. (2003) performed a molecular characterization of PrP^{Sc} of sheep and goats collected from a single Italian flock with iatrogenic scrapie and compared physicochemical properties of PrP^{Sc} types with Italian field scrapie. Polyacrylamide gel electrophoresis (SDS-PAGE) and immunoblotting were used to characterize prion proteins and estimate their molecular weights. In five animals with iatrogenic scrapie, a PrP^{Sc} type with a 20-kDa core fragment was found in all areas of the brain investigated. In three sheep and one goat, this isoform co-occurred with a fully glycosylated isoform that had a protease-resistant backbone of 17 kDa, whereas in two sheep and four goats, the two PrP^{Sc} types were detected in different regions of the brain. In sheep with natural field scrapie, a PrP^{Sc} type with physicochemical properties indistinguishable from the 20-kDa isoform was found. The results suggested the copresence of two prion strains in mammary gland and brain homogenates used for vaccination.

13.1.2   Animal reservoirs

Animal reservoirs of disease agents include (1) carrier animals, animals (and human beings) with inapparent infections that are also transmitters (or potential transmitters) of the infectious agent, and (2) intermediate hosts and vectors. **Amplifying hosts** may play a role in creating conditions favorable for epidemics of a disease by increasing the abundance of a disease agent in the vicinity of susceptibles.

Animals that have been exposed to an agent may become carriers. **Incubatory carriers** may serve as a source of infection while incubating the disease. This is a characteristic of many viral respiratory infections. **Convalescent carriers** continue to shed infectious organisms after the animal has recovered from disease signs and symptoms. This is seen with many parasitic infections caused by protozoa and helminths. Being a carrier does not necessarily mean that an animal is a **reservoir** of infection for others. The pathogen density or location in the carrier may preclude efficient transfer to susceptibles. The reservoir mechanism of *Ehrlichia canis* (discussed below) illustrates this point.

We tend to look at nature anthropocentrically, i.e., regarding humans as the central fact or final aim of the universe. In the case of zoonotic diseases, this means viewing animals as a source of infection for humans. In some cases, humans may be an important source of infection for other animals.

Example 13.2

Humans are the only definitive hosts of **Taenia saginata** (beef tapeworm) and **Taenia solium** (pork tapeworm). The beef tapeworm is associated with cattle husbandry and is the more widespread of the two (CDC, 1993). Cattle are intermediate hosts, while humans are the source of infection for cattle (Figure 13.1).

From January to March 1981, 37 slaughter cattle from a single Ohio feeding operation were determined, at postmortem inspection, to be infected with *T. saginata* cysticerci (Fertig and Dorn, 1985). A subsequent outbreak on the same

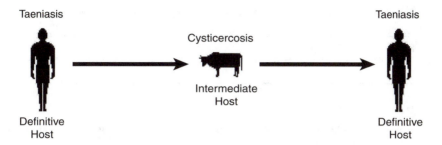

Figure 13.1 Taeniasis and cycticercosis (*T. saginata*) — transmission cycle. Humans are the only definitive hosts for *T. saginata* and *T. solium* and become infected by ingesting raw or undercooked infected meat. (From Acha, P.N. and Szyfres, B., *Zoonoses and Communicable Diseases Common to Man and Animals*, Pan American Health Organization, Washington, DC, 1980. With permission.)

farm in March 1983 involved seven slaughter cattle. By multiplying the prevalence rate of **cysticercosis** detected at federally inspected plants in Ohio by the number of cattle slaughtered at the Ohio Department of Agriculture (ODA)–inspected plants, eight cases per year would have been expected in ODA–inspected plants. Applying this same prevalence rate to the total number of cattle slaughtered from this farm in 1980, the expected number of cases was 0.005. The observed number, 37 cases, was 7400 times greater than expected and therefore constituted an outbreak.

An epidemiologic investigation was conducted of possible sources of the *T. saginata* ova; these included (1) leakage of raw sewage onto the pasture after a flood in 1980, (2) municipal sewage sludge application on the farm, (3) defecation in feed or water by farm workers, and (4) infection of cattle before arriving at the farm.

The farm consisted of approximately 243 hectares (1 hectare = approximately 2.5 acres), with 162 hectares for cropland and 81 hectares for pasture. Corn and hay were the only crops raised on this farm. A municipal sewage treatment plant was adjacent to the northeast corner of the farm, downstream from a 5- to 10-m wide creek that ran through pastures grazed by affected cattle. Following the creek was a sewer line that terminated at the sewage plant. There were nine manholes, covered with loose-fitting tops, along the sewer line in the pasture. These manholes were elevated approximately 30 cm above the pasture. The cattle had access to these manholes. On June 28, 1980, heavy rainfall occurred and much of the pasture and some croplands were flooded for approximately 4 to 5 days.

The farm had received applications of municipal sewage sludge intermittently for the last 20 years. The sludge originated only from the adjacent sewage treatment plant. During 1980 and 1982 (preceding the 1981 and 1983 cysticercosis outbreaks), sludge was applied to pastures.

Temporal and spatial observations implicated raw sewage contamination of pastures (from flooding) as the most likely source of infection in the 1981 outbreak. The outbreak in 1983 was more likely associated with sludge application.

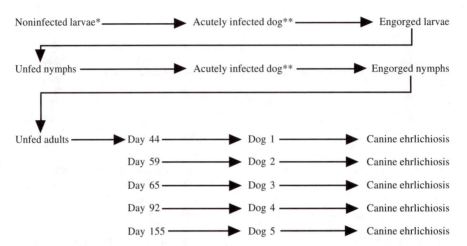

* Unfed *R. sanguineus* larvae, maintained for two previous generations on normal dogs.
** Acute canine ehrlichiosis: rectal temperature of 39.2°C, parasites in peripheral blood monocytes, and severe thrombocytopenia.

Figure 13.2 Evaluation of unfed adult *R. sanguineus* ticks, which fed as larvae and nymphs on acutely infected dogs, as reservoirs of *E. canis*. (From Lewis, G.E., Jr. et al., *Am. J. Vet. Res.*, 38, 1953–1955, 1977. With permission.)

The importance of invertebrate vectors vs. vertebrate hosts as reservoirs of disease agents depends on the life span of the respective hosts and the survival and infectivity of the disease agent in their tissues. Experimental studies may provide important information directly applicable to field situations.

Example 13.3

Ehrlichia canis, the etiologic agent of **canine ehrlichiosis**, is a tick-borne rickettsia that can persist in the blood of infected dogs for periods that far exceed the life span of the tick vector, *Rhipicephalus sanguineus*, the brown dog tick. Notwithstanding, experimental studies revealed that the period of infectivity of the dog for the tick is restricted to the febrile phase of infection, which does not exceed 2 weeks. The tick appears to remain infective for life (Figure 13.2).

Adult *R. sanguineus* ticks efficiently transmitted *E. canis* to susceptible dogs for 155 days after detachment as engorged nymphs from a dog in the acute phase of ehrlichiosis. Adult ticks that had similarly engorged on a dog in the chronic phase of ehrlichiosis failed to transmit *E. canis* to susceptible dogs. Infected but unfed adult ticks may thus be of greater importance than the chronically infected carrier dog as a natural reservoir of *E. canis* (Lewis et al., 1977).

Amplifying hosts are generally considered to be those intermediate hosts that do not suffer from disease, but in which the number of infectious units increases extensively and provides a source for epidemics in humans or domestic animals. **St. Louis encephalitis** provides an excellent example (Figure 13.3).

The basic cycle of the infection involves wild birds and ornithophilic mosquitoes. Peridomestic birds and domestic fowl serve as amplifiers of the virus.

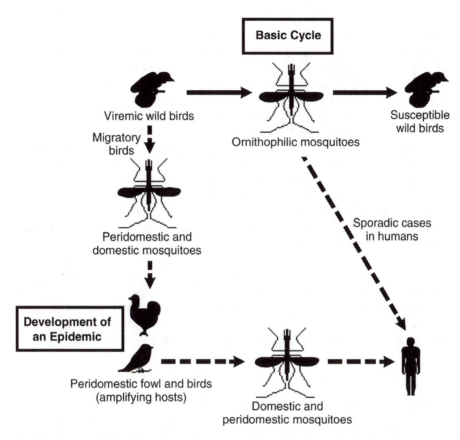

Figure 13.3 St. Louis encephalitis — probable cycle of virus and role of amplifying hosts in epidemics. (From Acha, P.N. and Szyfres, B., *Zoonoses and Communicable Diseases Common to Man and Animals*, Pan American Health Organization, Washington, DC, 1980. With permission.)

That, together with increased density of the human population, creates the conditions necessary for epidemics. How the virus gets into urban areas is not yet established, though it is suspected that migratory wild birds are responsible.

13.1.3   Environment

The environment may be considered a source of infection when the disease agent multiplies there, not requiring any animal host for its continued survival. *Histoplasma capsulatum*, causative agent of **histoplasmosis**, is an example of an infectious, nontransmissible disease agent. Infection results from inhalation of airborne conidia, which are produced during growth of organisms in the soil. See the next section for a further discussion of transmissible vs. nontransmissible diseases.

During the course of an outbreak investigation, a distinction should be made between those situations in which the environment is the ultimate source and reservoir of infection, and those in which the environment is a **fomite** or vehicle of transmission. In the latter case, even though the immediate source of a disease agent, such as parasite ova in the soil, is environmental, the ultimate source of infection is another host. From the standpoint of control, it may be unwise to restrict our view to only the immediate source of infection. Consider the following example.

Example 13.4

In the 3-month period from October 17, 1985 to January 9, 1986, 44 episodes of **pyoderma** occurred among 32 workers in an Oregon meat-packing plant. Most of the 44 reports involved impetigo-like lesions (pustules) on the hand, wrist, and forearm, but six episodes of cellulitis (inflammation of the cellular and subcutaneous tissue) and two of lymphangitis (inflammation of lymphatic vessels) were also reported. The same epidemic strain of **Group-A, -B hemolytic *Streptococcus*** (GAS) isolated from skin lesions was also isolated from meat in the plant. The attack rate for boners and killers was 74%, compared with 13% for workers who were never involved in killing or boning (relative risk = 5.7; 95% confidence interval = 2.9 to 11.3). The epidemic investigation suggested that though the infection was acquired from the environment, meat was a vehicle of transmission of GAS between workers, probably after initial contamination by an infected human. Knife use was probably the significant risk shared by killers and boners vs. other meat workers.

Recommendations to the meat-packing plant included an increased emphasis on worker safety; an increased emphasis on worker hygiene, e.g., covering skin lacerations; removal of workers with untreated skin infections from the meat-processing line; and improved surveillance of skin injuries and infections, including modifying sick leave benefits to encourage reporting (CDC, 1986).

13.2 Transmission

13.2.1 Mode of transmission vs. route of infection

A distinction must be made between the terms *mode of transmission* and *route of infection*. For example, if we say that the mode of transmission is via the respiratory tract, we have not indicated whether the organisms gained access via droplet transmission (direct) or droplet nuclei or dust (airborne). The respiratory route is really the route of infection. The **mode of transmission** refers to the way(s) in which an etiologic agent is transmitted from affected to susceptible individuals.

▼

Modes of transmission may be broadly classified as horizontal or vertical, and within horizontal as direct, indirect, or airborne. Routes of infection (and exit) include alimentary, respiratory, urogenital, anal, skin, and conjunctival.

▲

Modes of transmission may be broadly classified as horizontal or vertical, and within horizontal as direct, indirect, or airborne. The **route of infection** refers to the route by which an etiologic agent gains access to the body of a susceptible individual. Routes of infection (and exit) include alimentary, respiratory, urogenital, anal, skin, and conjunctival (Anderson and May, 1982) (Figure 13.4). **Mode of spread** or dissemination refers to how a disease agent is spread from one geographic region to another.

13.2.2 Transmissible vs. nontransmissible diseases

Diseases are broadly classified as **transmissible** (communicable) or **nontransmissible**. Transmissible disease may be due to a specific infectious agent or its toxic products (such

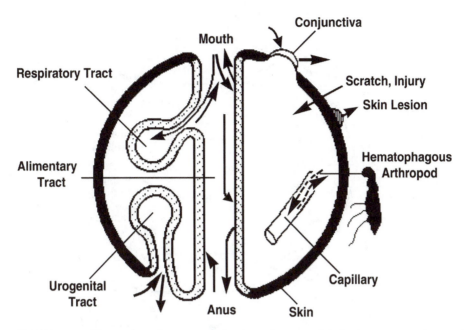

Figure 13.4 Diagram illustrating the routes of exit and entry of infectious agents in vertebrate animals. (From Anderson, R.M. and May, R.M., *Population Biology of Infectious Diseases*, Springer-Verlag, New York, 1982. With permission.)

as the carcass–maggot cycle of waterfowl botulism), which may arise through transmission of that agent or its products from a reservoir to a susceptible host. Transmission may occur directly, as from an infected person or animal, or indirectly, through an intermediate plant or animal host, vector, or the inanimate environment.

Nontransmissible diseases may be caused by infectious or noninfectious agents. Infectious agents may originate from environmental sources (such as the saprophytic fungi responsible for histoplasmosis, blastomycosis, and coccidioidomycosis, or infections caused by *Clostridium tetani*), or part of the normal flora, such as the bacterial secondary invaders responsible for pneumonia, wound infections, and abscesses. Noninfectious agents include poisons and environmental toxins, immunologic and metabolic mechanisms, nutritional deficiencies, and functional defects (such as congenital anomalies).

▼

Practically speaking, introduction into the herd of an animal afflicted with a nontransmissible disease does not increase the likelihood of disease in others.

▲

Contact with diseased animals is always viewed with some degree of apprehension. Practically speaking, introduction into the herd of an animal afflicted with a nontransmissible disease does not increase the likelihood of disease in others. Introduction into the herd of an individual with a transmissible disease increases the likelihood of disease for others. The degree of risk depends, in part, on the mode of transmission.

13.3 Modes of transmission

Transmission may occur **horizontally** by transmission of an infectious agent between contemporaries or animals of more or less the same generation directly, indirectly, or via

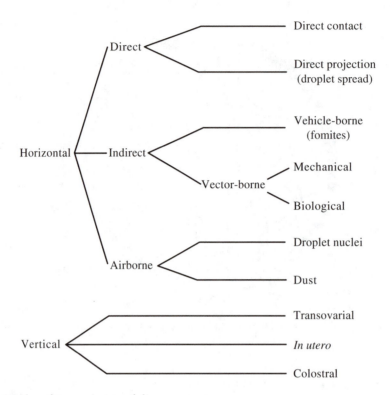

Figure 13.5 Modes of transmission of disease agents.

airborne routes. Transmission may also occur **vertically** by transmission from infected animals of one generation to animals of the succeeding generation (in utero or via colostrum). The modes of transmission of disease agents are depicted in Figure 13.5 and described in the following sections (Schwabe et al., 1977; Toma et al., 1999; Chin, 2000).

13.3.1   Horizontal transmission

Horizontal transmission describes the transmission of a disease agent among contemporaries. Modes of horizontal transmission may be direct, indirect, or airborne.

13.3.1.1   Direct transmission

Direct transmission implies direct and essentially immediate transfer of an agent from infected to susceptible hosts. This may occur by **direct contact**, as through touch, a scratch, lick, bite, or intercourse, or through **direct projection**, where atomized droplets are sprayed onto the conjunctiva or mucous membranes of the eye, nose, or mouth during coughing or sneezing. Direct projection, also known as **droplet spread**, is usually limited to a distance of 1 m or less.

Example 13.5

Human infection with *Toxocara canis*, a canine roundworm, may result in ocular larval migrans, visceral larval migrans, and covert toxocariasis. Human exposure from ingestion of contaminated soil has traditionally been considered the mode of transmission. Wolfe and Wright (2003) assessed the evidence for the soil contamination hypothesis and proposed that **direct contact** with dogs may provide a better explanation of the epidemiology of the disease. Hair was collected from 60 dogs from various places in Ireland and the U.K. and examined for the presence of *T. canis* eggs. They found that the maximum densities of embryonating and embryonated eggs on hair were much higher than densities reported for soil samples. Based on these findings, they propose that dogs infected with *T. canis* may infect people by direct contact. Simply patting a *T. canis*–infected dog that has eggs on its coat may be sufficient for transmission through ingestion.

▼

Direct transmission implies direct and essentially immediate transfer of an agent from infected to susceptible hosts. Indirect transmission implies the passage of infectious agents between individuals through the medium of inanimate or animate objects.

▲

13.3.1.2   Indirect transmission

Indirect transmission implies the passage of infectious agents between individuals through the medium of inanimate or animate objects. The period between contamination of the object and subsequent exposure of susceptible individuals is highly variable and may range from a few minutes to years. Indirect transmission may be vehicle-borne or vector-borne. Most parasitic diseases are transmitted indirectly, either from environmental contamination or via intermediate hosts.

13.3.1.2.1 Vehicle-borne transmission.   **Vehicle-borne transmission** occurs through exposure to contaminated inanimate objects (**fomites**) such as bedding, surgical instruments, soil, water, food, milk, and biological products (including blood, serum, plasma, tissues, or organs). The agent may or may not have multiplied or developed in or on the vehicle before being transmitted. The term *fomite* originates from the Latin word for tinder, *fomes* (Halpin, 1975). The equipment of sick animals has long been thought of as forms of smoldering tinder, which can ignite the fire of disease in others.

▼

The equipment of sick animals has long been thought of as forms of smoldering tinder, which can ignite the fire of disease in others.

▲

Example 13.6

A 37-year-old man became ill with signs and symptoms compatible with leptospirosis. Three days later, he entered a hospital with a temperature of 103.6°F, slightly abnormal liver function tests, leukopenia, and mild anemia. He was started on tetracycline, and 12 hours later his symptoms cleared. Thirty days later he again had a fever, headache, and myalgia. This time his symptoms were accompanied by bilateral orchitis. He was given oral ampicillin, and 3 days later his symptoms cleared. Paired serum samples collected after initial onset of disease showed increasing titers for *Leptospira ballum* in the microscopic agglutination test.

The patient had purchased two white mice at a local pet shop approximately 3 months before the initial illness. Both mice were sacrificed and found to have nephritis. Spirochetes were isolated from their kidneys. When inoculated into guinea pigs, the spirochetes caused a diagnostic titer rise in the guinea pigs for *L. ballum*. A mouse obtained from the mouse colony that was the source of these animals for the pet shop was also found to harbor *L. ballum* in its kidneys. Sera obtained from the patient's wife and three daughters, as well as the man and woman who owned the mouse colony, were all negative for leptospiral antibodies.

Because the patient had virtually no contact with the pet mice, the mode of transmission was uncertain. The patient speculated that one of his daughters, after an argument, had used his toothbrush to clean the mouse cage (Friedmann et al., 1971).

13.3.1.2.2 Vector-borne transmission.   **Vector-borne transmission** is generally understood to mean transmission by invertebrate vectors, such as flies, mosquitoes, or ticks. In some cases, vertebrate hosts such as dogs, foxes, or bats may serve as vectors, as in the case of rabies transmission. Transmission may be by injection of salivary gland fluid during biting or by regurgitation or deposition on the skin of feces or other body fluids that contaminate host tissues through the bite wound or through an area of trauma induced by scratching or rubbing. Vector-borne transmission may be either mechanical or biological.

Mechanical transmission results from simple mechanical carriage of the disease agent between hosts by crawling or flying arthropods. It does not require multiplication or development of the disease agent in the vector. The disease agent is transmitted between hosts on soiled appendages or the proboscis, or by passage of organisms through the gastrointestinal tract.

Biological transmission requires a period of multiplication, cyclic development, or both before the vector can transmit the infective form of the agent. This period is referred to as the **extrinsic incubation period**, as opposed to the **intrinsic incubation period** required for an infected vertebrate host to become infective. The disease agent may be transmitted vertically (**transovarially**) between generations of the vector or **transstadially** from one stage to another within a single generation.

▼

Horizontal transmission describes the transmission of a disease agent among contemporaries. Vertical transmission describes the transmission of a disease agent from animals of one generation to subsequent generations.

▲

13.3.1.3 Airborne transmission

Airborne transmission involves the dissemination of microbial aerosols. **Microbial aerosols** are suspensions of particles in the air consisting partially or wholly of microorganisms. They may remain suspended in the air for long periods and usually infect the host via the respiratory tract. Particle diameters range from less than 1 to 100 μm. Droplets and other large particles that promptly settle out of the air are not considered to be airborne. Airborne transmission may be affected by droplet nuclei or dust.

Droplet nuclei are the small residues that result from evaporation of fluid from droplets emitted by an infected host. They may also be created by atomizing devices, accidentally in microbiology laboratories, abattoirs, rendering plants, or necropsy rooms.

Droplet nuclei usually remain suspended in the air for long periods. **Dust** consists of the small particles of widely varying size that may arise from soil (as fungus spores separated from dry soil by wind or mechanical agitation), clothes, bedding, or contaminated floors.

13.3.2 Vertical transmission

Vertical transmission describes the transmission of a disease agent from animals of one generation to subsequent generations. Vertical transmission may be transovarial, e.g., between generations of invertebrate vectors via the egg, in utero, or transplacental (from parent to offspring within the uterus) or colostral (from parent to offspring at parturition via colostrum or milk). Vertical transmission provides an important reservoir or overwintering mechanism for certain vector-borne viruses, rickettsia, and protozoa.

13.4 Factors affecting communicability

Communicability may be defined as the ease with which a disease agent is spread within a population. One way of expressing communicability is the **intrinsic (or basic) reproductive number (R_o)**, which represents the average number of secondary infections generated by one primary case in a susceptible population, and can be used to estimate the level of immunization or other risk reduction strategy required to control an epidemic (Anderson and May, 1991; Pybus et al., 2001). It follows that as herd immunity (see Chapter 12) increases, the number of secondary cases declines by a factor roughly proportional to the fraction that is susceptible. This relationship is described by the equation $R = R_o \times (1 - P)$, where R is the **effective reproductive number** and P is the proportion of the population immune or resistant, e.g., herd immunity. If $R > 1$, then the number of infected individuals can increase, possibly leading to an epidemic. If R approximates 1, then conditions supporting endemic disease exist. If $R < 1$, then disease frequency will decline, possibly leading to eradication.

▼

Communicability may be defined as the ease with which a disease agent is spread within a population. One way of expressing communicability is the intrinsic (or basic) reproductive number (R_o), which represents the average number of secondary infections generated by one primary case in a susceptible population, and can be used to estimate the level of immunization or other risk reduction strategy required to control an epidemic.

▲

The value of R_o depends on three parameters: (1) the duration of the infectious period, (2) the probability that a contact between an infective and a susceptible individual will lead to an infection, and (3) the number of new susceptible individuals contacted per unit time (Dietz, 1993). The communicability of a disease agent is also determined by factors that are specific to the disease agent, its host, and the environment, e.g., the **agent–host–environment triad**. Some of these factors are discussed in the following sections.

13.4.1 Agent factors

13.4.1.1 Life cycle

The life cycle of a disease agent may be defined as the sequence of developmental stages from infection of one host to infection of a second host. Epidemiologically, the life cycle can be expressed as discrete periods. Included are the prepatent period, communicable period, and extrinsic incubation period.

The **prepatent period** (or **intrinsic incubation period**) is the time between infection of the vertebrate host and detectability of an agent in secretions, excretions, blood, or tissues. The **communicable period** is the time or times during which an infectious agent may be transferred directly or indirectly from one infected animal to another, including invertebrate vectors (Chin, 2000). The **extrinsic incubation period** is the time between infection of a biological vector and acquisition by the vector of the ability to transmit the agent to another susceptible vertebrate host. The extrinsic incubation period is a major determinant of the time between introduction of an infectious animal into a herd and occurrence of disease among susceptibles.

13.4.1.2   *Minimal infective dose*

Disease agents vary widely in their infectivity for a host. Generally speaking, the lower the **minimal infective dose**, the more readily the agent is transmitted.

13.4.2   *Host factors*

13.4.2.1   *Heterogeneity*

Within any population, individuals vary in their susceptibility to infection and disease, irrespective of their immune status. This phenomenon, generally referred to as **innate resistance**, is most likely an expression of the genetic composition of the host. By limiting infection, transmission is reduced. On the contrary, certain individuals may be particularly susceptible to infection and serve as a reservoir of infection for the rest of the herd. The term *lousy* refers to the propensity of certain individuals to develop heavy louse infestations, particularly in the winter. In cattle operations it is recommended that these animals be eliminated from the herd, rather than treated.

13.4.2.2   *Immunity*

Generally, vertebrate hosts develop a stronger immune response to microbial pathogens than they do to metazoans. This may be a result of the extensive multiplication of the former in the host, and the associated strong antigenic exposure. As a result, microbial infections tend to be of shorter duration and self-limiting, thus limiting the opportunity for secondary transmission.

13.4.3   *Environmental factors*

13.4.3.1   *Particle diameter*

13.4.3.1.1 *Droplets.*   The efficiency of transmission by direct projection is limited by the size of the **droplets**, which are greater than 100 μm in diameter. The typical settling velocity of the droplets is greater than 1 foot per second, and time of suspension is less than 3 seconds. Their flight range is restricted to about 1 m or less. Droplet spread can be effectively reduced through use of a face mask and by reducing crowding among animals (Schwabe et al., 1977).

13.4.3.1.2 *Dust particles.*   **Dust particles** are smaller than droplets, ranging from 10 to 100 μm in diameter. Their suspension time is limited by their settling velocity, which ranges from 1 foot per minute to 1 foot per second. They typically hover in clouds and

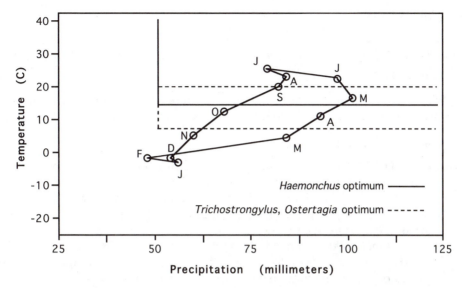

Figure 13.6 A bioclimatograph depicting months during which optimal conditions for pasture transmission of *Haemonchus*, *Trichostrongylus*, and *Ostertagia* occur in Urbana, IL, based on climatic data
from 1903 to 1954. Letters on the graphs are the first letters of the names of the months. (Adapted
from Levine, N.D., *Advanced Veterinary Science*, Vol. 8, Brandly, C.A. and Jungherr, E.L., Eds., Academic Press, New York, 1963, pp. 215–261. With permission.)

can be removed from the air by filtration and electrostatic precipitation. Dust-borne spread
can be reduced by air cleanliness and moistening or oiling contaminated sources.

    13.4.3.1.3 Droplet nuclei. **Droplet nuclei** are the smallest of the particles, ranging
from 2 to 10 µm in diameter. Their settling velocity is less than 1 foot per minute. They
are most efficiently dispersed throughout confined atmospheres, as in hog houses or
abattoirs, and their time of suspension is limited indoors by the degree of ventilation.
They can be removed from the air by electrostatic precipitation, and droplet spread can
be reduced through sanitary ventilation, e.g., air change and equivalent air disinfection.

13.4.3.2 Microclimate

Among environmental factors, desiccation plays a major role in reducing transmissibility
of infectious agents. Levine (1963, 1965) used **bioclimatographs** to predict the effect of
climate on the epidemiology of sheep nematodes. Climatographs are graphs in which total
precipitation is plotted against mean temperature for each month, and the resultant points
are joined in a closed curve. Bioclimatographs are climatographs on which lines indicating
the limits of climatic conditions most favorable for propagation of life, in this case free-
living stages of ruminant nematodes, have been superimposed.

    A climatograph for Urbana, IL, based on meteorologic data from 1903 to 1954 is presented
in Figure 13.6. Optimal conditions for pasture transmission of *Haemonchus*, *Trichostrongylus*,
and *Ostertagia* are superimposed. The resulting graph is a bioclimatograph. Urbana is suitable
for *Haemonchus* pasture transmission throughout the summer and for *Trichostrongylus* and
Ostertagia pasture transmission only during the spring and fall (Levine, 1965).

    The suitability of other regions for these three parasites can be compared by substi-
tuting monthly temperature and precipitation data for the Urbana data. The optimum
condition lines for each parasite remain unchanged.

13.5   Case study

13.5.1   An outbreak of Escherichia coli O157:H7 infections among visitors to a dairy farm

The ecology of an infectious agent in the farm environment and sources of infection for humans are defined (Crump et al., 2002).

13.5.1.1   Introduction

Escherichia coli **O157:H7** causes an estimated 60 deaths and 73,000 illnesses annually in the U.S. Healthy cattle are the main recognized animal reservoir and may harbor the organism as part of the bowel flora. Most reported human outbreaks are due to contaminated food or water. However, transmission of *E. coli* O157:H7 from animals and their environment to humans has been reported.

During September 2000, an unexpectedly large number of cases of *E. coli* O157:H7 infection occurred among visitors to a popular petting farm in Montgomery County, Pennsylvania. A joint investigation involving county, state, and federal (Centers for Disease Control (CDC)) agencies was initiated on November 2.

13.5.1.2   Purpose of the study

The goals of the investigation were to determine the magnitude of the outbreak, to identify risk factors for infection, to interrupt transmission, and to describe the ecology of *E. coli* O157:H7 in the farm environment.

13.5.1.3   Epidemiologic methodology

13.5.1.3.1   Epidemiologic investigation.   Physicians and medical microbiology laboratories across the country were asked to report outbreak-associated cases to the Montgomery County Health Department and to forward isolates to state health department laboratories for molecular subtyping. A case control study was conducted among farm visitors to identify specific risk factors for infection. A probable case was defined as acute diarrhea (three or more loose stools in a 24-hour period) in a person beginning within 10 days of visiting the farm after September 1. A confirmed case was defined as acute diarrhea in a person beginning within 10 days of visiting the farm after September 1, accompanied by either the hemolytic-uremic syndrome (HUS) or the isolation of *E. coli* O157:H7 from stool. Controls were persons who visited the farm after September 1 and did not have diarrhea within 10 days of the visit. In the process of obtaining controls, a survey was conducted to estimate the rate of illness among petting farm visitors.

The layout of the farm was determined, and a complete list of food and beverages available to visitors was compiled. A census of the animals present at the farm during September and October was conducted, and the farm's entire population of domestic animals was subjected to rectal or cloacal swab sampling between November 13 and 16. Swabs of the railings around animal enclosures were obtained. Water samples were collected at sites around the farm, and biofilm samples were collected from watering troughs.

13.5.1.3.2   Laboratory investigation.   All samples were processed for selective isolation of *E. coli* O157:H7, confirmed serologically, and tested for toxin production through the use of an enzyme immunoassay. Molecular subtyping of isolates was performed through the use of pulsed-field gel electrophoresis (PFGE). Shiga toxin genes were detected by multiplex polymerase chain reaction with the use of established primers.

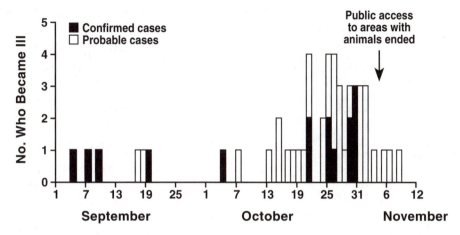

Figure 13.7 Onset of diarrheal illness among 49 visitors to a Pennsylvania farm, September to November 2000. (From Crump, J.A. et al., *N. Engl. J. Med.*, 347, 555–560, 2002. With permission.)

13.5.1.3.3   Statistical analysis.   Statistical analyses were conducted with the use of Epi Info, Version 6.04 (CDC), SAS System for Windows, Release 8.0 (SAS Institute), and LogXact for Windows, Version 4.1 (Cytel Software). Univariate analyses were performed to identify risk favors for inclusion in a multivariate logistic regression model. Factors considered for inclusion in the final model were demographic variables, direct contact with animals, environmental exposures, hand–mouth activities, foods and beverages, and hand-washing behavior. Where appropriate, combined exposure variables were defined. The analysis was stratified by age to account for possible age-related differences in exposure.

13.5.1.4   Assumptions inherent in the methodology

The presumed source and modes of transmission of the infectious agent were inferred based on (1) temporal relationship, (2) strength of association, (3) biologic plausibility, (4) consistency of findings with other studies, and (5) apparent reversible association.

13.5.1.5   Basic epidemiologic findings

13.5.1.5.1   Epidemiologic and clinical information.   As of November 12, 2000, 15 confirmed cases and 36 probable cases of *E. coli* O157:H7 had been identified. All were visitors; no residents or employees of the farm reported having diarrhea during the outbreak period. Dates of onset were known for 49 patients and ranged from September 4 through November 8, 2000. The epidemic curve is depicted in Figure 13.7. Cases ceased to occur a few days after access to animals was prohibited on November 4 (Figure 13.7).

Statistically significant ($p < 0.05$) variables identified through univariate analysis are listed in Table 13.1. Cases were more likely than controls to have direct or indirect contact with calves and other animals and their environment. Hand–mouth activities were also associated with greater risk of infection. Hand-washing behaviors and observing calves through a window were protective. Only two of the variables listed in Table 13.1 were retained (statistically significant) in the multivariate logistic regression analysis model (Table 13.2): viewing calves less than 6 weeks of age and viewing calves 6 to 35 weeks of age. Hand washing approached significance for protection ($p = 0.081$).

In the process of obtaining controls, 3497 households were contacted. Of these, 134 (4%) reported that a household member had visited the farm after September 1, and 22

Table 13.1 Univariate Analysis of Risk Factors for *E. coli* Infection among Farm Visitors

Category	Summary Odds Ratio (95% CI)[a]	*p* Value
Exposure to animals or their environment		
Viewing cattle or calves	10.9 (1.7–70.7)	0.012
Viewing calves <6 wk old	4.7 (1.6–13.6)	0.004
Viewing calves 6–35 wk old	3.8 (1.7–8.5)	0.001
Touching calf-hutch fence	3.8 (1.5–9.7)	0.007
Contact with cattle manure	2.5 (1.2–5.2)	0.013
Direct contact with animals		
Touching any animal	4.5 (1.8–11.0)	0.001
Touching any calf	2.3 (1.1–4.7)	0.021
Hand–mouth activities		
Purchasing food or drink at farm[b]	3.0 (1.4–6.1)	0.003
Nail biting	2.5 (1.1–5.7)	0.037
Hand-washing behaviors		
Washing hands in sink	0.19 (0.04–0.94)	0.042
Washing hands before eating	0.23 (0.08–0.74)	0.013
Washing hands after touching animals	0.27 (0.09–0.86)	0.027
Other behaviors		
Watching cattle through glass window	0.15 (0.03–0.75)	0.021

[a] CI = confidence interval.

[b] No individual food or drink item reached statistical significance by multivariate analysis.

Source: Crump, J.A. et al., *N. Engl. J. Med.*, 347, 555–560, 2002. With permission.

Table 13.2 Multivariate Analysis of Exposures among Patients and Controls Visiting the Farm

Exposure	Patients No./ Total No. (%)	Controls No./ Total No. (%)	Odds Ratio (95% CI)[a]
Viewing calves			
<6 wk old	47/51 (92)	63/91 (69)	3.9 (1.1–17.3)
6–35 wk old	41/51 (80)	47/91 (52)	3.3 (1.3–8.8)
Hand washing	3/20 (15)	18/40 (45)	0.5 (0.2–1.1)

[a] Adjusted odds ratios (conditional logistic regression analyses) were stratified according to age group. CI = confidence interval.

Source: Crump, J.A. et al., *N. Engl. J. Med.*, 347, 555–560, 2002. With permission.

of these (16%) reported that the household member had had diarrhea during the 10 days after the visit. This is more than twice the expected rate of diarrhea in the general population of 7% per 10 days.

13.5.1.5.2 Environmental investigation.   The farm was a small, working dairy farm. Calves younger than 6 weeks of age were kept in hutches, and calves 6 to 35 weeks of age were kept in a barn. Both areas were fully accessible to the public. Heifers and mature cows were kept separate from the calves and were less accessible to the public. In addition, pigs, donkeys, llamas, sheep, goats, peafowl, chickens, cats, and dogs were displayed. A store and concession stands sold food and drink that could be consumed in the animal areas. Raw milk was not served. Hand-washing facilities were limited, not configured for use by children, and unsupervised.

Table 13.3 Sources of *E. coli* O157:H7 and Pattern of Isolates
on Pulsed-Field Gel Electrophoresis (PFGE)

Source	*E. coli* O157:H7 Isolates No./Total No. (%)	PFGE Pattern No./Total No. (%)
Patients	8/51 (16)	8/8 (100)
All cattle	33/216 (15)	28/33 (85)
Calves, < 6 wk old	3/13 (23)	2/3 (67)
Calves, 6–35 wk old	5/38 (13)	5/5 (100)
Small heifers	10/25 (40)	9/10 (90)
Large heifers and dry cows	11/40 (28)	8/11 (73)
"Prefresh" cows (within 2 wk before parturition)	1/9 (11)	1/1 (100)
Lactating cows	3/91 (3)	3/3 (100)
Animals other than cattle	0/43	NA
Railings around animal enclosures	1/37 (3)	1/1 (100)
Biofilm samples from watering troughs	1/7 (14)	0/1
Water	0/7	NA

Note: NA = not applicable.

Source: Crump, J.A. et al., *N. Engl. J. Med.*, 347, 555–560, 2002. With permission.

Overall 15% of cattle were colonized with *E. coli* O157:H7, the prevalence varying with age/production group (Table 13.3). Most harbored isolates with the same PFGE pattern as isolates recovered from cases. Overall, calves and heifers were more often colonized than older cattle. No isolations were made from farm animals other than cattle. *E. coli* O157:H7 was occasionally isolated from the environment, but not from any water samples collected at sites around the farm (Table 13.3).

13.5.1.5.3 Laboratory results. The number of isolates of *E. coli* O157:H7 and the results of molecular subtyping are summarized in Table 13.3. All 8 *E. coli* O157:H7 isolates from patients and 29 (83%) of 35 isolates from nonhuman sources had the same rare PFGE pattern (EXHX01.0070, pattern 70) and produced both Shiga toxin 1 and Shiga toxin 2.

13.5.1.6 Conclusions and measures taken

High rates of carriage of *E. coli* O157:H7 among calves and young cattle on this farm most likely resulted in contamination of both the animals' hides and the environment. Farm visitors were exposed through direct contact with the animals and indirectly from their immediate environment. Among all farm visitors, the data showed a trend toward hand washing as providing protection. Other studies of *E. coli* O157:H7 prevalence in cattle herds have yielded values in the range of <0.5 to 2%. The high rate of colonization of cattle on this farm (15%) may indicate that the *E. coli* O157:H7 strain involved in the outbreak had recently been introduced to the farm, leading to the peak in prevalence that may occur when a new strain sweeps through a previously unexposed herd.

The household survey suggested that many illnesses escaped detection through routine case finding. Considering the mode of transmission revealed in this study, special precautions must be taken when bringing children, a group at increased risk for severe illness due to *E. coli* O157:H7 infection, together with cattle, major reservoirs of *E. coli* O157:H7, in an uncontrolled environment where eating is encouraged and hand-washing facilities are inadequate. Preventive strategies include the use of hand washing, controlled and supervised contact with animals, and clear separation of food-related activities from areas housing animals.

13.6 Summary

Infections may originate (1) iatrogenically, (2) from animal reservoirs, or (3) from the environment. Iatrogenic illnesses are those that are induced in a patient by a clinician's actions. Animal reservoirs of disease agents include (1) carrier animals, animals (including humans) with inapparent infections that are also transmitters (or potential transmitters) of the infectious agent, and (2) intermediate hosts and vectors. Amplifying hosts are intermediate hosts that do not suffer from disease, but in which the number of infectious units increases extensively and provides a source for epidemics in humans or domestic animals. Animals that have been exposed to an agent may become carriers. Incubatory carriers are capable of serving as a source of infection while incubating the disease. Convalescent carriers continue to shed infectious organisms after the signs and symptoms of disease have disappeared. The environment may be considered a source of infection when the disease agent multiplies there, not requiring any animal host for its continued survival.

Diseases are broadly classified as transmissible (communicable) or nontransmissible. Practically speaking, introduction into the herd of an animal afflicted with a nontransmissible disease does not increase the likelihood of disease in others. Horizontal disease transmission between contemporaries, or animals of more or less the same generation, may occur directly, indirectly, or via airborne routes. Direct transmission implies direct and essentially immediate transfer of an agent from infected to susceptible hosts. This may occur by direct contact, as through touch, a scratch, lick, bite, or intercourse. A second mode of direct transmission is through direct projection (droplet spread), where atomized droplets are sprayed onto the conjunctiva or mucous membranes of the eye, nose, or mouth during coughing or sneezing.

Indirect transmission may be vehicle-borne or vector-borne. Vehicle-borne transmission occurs through exposure to contaminated inanimate objects (fomites), such as bedding, surgical instruments, soil, water, food, milk, and biological products (including blood, serum, plasma, tissues, or organs). The agent may or may not have multiplied or developed in or on the vehicle before being transmitted. Vector-borne transmission is generally understood to mean transmission by invertebrate vectors, such as flies, mosquitoes, or ticks. It may be mechanical or biological. Mechanical transmission results from simple mechanical carriage of the disease agent between hosts by crawling or flying arthropods. It does not require multiplication or development of the disease agent in the vector. Biological transmission requires a period of multiplication, cyclic development, or both before the vector can transmit the infective form of the agent. The disease agent may be transmitted vertically (transovarially) between generations of the vector or transstadially from one stage to another within a single generation.

Airborne transmission involves the dissemination of microbial aerosols in the form of droplet nuclei or dust. Droplet nuclei are the small residues that result from evaporation of fluid from droplets emitted by an infected host. They may also be created by atomizing devices, accidentally in microbiology laboratories, abattoirs, rendering plants, or necropsy rooms. Droplet nuclei usually remain suspended in the air for long periods. Dust consists of the small particles of widely varying size that may arise from soil (as fungus spores separated from dry soil by wind or mechanical agitation), clothes, bedding, or contaminated floors.

Disease transmission may also occur vertically from animals of one generation to another. Vertical transmission may be transovarial, e.g., between generations of invertebrate vectors via the egg, in utero, or transplacental (from parent to offspring within the uterus) or colostral (from parent to offspring at parturition via colostrum or milk).

Communicability may be defined as the ease with which a disease agent is spread within a population. One way of expressing communicability is the intrinsic (or basic) reproductive number (R_o), which represents the average number of secondary infections generated by one primary case in a susceptible population and can be used to estimate the level of immunization or other risk reduction strategy required to control an epidemic. Communicability is affected by agent, host, and environmental factors. Agent factors include the nature of the agent's life cycle and the minimal infective dose. Host factors may appear as heterogeneity in susceptibility to disease due to innate or immune factors. Environmental factors include particle diameter and the microclimate in which the infectious agent resides.

chapter 14

The cost of disease

14.1 Defining disease in economic terms

Earlier in the text we discussed how disease could be defined in a variety of ways, including animal performance. A producer's decision as to whether to institute any sort of disease control program will be based, in large part, on economic considerations. Similarly, the relative merits of alternative regional or national disease control strategies are usually evaluated on the basis of expected short- and long-term economic impacts.

In order to better target a disease control program, some sort of economic analysis is usually necessary. A variety of economic modeling approaches have been used in veterinary medicine. Partial budgeting, cost–benefit analysis, and decision analysis are among the most common (Bennett, 1992; Huirne and Dijkhuizen, 1997). In the next section the measures-of-effect approach is used to introduce the topic and illustrate how the relative importance of risk factors can be compared in economic terms. Subsequent sections use more complex models to evaluate disease control programs based on their benefits and costs.

14.1.1 The measures-of-effect approach to estimating disease impact

The following example takes advantage of the concept of **measures of effect** for expressing risk developed in Chapter 6. In this case, risk is expressed in economic terms to determine which risk factors have the greatest economic impact. The history is that of a swine herd experiencing less than optimal performance.

▼

A producer's decision as to whether to institute any sort of disease control program will be based, in large part, on economic considerations.

▲

Example 14.1

A review was made of a year's records and of the relationship of animal performance and management procedures at a swine feedlot in central Kansas (Straw et al., 1985). Aspects of performance that were considered unsatisfactory included (1) slow growth rate of finishing pigs, (2) poor feed conversion, (3) high death rate (especially due to *Haemophilus pneumonia*), and (4) excessive carcass trim at the time pigs were slaughtered. During the year, there was a continuous flow of pigs into and out of the feedlot. Data were used from all groups that had been sold that year.

Table 14.1 Veterinary Expenses for Pigs Entered into a Feedlot at Two Times during the Year

Time Pigs Entered the Feedlot	No. of Groups	At Risk (%)	Mean Veterinary Expense per Pig[a]
April to September	15	39	$2.92
October to February	23	61	$4.73
Total	38	Mean	$4.02[b]

[a] Total costs of treatment for internal and external parasites, vaccinations, and antibiotics.

[b] Weighted mean.

Source of data: Straw, B.E. et al., *J. Am. Vet. Med. Assoc.*, 186, 986–968, 1985.

Table 14.2 Carcass Trim in Pigs Given Various Amounts of Injectable Antibiotics

Mean Amount of Injected Antibiotic per Pig	No. of Pigs	At Risk (%)	Carcass Trim Cost per Pig
<4 ml	1249	46	$0.56
>4 ml	1441	54	$3.06
Total	2690	Mean	$1.90[a]

[a] Weighted mean.

Source of data: Straw, B.E. et al., *J. Am. Vet. Med. Assoc.*, 186, 986–968, 1985.

Analyses were performed on 38 groups containing 9988 pigs. Although overall performance was low, certain groups of pigs (defined as **noncases**) performed considerably better than others (defined as **cases**). Comparisons were made between groups in an effort to identify management inputs (**risk factors**) that could be used to improve overall performance.

Due to the large number of pigs (4400) that could be housed at the feedlot at any one time, certain sound management procedures (all-in/all-out, single source of feeder pigs) could not be implemented. The effects of other management procedures (purchase weight, purchase time, vaccinations, treatment regimens) on growth rate, feed conversion, death rate, and carcass trim were compared among groups of pigs.

Daily death rates (incidences) were calculated by dividing the number of pigs that died on a given day by the total number of pigs present in the lot on the same day. Student's t-test was used to compare performance between groups of pigs. The chi-square test was used to compare mortality rates.

The factor having the greatest influence on performance was the month of entry of pigs into the feedlot. Pigs that entered the feedlot between April and September performed better than did pigs entering between October and February (Table 14.1). The amount of carcass trim per pig was significantly less ($p < 0.001$) in pigs that were treated with less than 4 ml of antibiotic by injection vs. pigs that were treated with more than 4 ml of antibiotic ($0.56 vs. $3.06 per pig slaughtered, respectively; Table 14.2).

Single-source pigs did not perform better than multiple-source pigs, nor did heavier pigs vs. lighter pigs. However, total veterinary costs per pig were lower for pigs that weighed more than 27 kg on entry into the feedlot than for pigs that weighed 27 kg or less ($3.53 vs. $4.70, respectively; $p < 0.01$). The average daily death rate among pigs that failed to reach market weight within 150 days of entry into the feedlot (0.0104) was nearly twice that of the pigs that reached market weight before 150 days (0.0054) (see Figure 5.3).

The investigators recommended that the producer (1) start pigs only during spring and summer months, (2) use oral antibiotic therapy if possible to avoid carcass trim at slaughter, (3) market all animals by 150 days after entry into the feedlot (regardless of age), and (4) use a *Haemophilus* vaccine of proven efficacy. However, the actual economic benefit of adopting these recommendations was not estimated.

An analysis of veterinary costs and carcass trim based on presence or absence of risk factors (time of entry into feedlot and volume of antibiotic used, respectively) appears in Table 14.3 and Table 14.4. Cost figures are drawn from Table

Table 14.3 Economic Effect of Time That Pigs Entered a Feedlot Using the Measures-of-Effect Approach

Simple Risks
Veterinary costs/pig in exposed[a] = $4.73
Veterinary costs/pig in unexposed[a] = $2.92
Veterinary costs/pig overall = $4.02
Prevalence of exposure = 61%

Compared Risks
Relative risk = 1.62
Attributable risk/pig = $1.81
Population attributable risk/pig = $1.10
Population attributable fraction = 27%

[a] Exposed pigs entered feedlot October to February; unexposed pigs entered feedlot April to September.
Source of data: Table 14.1.

Table 14.4 Economic Effect of Amount of Injected Antibiotic Used Upon Carcass Trim Using the Measures-of-Effect Approach

Simple Risks
Carcass trim/pig in exposed[a] = $3.06
Carcass trim/pig in unexposed[a] = $0.56
Carcass trim/pig overall = $1.90
Prevalence of exposure = 54%

Compared Risks
Relative risk = 5.46
Attributable risk/pig = $2.50
Population attributable risk/pig = $1.34
Population attributable fraction = 71%

[a] Exposed pigs injected with >4 ml of antibiotic; unexposed pigs injected with <4 ml of antibiotic.
Source of data: Table 14.2.

14.1 and Table 14.2, respectively. The prevalence of exposure to the risk factor in Table 14.3 is calculated from group data, whereas for Table 14.4 it is based on actual pig numbers. From Table 14.3 it can be seen that by starting pigs during spring and summer months, veterinary costs per pig can be reduced by $1.10, or 27% (**population attributable fraction**). The analysis in Table 14.4 shows that by reducing the amount of injected antibiotic below 4 ml, carcass trim per pig can be reduced by $1.34, or 71%.

A similar analysis could be performed on feed efficiency based on the cost per pound of gain. This sort of analysis gives the veterinarian or producer a better idea of where to start first in reducing economic losses due to endemic disease. However, the analysis does not include the cost of the disease control program. Partial budget analysis (discussed below) can be used to compare the benefits of disease control with the costs of control.

14.1.2   Partial budgeting and cost–benefit analysis

14.1.2.1   Partial budgeting

In order to estimate benefits and costs to producers of a specific disease control program, **partial budget analysis** rather than **enterprise budget analysis** may be used. The part of the enterprise budget affected by the disease is separated out so that the effect of the disease is not overshadowed by some other factor or disease. Fixed costs (such as labor costs, machinery and building operating costs and depreciation, rent, and interest) are excluded from the analysis. Determining costs specific to a single disease outbreak requires partial budget analysis.

Partial budgeting usually places farm budget items into one of four categories (Martin et al., 1987; Huirne and Dijkhuizen, 1997):

1. **Additional returns** due to adoption of a proposed control program
2. **Forgone returns**, such as income lost from a reduced number of culled animals
3. **Additional costs incurred** due to the control procedure, such as drugs and management procedures
4. **Costs no longer incurred**, such as veterinary expenses

The disease control program should be adopted if the sum of 1 and 4 above is greater than that of 2 and 3.

14.1.2.2   Cost–benefit analysis

Cost–benefit analysis is a method for estimating the profitability of disease control programs over an extended period. There are three main elements involved: (1) enumeration of benefits and costs (as described above), (2) selection and application of a discount rate to benefits and costs, and (3) specification of a decision criterion. **Cost-effectiveness analysis** is a variant of cost–benefit analysis that is used when the expected benefits are difficult to quantify in economic terms. A training workshop might be evaluated based on how many participants adopt the new technology. Preference is given to the program that, given its costs, benefits the largest number within the target population (Huirne and Dijkhuizen, 1997).

14.1.2.3   Discounting and present and future value of money

Veterinarians are familiar with interest rates on investments or loans as an indicator of the **time value of money**. In contrast, the **discount rate** and the process of discounting used in calculating **present values** for a cost–benefit analysis are less familiar. Because benefits and costs of a long-term disease control program do not occur simultaneously, they cannot be compared without adjusting for the time value of money. Further, costs may accrue during the relatively short life of the program. Benefits may accrue indefinitely into the future.

> Because benefits and costs of a disease control program do not occur simulta-
> neously, they cannot be compared without adjusting for the time value of
> money.

The interest rate determines the value of the principal of an investment at a future date. The discount rate is the reverse of interest rate. If, for example, we were to invest $500 in a disease control program that would yield a $1000 return 5 years from now, the current benefit of the program would not be $1000. This is because $1000 invested today would be worth considerably more than $1000 5 years from now. If, for example, we assume a 10% interest rate over the next 5 years, $1000 5 years from now would be equivalent to $620.90 invested today.

Using a discount rate, disease control program benefits and costs that accrue in the future are discounted to present values. The formula for calculating present value is

$$PV = \frac{1}{(1+r)^n} \times FV$$

where PV is present value, FV is **future value** (i.e., the value of a benefit or cost), r is discount rate (usually the prevailing interest rate paid by loan institutions), and n is the interest compounding interval, usually expressed in years. As the time (n) before a benefit accrues increases, the present value of future benefits decreases.

14.1.2.4 Decision criteria in cost–benefit analysis

Three measures are commonly used to interpret the results of a cost–benefit analysis and arrive at a decision (Huirne and Dijkhuizen, 1997).

14.1.2.4.1 Net present value (NPV). The **net present value** expresses the difference between the total present value of benefits and costs. Stated another way, it is the present value of net benefits. It represents the value of the program at today's prices. It indicates the scale of the net benefits, but does not show the relative size of the benefits and costs. Expensive programs will tend to have a high NPV, even if the return on investment is small.

14.1.2.4.2 Benefit–cost ratio (B/C ratio). The ratio of total present benefits to costs is the **benefit–cost ratio** and represents the relative size of benefits and costs. It provides an index of the dollar value of benefits that can be expected from a given cost investment, but gives no indication of the scale of investment, which should be considered if alternative control programs are to be compared.

14.1.2.4.3 Internal rate of return (IRR). The **internal rate of return** is the interest rate that would make the total present value of the benefits equal to that of the costs, e.g., to reduce the NPV to zero. The IRR can be easily compared with current interest rates without the necessity of selecting a discount rate. However, the IRR is difficult to calculate and is usually estimated empirically through trial and error.

14.2   Decision analysis

In most cases in veterinary practice, the prognosis or economic impact of medical decisions is not certain. The best option, e.g., defer treatment, treat empirically, or administer treatment based on the results of diagnostic tests, may not be readily apparent because of the interaction of a number of variables. If there are multiple possible outcomes of the proposed courses of action, and chance is an important factor in determining which outcome occurs, then **decision analysis** is the approach of choice.

At least four approaches to decision analysis have been described: (1) mathematical equations, (2) payoff matrices, (3) process diagrams or process flowcharts, and (4) decision trees. Decision tree analysis is probably the most frequently used technique of decision analysis (Huirne and Dijkhuizen, 1997). A decision tree provides the decision maker with a graphic approach to the decision-making process.

14.2.1   Steps in building a decision tree

Decision tree analysis is a process for analyzing complex choices by the use of decision trees (Pauker and Kassirer, 1987; Kassirer et al., 1987; Smith, 1993; Huirne and Dijkhuizen, 1997). There are three basic steps in building a decision tree. The first step is to specify the **decision context**, that is, the real-world situation in which a particular decision is to be made. The second step is the development of a **decision model** that includes the management options, the consequences of each option, and how likely and desirable each possible outcome is. The third step is to represent the decision model as a **decision tree** (Figure 14.1), with the consequences of each decision represented by nodes linked by branches.

14.2.1.1   Nodes
There are three basic types of **nodes**: decision, chance, and terminal. A **decision node** represents a choice between two or more options, such as the decision to test or not to test. **Chance or probability nodes** represent events that are at least partially determined by chance, such as the likelihood that disease is present or that a test result is correct. These probabilities can be assessed from literature, experimental data, or expert opinion. A **terminal node** represents a final outcome with no further significant options or consequences.

14.2.1.2   Utilities
The desirability of a final outcome is expressed as the **utility of a terminal node**. Utility is any measurement that can be used to compare outcomes and determine which outcome is more desirable. The value of each utility is expressed relative to a numerical scale common to all the terminal nodes in the tree. Examples are financial gain (value of the animal minus costs incurred for a particular intervention) and prognosis. The latter is frequently expressed as the probability of short-term survival without sequelae.

14.2.1.3   Variables
Each **variable** in a decision tree must be assigned a baseline value, and the baseline value should approximate the average condition as closely as possible. Two types of variables are found in all decision trees: probability variables and utility. Each of the possible

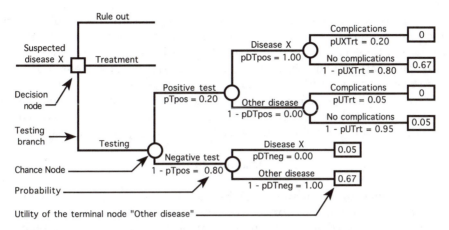

Figure 14.1 Diagram of a portion of a decision tree for Disease X to illustrate basic concepts of decision analysis. The decision node is designated by a square, chance nodes by circles, and terminal nodes by rectangles. Each of the three branches leading from the decision node represents a different strategic option. The probabilities are located beneath each chance node branch, and utilities are within the terminal nodes. For this example, the prior probability of Disease X has been assumed to be 0.20. Test sensitivity and specificity have been assumed to be 100%, simulating a perfect diagnostic test. Therefore, the probability of a positive test (pTpos) is 0.20, the predictive value of a positive test result (probability of disease given a positive test result, pDTpos) is 1.0, and the predictive value of a negative test result (probability of not having the disease given a negative test result, 1 – pDTneg) is 1.0. Baseline values for probabilities and utilities were chosen to approximate average clinical conditions. pUXTrt = probability of complications from treatment of Disease X leading to death; pUTrt = probability of complications leading to death from administering treatment for Disease X to animals suffering from other diseases. By fold-back of the tree, the expected utility of a negative test result would be (0.0 * 0.05) + (1.0 * 0.67) = 0.67. By risk analysis, the probability of death (utility = 0) for the testing branch of this decision tree is (0.2 * 1.0 * 0.2) + (0.2 * 0.0 * 0.05) = 0.04. (From Smith, R.D., *J. Am. Vet. Med. Assoc.*, 203, 1184–1192, 1993. With permission.)

outcomes of a chance node is expressed as a certain probability of occurrence. The sum of the probabilities from each chance node must be 100%, or 1.0.

14.2.2   Analysis of the decision tree

Once a decision tree is constructed, it can be analyzed by use of techniques for fold-back of the tree, sensitivity analysis, and risk profile analysis.

14.2.2.1   Fold-back

In a **fold-back**, the **expected utility** for each decision is calculated by adding the values obtained when the utility of each possible outcome of that decision (terminal node) is multiplied by the probability that the outcome will occur. Every fold-back starts from some node in the tree, which is referred to as the **root node for the fold-back**. In most cases, the root node for a fold-back is a decision node. The expected utility expresses the average utility of each management option when that option is chosen for a large number of animals. The management option with the highest expected utility is usually the option of choice.

14.2.2.2   Sensitivity analysis

Sensitivity analysis, which expresses the degree of confidence one can have in a particular decision, is simply a series of fold-backs over a range of values for one or more variables.

One-way sensitivity analysis is used to calculate the changes in expected utility that occur when the value for only one variable is varied. **Two- and three-way sensitivity analyses**, in which two or three values are varied simultaneously, result in a series of **thresholds**, or **break-even points**, at which the expected utility for each decision is equal. The resulting curves are referred to as indifference curves (Madison et al., 1984; Fetrow et al., 1985). Threshold values indicate whether a change in a given variable would change the optimal decision (i.e., would result in a different management option being the option of choice), but do not indicate how much would be gained or lost by choosing a given management option.

Example 14.2

Equine monocytic ehrlichiosis (EME) was discussed in Chapter 12 in the context of confounding. Prior to elucidating the mode of transmission and reservoir mechanism of the causative agent, *Neorickettsia (Ehrlichia) risticii*, in 1998, the only preventive measure available was immunization with killed *N. risticii* bacterins. Atwill and Mohammed (1996) conducted a cost–benefit analysis of vaccination as a control strategy for horses in the state of New York. At issue was how vaccine cost, efficacy, and risk of disease interacted to determine whether vaccination was a cost-effective control strategy.

Decision tree analyses were performed to estimate the **expected monetary loss** per horse attributable to EME, with or without vaccination, while varying the values of the above input variables (Figure 14.2). Input values for the decision tree were derived from data previously gathered through cross-sectional and case control studies of equine operations in New York State. The risk of being seropositive was dependent on the county in which the horse was located, farm elevation, and use of each horse, so decision tree analyses were stratified by these factors. Vaccine efficacy was set at 78% (95% confidence interval, 58 to 91%).

Fold-back of the decision tree revealed that regardless of the combination of risk region and farm elevation, and regardless of the price of vaccination, the annual expected monetary loss for nonvaccinated horses was considerably less than the annual expected monetary loss for vaccinated horses. **Sensitivity analysis** revealed that even among groups at highest risk of infection, the annual expected monetary loss associated with not vaccinating against EME was considerably lower than that associated with vaccination, regardless of the proportion of horses that developed protective immunity after vaccination (Figure 14.3). Annual expected monetary loss per horse attributable to EME for horses vaccinated by veterinarians ranged from $21 to $21.83/horse/year; for horses vaccinated by owners, it ranged from $10 to $10.83/horse/year; and for nonvaccinated horses, it ranged from $0 to $4.03/horse/year. Assuming 78% of vaccinated horses were protected and mean losses associated with EME included costs for horses that died, annual incidence density at which expected monetary loss for vaccinated horses was equal to that for nonvaccinated horses was 12 cases/1000 horses/year and 25 cases/1000 horses/year for horses vaccinated by owners or by veterinarians, respectively (Figure 14.4). Based on their analysis, the authors conclude that annual vaccination minimizes monetary losses attributable to EME only when the annual incidence density exceeds 12 to 25 cases/1000 horses/year. In New York, expected monetary losses are minimized when horses are not vaccinated because of the low annual incidence density in most regions.

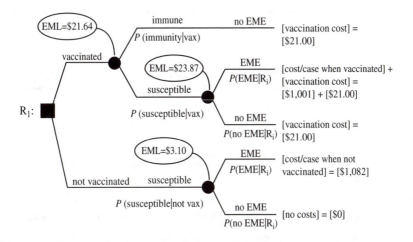

Figure 14.2 Components of the decision tree, where R_i is a specific set of risk factors for a population of horses; P (immunity | vax) is the probability that the horse developed vaccinal immunity after vaccination; P (susceptible | vax) is the probability that the horse failed to develop vaccinal immunity after vaccination, (P [susceptible | vax] = [1 − P (immunity | vax)]); P (EMEIR$_i$) is is the probability that the horse developed equine monocytic ehrlichiosis (EME) given the specific set of risk factors (R_i); P (no EMEIR$_i$) is is the probability that the horse did not develop EME given the specific set of risk factors(R_i); (P [no EMEIR$_i$] = 1 − P [EMEIR$_i$]); P (susceptibility | not vax) is the probability that nonvaccinated horses did not develop immunity. For each outcome, associated costs were calculated. Values used for the analysis were for a high-risk group of horses (horses located in risk region 2 or 3, farm elevation of of 150 to 300 m above mean sea level) and in which: P (immunity | vax) = 0.78; P (susceptible | vax) = 0.22; P (susceptible | not vax) = 1.00; P (EMEIR$_i$) = 0.003; P (no EMEIR$_i$) = 0.997; vaccination administered by a veterinarian ($21.00/dose); cost per case included values for horses that died. EML = expected monetary losses; ■ = decision node (to vaccinate or not to vaccinate); ● = chance nodes for the indicated outcomes. From Atwill, E.R. and Mohammed, H.O., Benefit-cost analysis of vaccination of horses as a strategy to control equine monocytic ehrlichiosis, *J. Am. Vet. Med. Assoc.*, 208, 1295–1299, 1996.

14.2.2.3 Risk profile analysis

Fold-back of the decision tree does not express how likely each result is. One may be more concerned with reducing the likelihood of a particular adverse outcome, such as death of the patient, than with obtaining the highest expected utility. **Risk profile analysis** expresses the probability of occurrence of each of the possible outcomes of a particular set of decisions in a decision tree. Starting at the root node, probabilities for each outcome are multiplied consecutively down to each terminal node. The resulting probabilities can be compared to find the set of decisions associated with the lowest risk of an unfavorable outcome.

14.3 Strategies to reduce the frequency of disease

Ultimately the practitioner must devise a plan for the reduction of disease in the population. This may be accomplished through disease prevention, control (treatment), or eradication. The choice of a particular strategy must be based on an economic evaluation of alternative actions. Most analyses rely on the decision criteria described above. Additional considerations are discussed below.

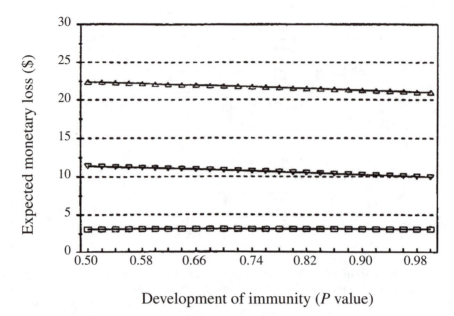

Development of immunity (*P* value)

Figure 14.3 Sensitivity analysis among a high-risk group of horses (horses located in risk region 2 or 3, farm elevation of of 150 to 300 m above mean sea level). The probability that the horse developed immunity after vaccination was varied from 0.50 to 1.00 to determine its effect on annual expected monetary loss per horse per owner when all other factors were kept constant. The analysis was conducted with the assumption that the financial losses associated with EME included the value of horses that died. □ = not vaccinated; ∇ = horses vaccinated by owners; △ = horses vaccinated by veterinarians. From Atwill, E.R. and Mohammed, H.O., Benefit-cost analysis of vaccination of horses as a strategy to control equine monocytic ehrlichiosis, *J. Am. Vet. Med. Assoc.*, 208, 1295–1299, 1996.

14.3.1   Disease prevention

The objective of **disease prevention** is to forestall disease transmission or the occurrence of clinical signs. One way to achieve this is by preventing contact of the host with the agent through isolation, e.g., the removal of a known infected individual from the population, or through quarantine, the confinement of individuals exposed to an infectious agent from other susceptibles. Additionally, animals may be treated prophylactically with antibiotics or immunized to increase their resistance to the agent. Ultimately, disease prevention focuses on the risk factors for disease.

Risk analysis is the formal process for evaluating, managing, determining, and communicating the impact of a risk in a population (Toma et al., 1999). It draws on the quantitative measures of risk assessment discussed in Chapter 6 and applies them to the prevention of disease at the population level. Risk analysis has become increasingly important in veterinary medicine to identify, evaluate, and mitigate food safety risks, and for decision making related to international trade and imports. The decision as to whether to allow the importation of cattle and their products from countries in which bovine spongiform encephalopathy (BSE) has been diagnosed is a classic example.

A risk analysis includes three components (Toma et al., 1999): (1) risk assessment, (2) risk management, and (3) risk communication. **Risk assessment** deals with identifying and quantifying the actual risks or hazards. **Risk management** is the pragmatic decision-making process aimed at the adoption of actions or policies to mitigate risks. **Risk communication** focuses on communicating risks and options for mitigating risks to the target audience. The objective is to accurately convey the information without overdiagnosing,

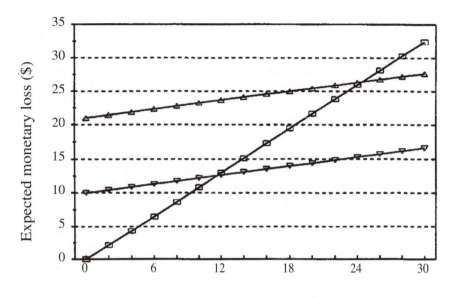

Annual incidence density (No. of cases/1,000 horses/y)

Figure 14.4 Graph in which the annual incidence density was varied from 0 to 35 cases/1,000 horses/y to illustrate the relationship between incidence density of EME and the annual expected monetary loss per horse. Values for annual incidence density at which expected monetary loss for vaccinated horses was equal to that for nonvaccinated horses was determined. The analysis was conducted with the assumption that the probability that vaccination resulted in protective immunity was 0.78 and that the financial losses associated with EME included values for horses that died. □ = not vaccinated; ▽ = horses vaccinated by owners; △ = horses vaccinated by veterinarians. From Atwill, E.R. and Mohammed, H.O., Benefit-cost analysis of vaccination of horses as a strategy to control equine monocytic ehrlichiosis, *J. Am. Vet. Med. Assoc.*, 208, 1295–1299, 1996.

overalarming, overreassuring, or overplanning. It requires a free, unambiguous exchange of information with the affected audience that defines limits of certainty and acknowledges uncertainties involved.

14.3.2   Disease control

Disease control is aimed at reducing the frequency of disease to a tolerable level. It is usually accomplished through treatment of affected individuals, as during a routine mastitis control program in a dairy. Disease control focuses primarily on the source and mode of transmission of a disease agent.

The level of a disease that is considered tolerable depends on the criteria being used, e.g., whose interests are at stake. Thus, a producer may be striving for certain production indices, the bank manager who loaned money to the producer may be looking at financial returns, and regulatory agencies who inspect the producer's animals or animal products must consider public health risks of the disease.

14.3.3   Disease eradication

Eradication is the complete elimination of a disease agent from the environment. Eradication may be considered in an individual herd, where the potential for reintroduction of the disease agent can be effectively controlled, or over wide geographic areas.

14.3.3.1   *Test and removal vs. herd depopulation*

Regional or national programs for animal disease eradication may have to decide whether to implement a **test and removal strategy**, where test-positive animals only are removed from the herd, or a **herd depopulation strategy**, where the detection of any test-positive animal results is condemnation of the entire herd. This decision is often based on the sensitivity of the test or test strategy being employed and the likelihood of false negative test results (see the Michigan tuberculosis program described by Norby et al., 2004, in Chapter 4 for an example).

14.3.3.2   *Necessary conditions for eradication*

Twelve major livestock diseases and pests have been eradicated from the U.S. since 1884. These are contagious bovine pleuropneumonia, Texas cattle fever, foot-and-mouth disease, dourine, glanders, fowl plague, vesicular exanthema, screwworms, sheep scabies, Venezuelan equine encephalitis, exotic Newcastle disease, and hog cholera. The feasibility of eradication depends on meeting one or more of the following conditions:

1. An effective means (diagnostic test) for identification of reservoirs (carriers)
2. An effective method for destruction of the agent in reservoirs (or the reservoirs themselves)
3. A small host range (preferably a single host)
4. A single or limited spectrum of disseminating mechanisms that can be readily manipulated
5. Acceptability to the industry

The level of artificially induced herd immunity required to eradicate disease is inversely related to the etiologic agent's intrinsic reproductive number (see Table 12.1). Even highly effective vaccines may be insufficient to eradicate or even control disease if vaccine coverage is inadequate.

▼

Twelve major livestock diseases and pests have been eradicated from the U.S. since 1884.

▲

Example 14.3

The effectiveness of vaccines in disease control programs may be limited by logistical, economic, political, or sociocultural factors. In India, for example, about 30,000 human rabies deaths occur yearly, accounting for 60% of the global human rabies incidence (Sudarshan et al., 2001). Most (96%) of these human rabies deaths are associated with dog bites. There are about 25 million dogs in India, but rabies incidence is sketchy, as canine rabies is not a reportable disease. In an effort to better understand community factors impeding rabies control, the authors surveyed 300 households in Bangalore through random sampling of households in 30 representative clusters (population units) throughout the city. About 12% of households had pet dogs, and 80.8% of these had received antirabies vaccination. Despite this relatively high level of vaccine coverage, about 61.5% of the city's estimated dog population are strays. Further, the estimated dog population had tripled from 1990 to 2001. The authors estimated the current yearly incidence of dog bites to be 1.9%, equivalent to 85,500 dog bites per year, or about 234 per day. Poor urban dwellers are particularly vulnerable to dog attacks and cannot afford lifesaving antirabies immunization and treatment. In 2000, in response to judicial decisions and pressure from animal welfare organizations, the city replaced the existing stray dog euthanasia program with an Animal Birth Control (ABC) program, which included capture, sterilization, deworming, vaccination, and release. However, the effectiveness of the program was limited by poor media publicity and lack of community participation and support. In its first year of implementation, the ABC program covered only about 10.4% of the stray dog population. A majority of those surveyed preferred that stray dogs be removed from their neighborhoods. The authors recommend an accelerated, better-planned, science-based stray dog elimination program that include sterilization, euthanasia of sick or rabid dogs, and enforcement of dog licensing.

14.4 Case study

14.4.1 Potential revenue impact of an outbreak of foot-and-mouth disease in the U.S.

An economic model is used to suggest how the impact of an FMD outbreak in the U.S. can be reduced (Paarlberg et al., 2002).

14.4.1.1 Introduction
The U.S. has been free of **foot-and-mouth disease (FMD)** since 1929. However, the 1997 outbreak of FMD in Taiwan and the 2001 outbreak of FMD in the U.K. raised concerns about the potential economic impact should FMD reappear in the U.S. Recent studies have estimated that the costs of an FMD outbreak in the U.S. would range from $0.2 to $27.6 billion, depending on the extent of the outbreak and control methods employed.

14.4.1.2 Purpose of the study
This study was conducted to estimate the potential farm revenue impact of an outbreak of FMD in the U.S. if it were similar to the 2001 outbreak in the U.K.

14.4.1.3 Epidemiologic methodology
Equilibrium values for the price, domestic supply and demand, and quantity of meat exports prior to the FMD outbreak were estimated. Next, an outbreak of FMD was assumed to occur in the U.S. An economic analysis of the combined effect of three components affecting markets was performed. First, animal inventories and milk production were reduced due to FMD-induced quarantine and slaughter of affected livestock. This reduced the domestic supply of meat and the quantity available for export, increased the price, and reduced domestic consumption. Second, an international embargo of all susceptible U.S. livestock and livestock products was added. As a result, domestic supply increased, depressing the price. Third, consumption of meat and milk in the U.S. was reduced to account for anticipated consumer fears of contracting FMD. Although there is no scientific basis for this concern, the effect would be to reduce consumption and further decrease prices.

An empirical partial-equilibrium model of the U.S. agricultural sector was used to quantify 1-year impacts of the preceding three components based on 1999 to 2000 data from various U.S. Department of Agriculture (USDA) reports. The model estimated potential percentage

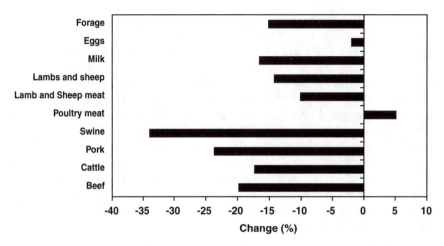

Figure 14.5 Potential percentage change in livestock-related gross revenues as a result of an outbreak of FMD in the U.S. (From Paarlberg, P.L. et al., *J. Am. Vet. Med. Assoc.*, 220, 988–992, 2002. With permission.)

change in livestock-related gross revenues as a result of an FMD outbreak, as well as potential change in gross revenues for grains and oilseed used in livestock production.

14.4.1.4 Assumptions inherent in the methodology
It was assumed that an outbreak in the U.S. would be similar to the spring 2001 outbreak in the U.K. Percentage reductions in livestock used in the model were slightly larger than those calculated for the U.K. because FMD had not been fully eliminated from the U.K. by May 21, 2001, when this analysis was conducted. It was further assumed that all exports of cattle, beef, swine, pork, poultry meat, lambs, sheep, lamb and sheep meat, and dairy products would be embargoed. Although the extent of consumer fears regarding FMD were unknown, it was assumed that 10% of consumers would stop eating red meat and dairy products, but would consume more poultry meat.

Because of the short period (1 year) over which impacts were calculated, livestock producers would have differing abilities to respond. Poultry and egg producers would be able to fully respond to price changes within a 1-year time frame, whereas swine producers would have a more limited ability to respond. Cattle and sheep producers would have almost no ability to adjust livestock numbers in response to price changes within such a short period.

14.4.1.5 Basic epidemiologic findings
In the baseline scenario the model predicted that an FMD outbreak would result in a decrease of $14 billion in U.S. farm income. This loss is equivalent to 6.2% of U.S. gross cash farm income and 9.5% in gross revenue for the commodities modeled. Percentage losses in gross revenue for each sector are summarized in Figure 14.5 and Figure 14.6 and were estimated to be live swine, –34%; pork, –24%; live cattle, –17%; beef, –20%; milk, –16%; live lambs and sheep, –14%; lamb and sheep meat, –10%; forage, –15%; and soybean meal, –7%.

The largest impacts on farm income of an FMD outbreak were from the loss of export markets and reductions in domestic demand arising from consumer fears, rather than output losses from FMD-induced removal of livestock. Outputs from the model were most sensitive to the assumed consumer reaction. If consumption of red meat and dairy products

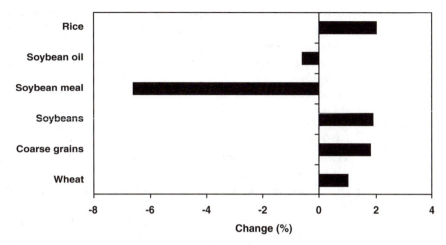

Figure 14.6 Potential percentage change in gross revenues for grains and oilseed as a result of an outbreak of FMD in the U.S. Coarse grains include corn, sorghum, barley, oats, rye, millet, and mixed grains, with corn being the dominant coarse grain in the U.S. (From Paarlberg, P.L. et al., *J. Am. Vet. Med. Assoc.*, 220, 988–992, 2002. With permission.)

were to decrease from 10% (used in the model) to 20%, the loss in farm income would increase from $14 billion to $20.8 billion. Conversely, if there were no adverse consumer reaction, loss of farm income would be only $6.8 billion.

14.4.1.6   *Conclusions and measures taken*
Based on their findings, the authors propose two approaches to help reduce the impact of an FMD outbreak in the U.S.: (1) development of procedures to contain an outbreak of FMD to specific regions of the U.S. (risk-based regionalization of the U.S.), thereby permitting continued export of livestock and livestock products from unaffected areas, and (2) mitigation of adverse consumer reactions to an outbreak through consumer education on the negligible risk posed to humans by FMD through the consumption of red meat and dairy products.

14.5   Summary

A producer's decision as to whether to institute any sort of disease control program will be based, in large part, on economic considerations. In order to better target a disease control program, some sort of economic analysis is usually necessary. The measures-of-effect approach is similar to that used to express risk, with the exception that cost figures are substituted for incidence rates. This sort of analysis gives the veterinarian and producer a better idea of which risk factors have the greatest economic impact. However, the cost of the disease control program is not included in the analysis.

In order to estimate benefits and costs to producers of a specific disease control program, partial budgeting and cost–benefit analyses may be used. Partial budgeting places disease-related expenses into one of four categories: (1) additional returns due to adoption of a proposed control program; (2) forgone returns, such as income lost from a reduced number of culled animals; (3) additional costs incurred due to the control procedure, such as drugs and management procedures; and (4) costs no longer incurred, such as veterinary expenses. The disease control program should be adopted if the sum of 1 and 4 is greater than that of 2 and 3.

Cost–benefit analysis is a method for estimating the profitability of disease control programs over an extended period. There are three main elements involved: (1) enumeration of benefits and costs (as described above), (2) selection and application of a discount rate to benefits and costs, and (3) specification of a decision criterion. Because benefits and costs of a disease control program do not occur simultaneously, they cannot be compared without adjusting for the time value of money. The interest rate determines the value of the principal of an investment at a future date. The discount rate is the reverse of interest rate. Using a discount rate, disease control program benefits and costs that accrue in the future are discounted to present values.

Finally, one must decide on the most appropriate decision criterion. Three measures are commonly used to interpret the results of a cost–benefit analysis and arrive at a decision. The net present value expresses the difference between the total present value of benefits and costs. The ratio of total present benefits to costs is the benefit–cost ratio and represents the relative size of benefits and costs. The internal rate of return is the interest rate that would make the total present value of the benefits equal to that of the costs, e.g., to reduce the NPV to zero.

In most cases in veterinary practice, the prognosis or economic impact of medical decisions is not certain. Decision tree analysis is a process for analyzing complex choices by the use of decision trees. There are three basic steps in building a decision tree. The first step is to specify the decision context, that is, the real-world situation in which a particular decision is to be made. The second step is the development of a decision model that includes the management options, the consequences of each option, and how likely and desirable each possible outcome is. The third step is to represent the decision model as a decision tree, with the consequences of each decision represented by nodes linked by branches.

After the tree is constructed, the expected utility of a particular decision may be computed by folding back the tree. In a fold-back, the expected utility for each decision is calculated by adding the values obtained when the utility of each possible outcome of that decision (terminal node) is multiplied by the probability that the outcome will occur. The branch with the highest expected utility will maximize favorable outcomes over a series of such choices.

Since a fold-back does not give the distribution of how likely each result is, the best choice may not be the branch with the highest expected utility. In this case, a risk profile can be used to estimate the risk of unfavorable outcomes for each branch on the decision tree. One of the principal benefits of decision tree analysis is that the sensitivity of a choice to its underlying assumptions can be tested. At the break-even point, the expected values for two or more interventions are equal. In this case, the decision about which approach to use can be made on grounds other than the prognosis.

Ultimately the practitioner must devise a plan for the reduction of disease in the population. This may be accomplished through disease prevention, control (including treatment), or eradication. The objective of disease prevention is to forestall disease transmission or the occurrence of clinical signs. Disease control is aimed at reducing the frequency of disease to a tolerable level. Eradication is the complete elimination of a disease agent from the environment. The feasibility of eradication depends on meeting one or more of the following conditions: (1) an effective means for identification of reservoirs (carriers), (2) an effective method for destruction of the agent in reservoirs (or the reservoirs themselves), (3) small host range (preferably a single host), and (4) single or limited spectrum of disseminating mechanisms that can be readily manipulated.

Glossary

Accuracy — Test accuracy is the proportion of all tests, both positive and negative, that are correct. It is often used to express the overall performance of a diagnostic test.

Alpha (type I) error — Concluding that outcomes are different when in fact they are not. Alpha error is analogous to the false positive result of diagnostic tests. *See* beta error and *p* value.

Alternative hypothesis — The alternative to the null hypothesis, i.e., that the observed difference between groups could not have arisen by chance and therefore is real.

Amplifying host — Generally considered to be those intermediate hosts that do not suffer from disease, but in which the number of infectious units increases extensively and provides a source for epidemics in humans or domestic animals.

Apparent prevalence — The prevalence of disease estimated on the basis of diagnostic tests. *Compare with* true prevalence.

Attack rate — The proportion of a defined population affected during a particular outbreak. It is equal to the total number of cases during the outbreak period divided by the number of individuals initially exposed, i.e., those present at the beginning at the outbreak.

Attributable risk (risk difference) — The additional incidence of disease attributable to a risk factor itself. It is calculated by subtracting incidence among those not exposed to a risk factor from incidence among exposed individuals.

Beta (type II) error — Concluding that outcomes are not different when in fact they are. Beta error is analogous to the false negative result of diagnostic tests. *See* alpha error.

Bias — A preference, inclination, process, or systematic error that inhibits impartial judgment or leads to deviations of results or inferences from the truth.

Carrier state — A state of infection in which an infected host can communicate the infection in the absence of manifest disease.

Carrion — Dead or decaying flesh.

Case control (retrospective) study — Subjects are followed backward in time, from effects to possible causes: cases and noncases are not necessarily members of the same population group.

Case definition — The combination of history, physical, and laboratory findings that are characteristic of a particular disease syndrome. It should include all true cases of the disease and exclude similar, but unrelated conditions. The case definition is the starting point for determining risk, prognosis, or the effectiveness of therapeutic regimens.

Case fatality rate — Number of deaths attributable to a disease during an outbreak divided by the number of cases of that disease during the outbreak period.

Case finding — A strategic form of screening targeted at individuals or groups suspected to be at high risk of infection or disease because of association with known infected or diseased individuals or groups, or through other forms of exposure.

Case report — Detailed presentation of a single case or a handful of cases (<10); may be either cross-sectional or longitudinal.

Case series — Cross-sectional study with no defined population and no comparison group.

Censored data — Data on individuals in a survival analysis with incomplete follow-up due to individuals leaving the study before its conclusion or having been followed for a shorter period than others that have experienced the outcome of interest.

Censored observations — Data on patients with incomplete follow-up.

Climatograph — Graphs in which total precipitation is plotted against mean temperature for each month, and the resultant points are joined in a closed curve.

Clinical course of disease — The progression of disease once it has come under medical care. *Compare with* natural history of disease.

Clinical epidemiology — Clinical epidemiology focuses on the sorts of questions asked in the practice of medicine. Consequently, the findings have a direct application in medical decision making. Studies may be observational or experimental.

Coefficient of determination (r^2) — The square of the correlation coefficient. A measure of closeness of fit of the data to the linear regression line. The value for r^2 expresses the amount of variation in the data that are accounted for by the linear relationship between two variables and may take any value between 0 and 1. As the amount of variability, or scatter, around the fitted regression line increases, the value of r^2 decreases. An r^2 value of 1 means that all values fall on the regression line.

Cohort — A group of individuals who have something in common when they are first assembled, and who are then observed for a period of time to see what happens to them. *See* survival cohort.

Cohort (prospective) study — Subjects are followed forward in time, from possible causes to effects. In a concurrent cohort study the cohort is assembled in the present and followed into the future. In a historical cohort study the cohort is identified from past records and followed forward from that time up to the present.

Communicable disease — An illness due to a specific infectious agent or its toxic products that arises through transmission of that agent or its products from an infected person, animal, or inanimate reservoir to a susceptible host, either directly or indirectly, through an intermediate plant or animal host, vector, or the inanimate environment (Chin, 2000).

Communicable period — The time or times during which an infectious agent may be transferred directly or indirectly from an infected person to another person, from an infected animal to humans, or from an infected person to an animal, including arthropods (Chin, 2000).

Compliance — The proportion of individuals (or their owners) that adhere to the prescribed treatment regimen. Thus, an efficacious treatment could be ineffective due to poor compliance.

Concordance — Test concordance is the proportion of all test results on which two or more different tests agree. As the number of different tests applied to the same sample increases, the likelihood of agreement on all tests decreases.

Conditional likelihood of a disease — An estimate of likelihood that the observed morphologic findings would occur in a disease. Basically, an expression of sensitivity data.

Confidence interval — The theoretical range over which there is a specified probability (usually 95%) of including the true value.

Confounding — When two or more variables found to be associated with an outcome (as disease) are also associated with each other. As a result, it is impossible, from a cursory examination, to determine which variable is responsible for the observed outcome. The confounder's association with the outcome may be causal, or it may simply be associated with the true cause.

Congenital transmission — Transmission occurring at, and usually before, birth transovarially, via the placenta, or via the colostrum.

Contagious infection — A transmissible infection that is spread only as the result of an intimate association or contact with infected animals or their excretions or secretions.

Correlation coefficient (r) — The square root of the coefficient of determination. A measure of the degree of linear association between two variables. The value of r may take any value between –1 and 1. If r is either –1 or 1, the variables have a perfect linear relationship. If r is near –1 or 1, there is a high degree of linear correlation. A positive correlation means that as one variable increases, the other increases. A negative correlation means that as one variable increases, the other decreases. If r is equal to 0, we say the variables are uncorrelated and that there is no linear association between them.

Covariance — The situation in which the initial values for animals in each experimental group will influence subsequent values. Covariance is of concern in regression analysis where variables, other than the one under consideration, may influence the outcome.

Cross-sectional study — A study in which all observations on a subject are made at essentially one point in time in the course of that subject's illness.

Crude death rate — Number of deaths during an outbreak/mean population during the outbreak period.

Crude rate — An overall rate defined by the formula: (number in entire population with characteristic of interest) ÷ (total number in entire population). *Compare with* specific rate.

Cyclical changes — Increases or decreases in rates (such as disease incidence) developing at intervals longer than a year.

Descriptive epidemiology — Descriptive epidemiology endeavors to describe and quantify the distribution of diseases and associated factors in terms of individuals, place, and time. Results are typically expressed as rates, which require numerator (affected individuals) and denominator (population at risk) data.

Diagnostic test — Use of a test to discriminate animals that have the disease in question from those that have other diseases that compete with the disease of interest in the differential diagnosis. Diagnostic testing begins with diseased individuals.

Dissemination — *See* mode of spread.

Double counting — A form of multiple testing bias that occurs when interpretation of a test finding is based, in part, on prior test findings. This may occur when two or more tests really measure the same thing (such as the same class of antibody), or when two or more specialists (as clinician and pathologist) interpret findings from the same clinical case.

Ecological epidemiology — Ecological epidemiology focuses on understanding the important factors that affect transmission of particular disease agents. These factors are frequently referred to as the host, agent, and environment triad.

Effectiveness — A measure of how well a treatment works among those to whom it is offered. *Compare with* efficacy.

Efficacy — The power to produce effects or intended results. A measure of how well a treatment works among those who receive it. *Compare with* effectiveness.

Endemic disease — A disease that occurs with predictable regularity in a population unit with only relatively minor fluctuations in its frequency. *See* epidemic disease and sporadic disease.

Epidemic (epizootic) disease — A disease whose frequency in a population during a given time interval is clearly in excess of its expected frequency, as during an outbreak. *Compare with* endemic disease and sporadic disease.

Epidemiology — The study of health and disease in populations. Epidemiology involves (1) the observational study of naturally occurring vs. experimentally induced disease, (2) the study of disease in the population vs. the individual, and (3) the detection of associations by inferential methods vs. the study of pathologic mechanisms.

Etiologic epidemiology — Etiologic epidemiology is primarily concerned with establishing causal relationships in diseases of undetermined origin. Other terms that have been used to describe this activity are medical detection and "shoe leather" epidemiology.

Evapotranspiration — The combined evaporation from the soil surface and transpiration from plants. It is the reverse of precipitation, since it represents the transport of water from the earth back to the atmosphere.

Experimental study — Epidemiologic study in which the researcher tries to alter the course of events by manipulating the conditions of the experiment. Experimental studies may evaluate the relative merits of various therapeutic, surgical, or preventative measures for a particular disease syndrome. *Compare with* observational study.

Extrinsic incubation period — The period of time between infection of a biological vector and acquisition by the vector of the ability to transmit the agent to another susceptible vertebrate host.

Extrinsic risk factors — Risk factors that are not properties of the host, i.e., agent and environment.

False negative rate — The likelihood of a negative test result in patients known to have the disease (pT–/D+). It equals (1 – sensitivity).

False positive rate — The likelihood of a positive test result in patients known to be free of the disease (pT+/D–). It equals (1 – specificity).

Gold standard — The gold standard refers to the means by which one can determine whether a disease is truly present. Its function is that of a quality control device.

Herd health/preventive medicine — Herd health/preventive medicine endeavors to use epidemiologic information to design optimal disease prevention strategies. Economic considerations, expressed either as cost-effectiveness or cost–benefit, frequently determine which strategy is most effective.

Herd immunity — The proportion of animals in a population that are resistant to infection or disease.

Herd retest — Herd retest is a modification of serial testing with the exception that test-negative animals, rather than test-positive animals, are retested. The net effect is to ask the herd to prove that it is free of the condition being sought, thereby increasing test sensitivity at the herd level.

Horizontal transmission — Transmission of an infectious agent between contemporaries, or animals of more or less the same generation. *See* vertical transmission.

Iatrogenic — Induced in a patient by a physician's words or actions.

Incidence — The proportion of individuals that develop a condition of interest over a defined period. Incidence takes into account new cases only, i.e., cases that have their onset during the period specified. It is therefore a measure of the risk of becoming a case over a defined period.

Incidence density — A way of expressing incidence where the denominator is not the number of animals at risk for a specific time period, but rather animal time at risk of the event. An incidence of this type is expressed as the number of new cases per total number of animal days or years at risk.

Interval data — Data that are ordered and for which the size of the intervals is known.

Intrinsic incubation period (incubation period) — The period of time between infection of the vertebrate host and the appearance of clinical signs.

Intrinsic reproductive number (basic reproductive number) — The average number of secondary infections generated by one primary case in a susceptible population; can be used to estimate the level of immunization or other risk reduction strategy required to reduce or eliminate disease.

Intrinsic risk factors — Risk factors that are properties of the host.

Irregular variation — Reflects random variation in disease occurrence among individuals in a population.

Latency — A state of infection in which an agent is quiescent in a host and therefore difficult to detect; implies a potential for activity.

Life table analysis — A method for analyzing the survival of a cohort of patients where the probability of surviving during each time interval is calculated as the ratio of the number of patients surviving to the number at risk of dying during the interval. The chance of surviving to any point in time is obtained by multiplying the probability of surviving during the time interval by the probability of surviving up to the beginning of that interval. The technique can be used to describe other outcomes of disease besides death, such as recurrence of tumor, remission duration, rejection of graft, or reinfection. *See* survivorship curve.

Likelihood ratio — A single measure that summarizes a test's performance. It expresses the likelihood that a given test result would occur in a patient with a disease, compared to the likelihood of the same result in a patient without that disease. The likelihood ratio for a positive test result is the ratio of the likelihood of a positive result in patients with disease to the likelihood of a positive result in patients without disease (true positive rate/false positive rate). The likelihood ratio for a negative test result is the ratio of the likelihood of a negative result in patients with disease to the likelihood of a negative result in patients without the disease (false negative rate/true negative rate).

Longitudinal study — Subjects are observed over a period, either retrospectively (patient history and medical records) or prospectively (through follow-up).

Mark recapture — A technique for estimating total population size (N) from the number sampled (n), based on the proportion of marked animals (M) that are recaptured (m), where $N = n(M/m)$.

Mass screening — The application of screening tests to large unselected populations. Identification of an affected population may then lead to case finding through testing of each animal in the herd.

Measures of effect — Measures of the association between exposure and disease. Included are relative risk, attributable risk, population attributable risk, and population attributable fraction.

Meta-analysis — A systematic, quantitative method for combining information from multiple studies in order to derive the most meaningful answer to a specific question.

Mode of spread — Refers to how a disease agent is spread from one geographic area to another. Synonymous with dissemination.

Mode of transmission — The way(s) in which an etiologic agent is transmitted from affected to susceptible individuals.

Monitoring — *See* surveillance.

Morbidity rates — Direct measures of the commonness of disease in a population. Examples are attack rate, incidence, and prevalence. *See* vital statistics.

Mortality rate — An incidence rate in which the numerator is the number of deaths occurring in a population over a defined period. The denominator is the population at risk over that period.

Moving average — A moving average is a series of data averages centered at each successive measurement point on the timescale.

Natural history of disease — The evolution of disease without medical intervention. *Compare with* clinical course of disease.

Negative correlation — *See* correlation coefficient.

Nominal data — Data that can only be placed into categories, without any inherent order. For analytic purposes, nominal data are treated as discrete variables.

Nonrandomized controlled clinical trial — Patients are allocated to concurrent comparison groups by means of some nonrandom process (e.g., convenience, clinical judgment, owner preference).

Nosocomial — Hospital-acquired infection or disease.

Null hypothesis — The hypothesis, or operational assumption, that no difference exists between treatment groups. Observed differences are due to chance.

Objective data — Measurable indices, such as temperature, pulse, respiration, results of parasitologic examinations, complete blood counts, radiographs, etc.

Observational study — Epidemiologic study in which the researcher is merely an observer and does not interfere with the natural course of events. Observational studies focus on such things as assessment of risk, cause, or prognosis. *Compare with* experimental study.

Odds ratio — The odds that a case is exposed divided by the odds that a control is exposed to a risk factor. The odds ratio provides a measure of risk for case control studies that is conceptually and mathematically similar to the relative risk obtained in cohort studies; e.g., the stronger the association between exposure and disease, the higher the odds ratio.

Ordinal data — Data in which the order is known (small to large, good to bad, etc.), but the size of the intervals between values is not. For analytic purposes, ordinal data may be treated as continuous or discrete variables.

Outbreak — A sudden occurrence of a large number of cases of disease in a short period. The actual number of cases that constitutes an epidemic depends on the past history and seriousness of the condition.

Outbreak period — Period of time over which the first and last cases occurred in a population during an outbreak.

p **value** — The likelihood that an observed result could have arisen by chance alone.

Pandemic — A very large scale epidemic, usually involving several countries or continents.

Parallel testing — The performance of two or more tests on a patient or herd at the same time. The net effect of parallel testing is to ask the patient to prove that it is healthy.

Parenteral — Not through the alimentary canal, i.e., such as subcutaneous, intramuscular, intradermal, intravenous, etc.

Patency — A state of infection in which an agent can be recovered or identified from blood or tissues.

Pathogenicity — A measure of an agent's ability to induce disease. *See* virulence.

Pathognomonic — Specifically distinctive or characteristic of a disease or pathologic condition and rarely found in healthy individuals or those afflicted with clinically similar conditions; a sign or symptom on which a diagnosis can be made.

Period prevalence — Number of cases (old and new) detected over a period ÷ number of animals examined over the same period.

Placebo — In clinical trials, an intervention that is indistinguishable from the active treatment, but does not possess its specifically active component.

Point prevalence — Number of cases (old and new) detected at a particular point in time divided by the number of animals examined at the same point in time.

Population at risk — Population group in which an event could occur.

Population attributable fraction — The fraction of disease occurrence in a population that is associated with a particular risk factor. It is estimated by dividing the population attributable risk by the total incidence of disease in the population.

Population attributable risk — A measure of the excess incidence of disease in a population that is associated with the occurrence of a risk factor. It is the product of the attributable risk and the prevalence of the risk factor in a population.

Positive correlation — *See* correlation coefficient.

Posttest probability (or posterior likelihood) of disease — The likelihood that a patient has a disease or condition based on a particular test result. Besides the test result, the posttest probability is influenced by the pretest probability of disease and the sensitivity and specificity of the test being used.

Power of a study — The probability that a trial will find a statistically significant difference when a difference really exists. A powerful study has a higher probability of rejecting the null hypothesis when it should be rejected. Power is analogous to the sensitivity of a diagnostic test and is equal to 1 minus the probability of a beta error.

Predictive value — The probability of a disease, given the results of a test, is called the predictive value of the test. Positive predictive value is the probability of disease in an animal with a positive (abnormal) test result. Negative predictive value is the probability that an animal does not have the disease when the test result is negative (normal).

Prepatent period — The period of time between infection of the vertebrate host and detectability of an agent in secretions, excretions, blood, or tissues.

Pretest probability (or prior likelihood) of disease — The likelihood that a patient has a disease or condition before a test is run. The pretest probability of disease may be based on a number of parameters, including a clinician's experience with similar patients, the prevalence of the condition in the population from with the individual was drawn, or the posttest probability estimated from one or more previous test results.

Prevalence — The proportion of sampled individuals possessing a condition of interest at a given point in time. It is measured by a single examination of each individual of the group. Prevalence can be likened to a snapshot of the population and includes both old and new cases. It is a measure of the risk of being a case at a given moment.

Prevalence survey — Cross-sectional study of a defined population; commonly used in outbreak investigations.

Prognosis — The prediction of the future course of disease following its onset.

Prognostic factors — Conditions that, when present in individuals already known to have disease, are associated with an outcome of the disease.

Proportional morbidity — Proportion of all morbidity represented by a particular disease.

Randomized controlled clinical trial — Subjects are randomly allocated into treatment and control groups.

Rate — A fraction in which the numerator is included in the denominator.

Ratio — A fraction in which the numerator is not included in the denominator.

Receiver operating characteristic (ROC) curve — A plot of the true positive rate (sensitivity) on the vertical axis against the false positive rate (1 – specificity) on the horizontal axis. The ROC curve provides a standard approach to the evaluation of diagnostic test performance.

Relative risk (risk ratio) — The ratio of incidence in exposed individuals to incidence in nonexposed individuals. Relative risk is an index of the strength of the association between exposure and disease. If no additional risk is associated with exposure, then both incidences should be equal and the ratio would be equal to 1.

Reliability — A measure of the repeatability or reproducibility of a clinical measurement. Reliability is sometimes referred to as precision.

Reproducibility — Test reproducibility refers to the degree to which repeated tests on the same sample(s) give the same result.

Revised likelihood of a disease — *See* posttest probability of disease.

Risk factors — Factors that are associated with an increased likelihood of acquiring disease.

Route of infection — The route by which an etiologic agent gains access to the body of a susceptible individual.

Screening — The presumptive identification of unrecognized disease or defect in apparently healthy populations.

Seasonal fluctuations — Regular changes in incidence rates with periods shorter than a year.

Secular trends — Overall long-term rises or declines in incidence rate that occur gradually over long periods.

Sensitivity — Test sensitivity is defined as the likelihood of a positive test result in individuals known to have the disease or condition being sought. Test sensitivity is sometimes referred to as operational sensitivity to distinguish it from absolute sensitivity, a term used to express the detection limits of an assay.

Serial testing — The retesting of animals that initially tested positive. The net effect is to ask the individual to prove that it is truly affected by the condition being sought.

Sign — An indication of the existence of something; any objective evidence of a disease, i.e., such evidence as is perceptible to the examining physician, as opposed to the subjective sensations (symptoms) of the patient.

Signalment — The systematic description of an individual for purposes of identification (age, breed, sex, identifying marks, etc.).

Specific rate — A rate for a specific subgroup of a population of interest (e.g., 3- to 5-year age group). *Compare with* crude rate.

Specific seasonals — A ratio in which the observed monthly disease incidence rate is divided by the 12-month moving average value centered on the middle of that month.

Specificity — Test specificity is defined as the likelihood of a negative test result in individuals known to be free of the disease or condition being sought.

Sporadic disease — A disease that occurs rarely and without regularity in a population unit. *Compare with* endemic disease and epidemic disease.

Standard population — A population in which the population characteristics of age, breed, sex, etc., are known and used as a standard. When populations are to be compared, they should have similar components, and so usually they are mathematically adjusted to have the same proportions as a standard population.

Statistically significant — A level of confidence in the results of a study based on a predefined p value. Generally refers to p values falling below 0.05; i.e., we are willing to be wrong 5% of the time.

Subjective data — Findings such as general condition, alertness, appetite, bowel movements, urination, evidence of pain, etc., which are based on our own observations and those of the owner.

Surveillance (epidemiologic surveillance, monitoring) — The ongoing systematic and continuous collection, analysis, and interpretation of health data for the purpose of monitoring the spatial and temporal patterns of one or more diseases and their associated risk factors.

Survival cohort — A group of patients who are assembled at various times in the course of their disease, rather than at the beginning, and who are then observed for a period to see what happens to them. Generally not considered a true cohort. *See* cohort.

Survivorship curve — Graphic representation of the number or proportion of a cohort of patients with a particular condition remaining at different points throughout the course of their illness. The technique can be used to describe other outcomes of disease besides death, such as recurrence of tumor, remission duration, rejection of graft, or reinfection. *See* life table analysis.

Sylvatic — Affecting wild animals.

Symptom — Any subjective evidence of disease or of a patient's condition, i.e., such evidence as perceived by the patient; a change in a patient's condition indicative of some bodily or mental state.

Synanthropic — Together with or accompanying human beings.

Type I error — *See* alpha error.

Type II error — *See* beta error.

Transmissible (communicable) infection — An infection that can be passed from infected to susceptible animals.

True prevalence — The prevalence of disease estimated through use of an appropriate gold standard. *Compare with* apparent prevalence.

Typical seasonals — Indices of the amount of variation attributable to seasonal influences obtained by averaging (by mean or median) the specific seasonals for each month.

Unapparent infection — The presence of infection in a host without recognizable clinical signs or symptoms. Unapparent infections may be identified by laboratory means, including immunologic tests. *Synonyms*: asymptomatic, subclinical, occult infection.

Uncontrolled clinical trial — Clinical trial with no concurrent comparison group.

Validity — The degree to which a measurement reflects the true status of what is being measured. Another name for validity is accuracy.

Vertical transmission — Transmission of an infectious agent from animals of one generation to animals of the succeeding generation, sometimes transovarially, in utero, or with colostrum. *See* horizontal transmission.

Veterinarian–client–patient relationship — Recognized by the Food and Drug Administration when a veterinarian in a practice (1) has seen the animals to be treated, (2) is familiar with the premises and management system, and (3) has established a tentative diagnosis for the condition to be treated.

Virulence — A measure of an agent's ability to induce severe disease. *See* pathogenicity.
Vital statistics — Rates or population indices that provide indirect evidence of the health status of a population. Examples are birth, fertility, and death rates. *See* morbidity rates.

References

Acha, P.N. and Szyfres, B., *Zoonoses and Communicable Diseases Common to Man and Animals*, Pan American Health Organization, Washington, DC, 1980.

Anderson, R.M. and May, R.M., *Population Biology of Infectious Diseases*, Springer-Verlag, New York, 1982.

Anderson, R.M. and May, R.M., *Infectious Diseases of Humans: Dynamics and Control*, Oxford University Press, Oxford, 1991.

Anonymous, Opie on the heart, *Lancet*, 1, 692, 1980.

Armstead, W.W., Analytical epidemiology and veterinary economics, in *Veterinary Medicine and Human Health*, 3rd ed., Schwabe, C.W., Ed., Williams & Wilkins, Baltimore, 1984, chap. 17.

Atwill, E.R. and Mohammed, H.O., Benefit-cost analysis of vaccination of horses as a strategy to control equine monocytic ehrlichiosis, *J. Am. Vet. Med. Assoc.*, 208, 1295–1299, 1996.

AVMA, Student enrollment (1985–1986) favors women, *J. Am. Vet. Med. Assoc.*, 188, 573–575, 1986.

AVMA, AVMA guidelines for complementary and alternative veterinary medicine, *J. Am. Vet. Med. Assoc.*, 218, 1731, 2001.

Bennett, R.M., The use of "economic" quantitative modelling techniques in livestock health and disease-control decision making: a review, *Prev. Vet. Med.*, 13, 63–76, 1992.

Blair, A. and Hayes, H.M., Jr., Mortality patterns among U.S. veterinarians, 1947–1977: an expanded study, *Int. J. Epidemiol.*, 11, 391–397, 1982.

Boutilier, P., Carr, A., and Schulman, R.L., Leptospirosis in dogs: a serologic survey and case series 1996 to 2001, *Vet. Ther.*, 4, 178–187, 2003.

Bowman, G.L., Hueston, W.D., Boner, G.J., Hurley, J.J., and Andreas, J.E. *Serratia liquefaciens* mastitis in a dairy herd. *J. Am. Vet. Med. Assoc.*, 189, 913–915, 1986.

Bronson, R.T., Variation in age at death of dogs of different sexes and breeds, *Am. J. Vet. Res.*, 43, 2057–2059, 1982.

Carter, J.D., Hird, D.W., Farver, T.B., and Hjerpe, C.A., Salmonellosis in hospitalized horses: seasonality and case fatality rates, *J. Am. Vet. Med. Assoc.*, 188, 163–167, 1986.

Cates, S.C., Anderson, D.W., Karns, S.A., and Brown, P.A. Traditional versus hazard analysis and critical control point-based inspection: results from a poultry slaughter project, *J. Food Prot.*, 64, 826–832, 2001.

CDC, Group-A, -B hemolytic *Streptococcus* skin infections in a meat-packing plant: Oregon, *MMWR*, 35 (October 10, No. 40), 629–630, 1986.

CDC, Recommendations of the international task force for disease eradication, *MMWR*, 42 (December 31, No. RR-16), 1993.

Center, S.A., Baldwin, B.H., Dillingham, S., Erb, H.N., and Tennant, B.C., Diagnostic value of serum gamma-glutamyl transferase and alkaline phosphatase activities in hepatobiliary disease in the cat, *J. Am. Vet. Med. Assoc.*, 188, 507–510, 1986.

Chin, J., *Control of Communicable Diseases Manual*, 17th ed., American Public Health Association, Washington, DC, 2000.

Christley, R.M. and Reid, S.W., No significant difference: use of statistical methods for testing equivalence in clinical veterinary literature, *J. Am. Vet. Med. Assoc.*, 222, 433–437, 2003.

Christopher, M.M. and Hotz, C.S., Cytologic diagnosis: expression of probability by clinical pathologists, *Vet. Clin. Pathol.*, 33, 84–95, 2004.

Cochran, W.G., *Sampling Techniques*, 3rd ed., Wiley & Sons, New York, 1977.

Collins, M.T. and Sockett, D.C., Accuracy and economics of the USDA-licensed enzyme-linked immunosorbent assay for bovine paratuberculosis, *J. Am. Vet. Med. Assoc.*, 203, 1456–1463, 1993.

Cooper, V.L. and Helman, R.G., Selecting the best specimens for diagnosing disease, *Vet. Med.*, 94, 968–973, 1999.

Courtney, C.H. and Cornell, J.A., Evaluation of heartworm immunodiagnostic tests, *J. Am. Vet. Med. Assoc.*, 197, 724–729, 1990.

Courtney, C.H., Zeng, Q.Y., and Bean, E.S., Sensitivity and specificity of the Dirochek heartworm antigen test for immunodiagnosis of canine dirofilariasis and a comparison with other immunodiagnostic tests, *J. Am. Anim. Hosp. Assoc.*, 24, 27–32, 1988.

Courtney, C.H., Zeng, Q.Y., and Tonelli, Q., Sensitivity and specificity of the CITE heartworm antigen test and a comparison with the DiroChek heartworm antigen test, *J. Am. Anim. Hosp. Assoc.*, 26, 623–628, 1990.

Crow, S.E., Usefulness of prognoses: qualitative terms vs. quantitative designations, *J. Am. Vet. Med. Assoc.*, 187, 700–703, 1985.

Crump, J.A., Sulka, A.C., Langer, A.J., Schaben, C., Crielly, A.S., Gage, R., Baysinger, M., Moll, M., Withers, G., Toney, D.M., Hunter, S.B., Hoekstra, R.M., Wong, S.K., Griffin, P.M., and Van Gilder, T.J., An outbreak of *Escherichia coli* O157:H7 infections among visitors to a dairy farm, *N. Engl. J. Med.*, 347, 555–560, 2002.

Dargatz, D.A., Byrum, B.A., Hennager, S.G., Barber, L.K., Kopral, C.A., Wagner, B.A., and Wells, S.J., Prevalence of antibodies against *Mycobacterium avium* subsp. *paratuberculosis* among beef cow-calf herds, *J. Am. Vet. Med. Assoc.*, 219, 497–501, 2001.

Davis, S., Begon, M., De Bruyn, L., Ageyev, V.S., Klassovskiy, N.L., Pole, S.B., Viljugrein, H., Stenseth, N.C., and Leirs, H., Predictive thresholds for plague in Kazakhstan, *Science*, 304, 736–738, 2004.

Dean, A.G., Dean, J.A., Coulombier, D., Brendel, K.A., Smith, D.C., Burton, A.H., Dicker, R.C., Sullivan, K., Fagan, R.F., and Arner, T.G., *Epi Info*, Version 6, Centers for Disease Control and Prevention, Atlanta, 1995 (word processing, database and statistics program for public health on IBM-compatible microcomputers).

Dean, A.G., Arner, T.G., Sangam, S., Sunki, G.G., Friedman, R., Lantinga, M., Zubieta, J.C., Sullivan, K.M., and Smith, D.C., *Epi Info 2000*, Centers for Disease Control and Prevention, Atlanta, 2000 (database and statistics program for public health professionals for use on Windows 95, 98, NT, and 2000 computers).

Dey, B.P. and Parham, G.L., Incidence and economics of tuberculosis in swine slaughtered from 1976 to 1988, *J. Am. Vet. Med. Assoc.*, 203, 516–519, 1993.

DiBartola, S.P., Rutgers, H.C., Zack, P.M., and Tarr, M.J., Clinicopathologic findings associated with chronic renal disease in cats: 74 cases (1973–1984), *J. Am. Vet. Med. Assoc.*, 190, 1196–1202, 1987.

Dietz, K., The estimation of the basic reproduction number for infectious diseases. *Stat. Methods Med. Res.*, 2, 23–41, 1993.

Dohoo, I.R., Morris, R.S., Martin, S.W., Perry, B.D., Bernardo, T., Erb, H., Thrusfield, M., Smith, R., and Welte, V.R., Epidemiology, *Nature*, 368, 284, 1994 (letter).

Dohoo, I.R. and Waltner-Toews, D., Interpreting clinical research. Part I. General considerations., *Compend. Contin. Educ. Pract. Vet.*, 7, S473–S478, 1985a.

Dohoo, I.R. and Waltner-Toews, D., Interpreting clinical research. Part II. Descriptive and experimental studies, *Compend. Contin. Educ. Pract. Vet.*, 7, S513–S520, 1985b.

Dohoo, I.R. and Waltner-Toews, D., Interpreting clinical research. Part III. Observational studies and interpretation of results, *Compend. Contin. Educ. Pract. Vet.*, 7, S605–S613, 1985c.

Drobatz, K.J, and Smith G., Evaluation of risk factors for bite wounds inflicted on caregivers by dogs and cats in a veterinary teaching hospital, *J. Am. Vet. Med. Assoc.*, 223, 312–316, 2003.

Dubensky, R.A. and White, M.E., The sensitivity, specificity and predictive value of total plasma protein in the diagnosis of traumatic reticuloperitonitis, *Can. J. Comp. Med.*, 47, 241–244, 1983.

Dwyer, R.M., Garber, L.P., Traub-Dargatz, J.L., Meade, B.J., Powell, D., Pavlick, M.P., and Kane, A.J., Case-control study of factors associated with excessive proportions of early fetal losses associated with mare reproductive loss syndrome in central Kentucky during 2001, *J. Am.Vet. Med. Assoc.*, 222, 613–619, 2003.

Erskine, R.J., Eberhart, R.J., Hutchinson, L.J., Spencer, S.B., and Campbell, M.A., Incidence and types of clinical mastitis in dairy herds with high and low somatic cell counts, *J. Am. Vet. Med. Assoc.*, 15, 192, 761–765, 1988.

Evans, G.O., Plasma lactate measurements in healthy beagle dogs, *Am. J. Vet. Res.*, 48, 131–132, 1987.

Fagan, T.J., Nomogram for Bayes's theorem, *N. Engl. J. Med.*, 293, 257, 1975 (letter).

Fertig, D.L. and Dorn, C.R., *Taenia saginata* cysticercosis in an Ohio cattle feeding operation. *J. Am. Vet. Med. Assoc.*, 186, 1281–1285, 1985.

Fetrow, J., Madison, J.B., and Galligan, D., Economic decisions in veterinary practice: a method for field use, *J. Am. Vet. Med. Assoc.*, 186, 792–797, 1985.

Fettman, M.J., Evaluation of the usefulness of routine microscopy in canine urinalysis, *J. Am. Vet. Med. Assoc.*, 190, 892–896, 1987.

Fletcher, R.H., Fletcher, S.W., and Wagner, E.H., *Clinical Epidemiology: The Essentials*, Williams & Wilkins, Baltimore, 1982.

Fletcher, R.H., Fletcher, S.W., and Wagner, E.H., *Clinical Epidemiology: The Essentials*, 2nd ed., Williams & Wilkins, Baltimore, 1988.

Fletcher, R.H., Fletcher, S.W., and Wagner, E.H., *Clinical Epidemiology: The Essentials*, 3rd ed., Lippincott Williams & Wilkins, Baltimore, 1996.

Friedmann, C.T.H., Spiegel, E.R., Aaron, E., and McIntyre, R., *CDC Reports*, Centers for Disease Control, Atlanta, 1971, p. 10.

Gibbons-Burgener, S.N., Kaneene, J.B., Lloyd, J.W., Leykam, J.F., and Erskine, R.J., Reliability of three bulk-tank antimicrobial residue detection assays used to test individual milk samples from cows with mild clinical mastitis, *Am. J. Vet. Res.*, 62, 1716–1720, 2001.

Goodger, W.J. and Skirrow, S.Z., Epidemiologic and economic analyses of an unusually long epizootic of trichomoniasis in a large California dairy herd, *J. Am. Vet. Med. Assoc.*, 189, 772–776, 1986.

Gordon, J.C., Bech-Nielsen, S., Kohn, C., Farrar, W., Parsons, M., and Foster, W., An epidemiological investigation of farms with Potomac horse fever (equine monocytic ehrlichiosis), *Acta. Vet. Scand. Suppl.*, 84, 319–322, 1988.

Greiner, M., Pfeiffer, D., and Smith, R.D., Principles and practical application of the receiver-operating characteristic analysis for diagnostic tests, *Prev. Vet. Med.*, 45, 23–41, 2000.

Greiner, M., Sohr, D., and Gobel, P., A modified ROC analysis for the selection of cut-off values and the definition of intermediate results of serodiagnostic tests, *J. Immunol. Methods*, 185, 123–132, 1995.

Guptill, L., Glickman, L., and Glickman, N., Time trends and risk factors for diabetes mellitus in dogs: analysis of veterinary medical data base records (1970–1999), *Vet. J.*, 165, 240–247, 2003.

Halpin, B., *Patterns of Animal Disease*, Williams & Wilkins, Baltimore, 1975.

Hammer, A.S. and Buffington, C.A., Survey of statistical methods used in the veterinary medical literature, *J. Am. Vet. Med. Assoc.*, 205, 344–345, 1994.

Hannah, H.W., Promising a result, *J. Am. Vet. Med. Assoc.*, 186, 1166, 1985.

Hardy, W.D., Jr., McClelland, A.J., Zuckerman, E.E., Hess, P.W., Essex, M., Cotter, S.M., MacEwen, E.G., and Hayes, A.A., Prevention of the contagious spread of feline leukaemia virus and the development of leukaemia in pet cats, *Nature*, 263, 326–328, 1976.

Hart, B.L. and Miller, M.F., Behavioral profiles of dog breeds, *J. Am. Vet. Med. Assoc.*, 186, 1175–1180, 1985.

Hawkins, E.C. and Murphy, C.J., Inconsistencies in the absorptive capacities of the Schirmer tear test strips. *J. Am. Vet. Med. Assoc.*, 188, 511–513, 1986.

Hayes, H.M., Tarone, R.E., Cantor, K.P., Jessen, C.R., McCurnin, D.M., and Richardson, R.C., Case-control study of canine malignant lymphoma: positive association with dog owner's use of 2,4-dichlorophenoxyacetic acid herbicides, *J. Natl. Cancer Inst.*, 83, 1226–1231, 1991.

Holden, C., IOM sees need for autopsy policy, *Science*, 229, 539, 1985.

Holton, L.L., Scott, E.M., Nolan, A.M., Reid, J., and Welsh, E., Relationship between physiological factors and clinical pain in dogs scored using a numerical rating scale, *J. Small Anim. Pract.*, 39, 469–474, 1998.

Holton, L.L., Scott, E.M., Nolan, A.M., Reid, J., Welsh, E., and Flaherty, D., Comparison of three methods used for assessment of pain in dogs, *J. Am. Vet. Med. Assoc.*, 212, 61–66, 1998.

Hoskins, J.D., Hribernik, T.N., and Kearney, M.T., Complications following thi-acetarsamide sodium therapy in Louisiana dogs with naturally-occurring heartworm disease, *Cornell Vet.*, 75, 531–539, 1985.

House, J.A. and Baker, J.A., Comments on combination vaccines for bovine respiratory diseases. *J. Am. Vet. Med. Assoc.*, 152, 893–894, 1968.

Huirne, R.B.M. and Dijkhuizen, A.A., Basic methods of economic analysis, in *Animal Health Economics: Principles and Applications*, Dijkhuizen, A.A. and Morris, R.S., Eds., Post Graduate Foundation in Veterinary Science, University of Sydney, Sydney, 1997, chap. 3.

Hulley, S.B. and Cummings, S.R., *Designing Clinical Research*, Williams & Wilkins, Baltimore, 1988.

Hulley, S.B., Cummings, S.R., Browner, W.S., Grady, D., Hearst, N., and Newman, T.B., *Designing Clinical Research*, 2nd ed., Lippincott Williams & Wilkins, Philadelphia, 2001.

Jeglum, K.A., de Guzman, E., and Young, K.M., Chemotherapy of advanced mammary adenocarcinoma in 14 cats. *J. Am. Vet. Med. Assoc.*, 187, 157–160, 1985.

Jergens, A.E., Schreiner, C.A., Frank, D.E., Niyo, Y., Ahrens, F.E., Eckersall, P.D., Benson, T.J., and Evans, R.J., A scoring index for disease activity in canine inflammatory bowel disease, *Vet. Intern. Med.*, 17, 291–297, 2003.

Joly, D.O., Ribic, C.A., Langenberg, J.A., Beheler, K., Batha, C.A., Dhuey, B.J., Rolley, R.E., Bartelt, G., Van Deelen, T.R., and Samuel, M.D., Chronic wasting disease in free-ranging Wisconsin white-tailed deer, *Emerg. Infect. Dis.*, 9, 599–601, 2003.

Kasari, T.R. and Naylor, J.M., Clinical evaluation of sodium bicarbonate, sodium L-lactate, and sodium acetate for the treatment of acidosis in diarrheic calves, *J. Am. Vet. Med. Assoc.*, 187, 392–397, 1985.

Kassirer, J.P., Moskowitz, A.J., Lau, J., and Pauker, S.G., Decision analysis: a progress report, *Ann. Intern. Med.*, 106, 275–291, 1987.

Kent, M.S., Lucroy, M.D., Dank, G., Lehenbauer, T.W., and Madewell, B.R., Concurrence between clinical and pathologic diagnoses in a veterinary medical teaching hospital: 623 cases (1989 and 1999), *J. Am. Vet. Med. Assoc.*, 224, 403–406, 2004.

King, L.J., Unique characteristics of the National Animal Disease Surveillance System, *J. Am. Vet. Med. Assoc.*, 186, 35–39, 1985.

Kleinbaum, D.G. and Kleinbaum, A., *Adjusted Rates. The Direct Rate. A Self-Instructional Program*, Publication 122-00-004, Health Sciences Consortium, Chapel Hill, NC, 1976.

Kramer, M.S., *Clinical Epidemiology and Biostatistics*, Springer-Verlag, New York, 1988.

Lebeau, A., L'age du chien et celui de l'homme. Essai de statistique sur la mortalite canine, *Bull. Acad. Vet. France*, 26, 229–232, 1953.

Levine, N.D., Weather, climate, and the bionomics of ruminant nematode larvae, in *Advanced Veterinary Science*, Vol. 8, Brandly, C.A. and Jungherr, E.L., Eds., Academic Press, New York, 1963, pp. 215–261.

Levine, N.D., Bioclimatographs, evapotranspiration, soil moisture data and the free-living stages of ruminant nematodes and other disease agents, *Theoretical Questions of Natural Foci of Diseases*, Rosicky, B. and Heyberger, K., Eds., Czechoslovak Academy of Sciences, Prague, 1965.

Lewis, G.E., Jr., Ristic, M., Smith, R.D., Lincoln, T., and Stephenson, E.H., The brown dog tick *Rhipicephalus sanguineus* and the dog as experimental hosts of *Ehrlichia canis*, *Am. J. Vet. Res.*, 38, 1953–1955, 1977.

Losonsky, J.M. and Kneller, S.K. Variable locations of nutrient foramina of the proximal phalanx in forelimbs of Standardbreds, *J. Am. Vet. Med. Assoc.*, 193, 671–673, 1988.

Lund, E.M., Armstrong, P.J., Kirk, C.A., Kolar, L.M., and Klausner, J.S., Health status and population characteristics of dogs and cats examined at private veterinary practices in the United States, *J. Am. Vet. Med. Assoc.*, 214, 1336–1341, 1999.

MacMahon, B. and Pugh, T.F., 1970. *Epidemiology: Principles and Methods*, Little, Brown & Co., Boston, 1970.

Madison, J.B., Fetrow, J., and Galligan D., Economic decisions in food animal practice: to treat or not to treat? *J. Am. Vet. Med. Assoc.*, 185, 520–521, 1984.

Martin, S.W., Meek, A.H., and Welleberg, P., *Veterinary Epidemiology: Principles and Methods*, Iowa State University Press, Ames, 1987.

May, R.M., Parasitic infections as regulators of animal populations. *Am. Sci.*, 71, 36–45, 1983.

McClelland, A.J., Hardy, W.D., Jr., and Zuckerman, E.E., Prognosis of healthy feline leukemia virus infected cats, in *Feline Leukemia Virus*, Hardy, W.D., Jr., Essex, M., and McClelland, A.J., Eds., Elsevier, New York, 1980, pp. 121–126.

McMillan, F.D., The placebo effect in animals, *J. Am. Vet. Med. Assoc.*, 215, 992–999, 1999.

Merkal, R.S., Whipple, D.L., Sacks, J.M., and Snyder, G.R., Prevalence of *Mycobacterium paratuberculosis* in ileocecal lymph nodes of cattle culled in the United States, *J. Am. Vet. Med. Assoc.*, 190, 676–680, 1987.

Mischke, R. and Busse, L., Reference values for the bone marrow aspirates in adult dogs, *J. Vet. Med. A Physiol. Pathol. Clin. Med.*, 49, 499–502, 2002.

Moore, B.R., Reed, S.M., Biller, D.S., Kohn, C.W., and Weisbrode, S.E., Assessment of vertebral canal diameter and bony malformations of the cervical part of the spine in horses with cervical stenotic myelopathy, *Am. J. Vet. Res.*, 55, 5–13, 1994.

Morens, D., When was epidemiology born? *Epidemiol. Monitor*, 20, 3, 6, 9, 2003.

Morton, R.F., Hebel, J.R., and McCarter, R.J., *A Study Guide to Epidemiology and Biostatistics*, 3rd ed., Aspen, Rockville, 1990.

NLM, Medical Subject Heading (MeSH), U.S. National Library of Medicine, 8600 Rockville Pike, Bethesda, MD 20894, http://www.nlm.nih.gov/mesh/, 2004.

Norby, B., Bartlett, P.C., Fitzgerald, S.D., Granger, L.M., Bruning-Fann, C.S., Whipple, D.L., and Payeur, J.B., The sensitivity of gross necropsy, caudal fold and comparative cervical tests for the diagnosis of bovine tuberculosis, *J. Vet. Diagn. Invest.*, 16, 126–131, 2004.

O'Leary, D.R., Marfin, A.A., Montgomery, S.P., Kipp, A.M., Lehman, J.A., Biggerstaff, B.J., Elko, V.L., Collins, P.D., Jones, J.E., and Campbell, G.L., The epidemic of West Nile virus in the United States, 2002, *Vector Borne Zoonotic Dis.*, 4, 61–70, 2004.

Olivry, T. and Mueller, R.S., Evidence-based veterinary dermatology: a systematic review of the pharmacotherapy of canine atopic dermatitis, *Vet. Dermatol.*, 14, 121–146, 2003.

Owen, L.N., Ed., *TNM Classification of Tumours in Domestic Animals*, 1st ed., WHO, Geneva, 1980.

Oxender, W.D., Newman, L.E., and Morrow, D.A., Factors influencing dairy calf mortality in Michigan. *J. Am. Vet. Med. Assoc.*, 162, 458–460, 1973.

Paarlberg, P.L., Lee, J.G., and Seitzinger, A.H., Potential revenue impact of an outbreak of foot-and-mouth disease in the United States, *J. Am. Vet. Med. Assoc.*, 220, 988–992, 2002.

Padgett, G., New research unlocking genetic disease mysteries, *DVM*, 16, 30–32, 1985.

Pauker, S.G. and Kassirer, J.P., Decision analysis. *New Engl. J. Med.*, 316, 250–258, 1987.

Payne, J.M., Dew, S.M., Manston, R., and Faulks, M., The use of a metabolic profile test in dairy herds, *Vet. Rec.*, 87, 150–157, 1970.

Petrie, A. and Watson, P., *Statistics for Veterinary and Animal Science*, Blackwell, London, 1999, pp. 50–51.

Pion, P.D., Kittleson, M.D., Thomas, W.P., Delellis, L.A., and Rogers, Q.R., Response of cats with dilated cardiomyopathy to taurine supplementation. *J. Am. Vet. Med. Assoc.*, 201, 275–284, 1992.

Pusterla, N., Madigan, J.E., Chae, J.S., DeRock, E., Johnson, E., and Pusterla, JB., Helminthic transmission and isolation of *Ehrlichia risticii*, the causative agent of Potomac horse fever, by using trematode stages from freshwater stream snails, *J. Clin. Microbiol.*, 38, 1293–1297, 2000.

Pybus, O.G., Charleston, M.A., Gupta, S., Rambaut, A., Holmes, E.C., and Harvey, P.H., The epidemic behavior of the hepatitis C virus, *Science*, 292, 2323–2325, 2001.

Ramey, D., "Alternative" therapies: doing the right thing, *Vet. Forum*, 20, 30–31, 2003a.

Ramey, D.W., Regulatory aspects of complementary and alternative veterinary medicine, *J. Am. Vet. Med. Assoc.*, 222, 1679–1682, 2003b.

Ransohoff, D.F. and Feinstein, A.R., Problems of spectrum and bias in evaluating the efficacy of diagnostic tests, *N. Engl. J. Med.*, 299, 926–930, 1978.

Reichenbach, T., Aging in canine pets, *Calif. Vet.*, 43, 11, 13–15, 1989.

Reif, J.S., Maguire, T.G., Kenney, R.M., and Brodey, R.S., A cohort study of canine testicular neoplasia, *J. Am. Vet. Med. Assoc.*, 175, 719–723, 1979.

Reubel, G.H., Barlough, J.E., and Madigan, J.E., Production and characterization of *Ehrlichia risticii*, the agent of Potomac horse fever, from snails (Pleuroceridae: *Juga* spp.) in aquarium culture and genetic comparison to equine strains, *J. Clin. Microbiol.*, 36, 1501–1511, 1998.

Risco, C.A., Reynolds, J.P., and Hird, D., Uterine prolapse and hypocalcemia in dairy cows. *J. Am. Vet. Med. Assoc.*, 185, 1517–1519, 1984.

Rollin, B.E., The use and abuse of Aesculapian authority in veterinary medicine, *J. Am. Vet. Med. Assoc.*, 220, 1144–1149, 2002.

Ruble, R.P. and Hird, D.W., Congenital abnormalities in immature dogs from a pet store: 253 cases (1987–1988), *J. Am. Vet. Med. Assoc.*, 202, 633–636, 1993.

Sackett, D.L., The rational clinical examination. A primer on the precision and accuracy of the clinical examination, *J.A.M.A.*, 267, 2638–2644, 1992.

Sackett, D.L., Haynes, R.B., Guyatt, G.H., and Tugwell, P., *Clinical Epidemiology: A Basic Science for Clinical Medicine*, 2nd ed., Little, Brown & Co., Boston, 1991.

Sackett, D.L., Richardson, W.S., Rosenberg, W., and Haynes, R.B., *Evidence-Based Medicine: How to Practice and Teach EBM*, Churchill Livingston, New York, 1997.

Sandlow, L.J., Hammett, W.H., and Bashook, P.G., *Problem Oriented Medical Records: Guidelines for Format and Forms*, Michael Reese Medical Center, Chicago, 1974.

Sanford, S.E., Enteric cryptosporidial infection in pigs: 184 cases (1981–1985), *J. Am. Vet. Med. Assoc.*, 190, 695–698, 1987.

Scavelli, T.D., Patnaik, A.K., Mehlhaff, C.J., and Hayes, A.A., Hemangiosarcoma in the cat: retrospective evaluation of 31 surgical cases, *J. Am. Vet. Med. Assoc.*, 187, 817–819, 1985.

Schick, R.O. and Fadok, V.A., Responses of atopic dogs to regional allergens: 268 cases (1981–1984), *J. Am. Vet. Med. Assoc.*, 189, 1493–1496, 1986.

Schwabe, C.W., Riemann, H.P., and Franti, C.E., *Epidemiology in Veterinary Practice*, Lea & Febiger, Philadelphia, 1977.

Schwartz, B.S., Goldstein, M.D., Ribeiro, J.M.C., Schulze, T.L., and Shahied, S.I., Antibody testing in Lyme disease. A comparison of results in four laboratories., *J.A.M.A.*, 262, 3431–3434, 1989.

Sharp, V.F., *Statistics for the Social Sciences*, Little, Brown & Co., Boston, 1979.

Shott, S., Statistics in veterinary research, *J. Am. Vet. Med. Assoc.*, 187, 138–141, 1985.

Smith, R.D., Ehrlichiae, in *Parasitic Protozoa*, Vol. IV, Kreier, J.P., Ed., Academic Press, New York, 1977, pp. 295–328.

Smith, R.D., Veterinary clinical research: a survey of study designs and clinical issues appearing in a practice journal, *J. Vet. Med. Educ.*, 15, 2–7, 1988.

Smith, R.D., Decision analysis in the evaluation of diagnostic tests, *J. Am. Vet. Med. Assoc.*, 203, 1184–1192, 1993.

Spain, C.V., Scarlett, J.M., and Cully, S.M., When to neuter dogs and cats: a survey of New York state veterinarians' practices and beliefs, *J. Am. Anim. Hosp. Assoc.*, 38, 482–488, 2002.

Spain, C.V., Scarlett, J.M., and Houpt, K.A., Long-term risks and benefits of early-age gonadectomy in cats, *J. Am. Vet. Med. Assoc.*, 224, 372–379, 2004a.

Spain, C.V., Scarlett, J.M., and Houpt, K.A., Long-term risks and benefits of early-age gonadectomy in dogs, *J. Am. Vet. Med. Assoc.*, 224, 380–387, 2004b.

Spain, J.D., *BASIC Microcomputer Models in Biology*, Addison-Wesley, Reading, MA, 1982, p. 114.

Spangler, C., Bech-Nielsen, S., Heider, L.E., and Dorn, C.R., Interpretation of an enzyme-linked immunosorbent test using different cut-offs between positive and negative samples for diagnosis of paratuberculosis, *Prev. Vet. Med.*, 13, 197–204, 1992.

Stedman's Medical Dictionary, 27th ed., Lippincott William & Wilkins, Baltimore, 2000.

Stein, T.E. and Duffy, S.J., Parity-specific production values for 68 North American swine breeding herds, Proceedings of the 5th Int'l. Symposium on Veterinary Epidemiology and Economics, July 25–29, 1988, Copenhagen, Denmark, *Acta Vet. Scand.*, Supplementum 84, 522, 1988.

Stevens, J.B., Anderson, J.F., Olson, W.G., and Schlotthauer, J.C., Metabolic profile testing, in *Bovine Medicine and Surgery*, Vol. I, Amstutz, H.E., Ed., American Veterinary Publications, Santa Barbara, CA, 1980, pp. 597–614.

Straus, J.H., Anemia, in *Quick Reference to Veterinary Medicine*, Fenner, W.R., Ed., J.B. Lippincott Co., Philadelphia, 1982, pp. 383–398.

Straw, B.E., Henry, S.C., and Fleming, S.A., Interactions of management and animal performance in a swine feedlot. *J. Am. Vet. Med. Assoc.*, 186, 986–988, 1985.

Sudarshan, M.K., Mahendra, B.J., and Narayan, D.H., A community survey of dog bites, anti-rabies treatment, rabies and dog population management in Bangalore city, *J. Commun. Dis.*, 33, 245–251, 2001.

Swets, J.A., Measuring the accuracy of diagnostic systems, *Science*, 240, 1285–1293, 1988.

Tobias, K.M. and Rohrbach, B.W., Association of breed with the diagnosis of congenital portosystemic shunts in dogs: 2,400 cases (1980–2002), *J. Am. Vet. Med. Assoc.*, 223, 1636–1639, 2003.

Toma, B., Vaillancourt, J.-P., Dufour, B., Eloit, M., Moutou, F., Marsh, W., Bénet, J.-J., Sanaa, M., and Michel, P., *Dictionary of Veterinary Epidemiology*, Blackwell, Ames, 1999.

Turrel, J.M., Intraoperative radiotherapy of carcinoma of the prostate gland in ten dogs. *J. Am. Vet. Med. Assoc.*, 190, 48–52, 1987.

U.S. Census Bureau, Expectation of life and expected deaths by race, sex, and age: 2001, in *Statistical Abstract of the United States*, 2004–2005 ed., U.S. Department of Commerce.

Wells, D.L., Comparison of two treatments for preventing dogs eating their own faeces, *Vet. Rec.*, 153, 51–53, 2003.

White, M.E., Evaluating diagnostic test results, *J. Am. Vet. Med. Assoc.*, 188, 1141, 1986 (letter).

Wolfe, A. and Wright, I.P., Human toxocariasis and direct contact with dogs, *Vet. Rec.*, 152, 41–22, 2003.

Woodward, M., *Epidemiology: Study Design and Data Analysis*, Chapman & Hall/CRC, Boca Raton, FL, 1999.

Yamagami, T., Kobayashi, T., Takahashi, K., and Sugiyama, M., Prognosis for canine malignant mammary tumors based on TNM and histologic classification, *J. Vet. Med. Sci.*, 58, 1079–1083, 1996.

Zanusso, G., Casalone, C., Acutis, P., Bozzetta, E., Farinazzo, A., Gelati, M., Fiorini, M., Forloni, G., Sy, M.S., Monaco, S., and Caramelli, M., Molecular analysis of iatrogenic scrapie in Italy, *J. Gen. Virol.*, 84, 1047–1052, 2003.

Zweig, M.H. and Campbell, G., Receiver-operating characteristic (ROC) plots: a fundamental evaluation tool in clinical medicine, *Clin. Chem.*, 39, 561–577, 1993.

Index